ENDOSCOPY OF GI TRACT

Edited by **Somchai Amornyotin**

Endoscopy of GI Tract
http://dx.doi.org/10.5772/45916
Edited by Somchai Amornyotin

Contributors

Arjuna De Silva, Ghoshal, Waleed Al-Khyatt, Farhan Rashid, S Y Iftikhar, Hiroto Kita, Yasutoshi Ochiai, Shin Arai, Keiko Ishikawa, Masamitsu Nakao, Osamu Togawa, Makoto Nishimura, Takashi Shono, Kouichi Nonaka, Naohisa Yoshida, Naito, Maria Teresa Mascellino, Alessandra Oliva, Barbara Porowska, Michele Molinari, Karim Mohamed Eltawil, Bassam Abu Wasel, Akash Nabh, Muhammed Sherid, Marco Gasparetto, Graziella Guariso, David Gorard, Neil Rajoriya, Borislav Vladimirov, Radina Ivanova, Ivan Terziev, Urszula Grzybowska-Chlebowczyk, Ludwik Stołtny, Halina Woś, Anna Stołtny, Kin Fah Chin, Eng Hong Pok, Somchai Amornyotin

Published by InTech

Janeza Trdine 9, 51000 Rijeka, Croatia

Publishing Process Manager Iva Simcic
Technical Editor InTech DTP team
Cover InTech Design team

Additional hard copies can be obtained from orders@intechopen.com

Endoscopy of GI Tract, Edited by Somchai Amornyotin
p. cm.
ISBN 978-953-51-1034-7

For EU product safety concerns:
IN TECH d.o.o., Prolaz Marije Krucifikse Kozulić 3, 51000 Rijeka, Croatia,
info@intechopen.com or visit our website at intechopen.com.

Meet the editor

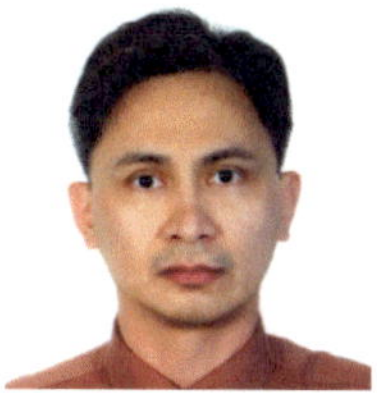

Dr. Somchai Amornyotin graduated at the Faculty of Medicine Siriraj Hospital, Mahidol University in 1989. He became the staff of the Department of Anesthesiology, Faculty of Medicine Siriraj Hospital, Mahidol University, Bangkok, Thailand in 1996. Until 2004 he became the associate professor of the Department of Anesthesiology, Faculty of Medicine Siriraj Hospital, Mahidol University. From 2005 until 2009 he was the chief of Anesthesiology Division of Siriraj GI Endoscopy Center, Faculty of Medicine Siriraj Hospital, Mahidol University. His first scientific paper was puplished in Thailand in 1999. He has practiced anesthesia for gastrointestinal endoscopy since 2002. He was the committee of Siriraj GI Endoscopy Center, Faculty of Medicine Siriraj Hospital in 2005. More than 50 of his articles have been published in Thai and international medical journals. Dr. Amornyotin is member of the Royal College of Anesthesiologists of Thailand and many scientific societies. He is the reviewer and editor of many international journals.

Contents

Preface

Endoscopy is a fast moving field, and new techniques are constantly emerging. Gastrointestinal endoscopy has a central role in the evaluation of gastrointestinal complaints and in the diagnosis and management of gastrointestinal diseases. It is a very safe procedure in the general population as demonstrated by numerous studies. Several data provide a better understanding of pathogenic mechanisms. In recent decades, gastrointestinal endoscopy has evolved and branched out from a visual diagnostic modality to impressive interventional capabilities. Some new endoscopic techniques will be too complex or expensive to make the leap into general gastroenterology practice, others already show major progress in the management of digestive diseases. In this chapter the authors will discuss some of the emerging techniques and technologies used to increase the diagnostic and therapeutic yield in the gastrointestinal tract. As in any field, demands of service delivery by conventional equipment and newer, more glamorous, and usually more expensive technologies are often in competition.

Modern endoscopic equipment provides us with the benefit of many technical advances. New videoendoscopes, magnification endoscopes and confocal of narrow band imaging endoscopes emerged. An increased knowledge of normal and pathologic endoscopic patterns has been increasing in the last decades. Endoscopy is an effective and safe procedure even in special populations including pediatric patients, geriatric patients, pregnant patients and liver transplant patients. In addition, many diagnostic techniques and therapeutic interventions documented real improvement.

The contributions in this book are very valuable. InTech Open Access Publisher selected several known names from many countries with different levels of development. Multiple specific points of view were presented together with various topics regarding diagnostic or therapeutic endoscopy. The readers can take into consideration of practical knowledge in the gastroenterology field. This book actually represents a valuable tool for formation and continuous medical education in the gastrointestinal endoscopy procedure considering the performances or technical possibilities in different parts of the world.

I very much appreciate and thank to all authors of this book. Many thanks to InTech Open Access Publisher which offered me the possibility of editing this attractive book. It was a real pleasure to read such interesting works by so many experts from all over the world. Finally, I also thank Ms. Iva Simcic for her perfect, prompt and efficient co-operation.

Assoc. Prof. Somchai Amornyotin MD, FRCAT
Department of Anesthesiology and Siriraj GI Endoscopy Center
Faculty of Medicine Siriraj Hospital
Mahidol University, Bangkok
Thailand

Section 1

General Aspects

Chapter 1

Pediatric Sedation Related to Endoscopy

Ludwik Grzegorz Stołtny,
Urszula Grzybowska–Chlebowczyk, Halina Woś and
Anna Agata Stołtny

Additional information is available at the end of the chapter

http://dx.doi.org/10.5772/52536

1. Introduction

Nowadays, the endoscopy is the basic diagnostic and therapeutic examination in cases of the gastrointestinal diseases, growth and weight gain disorders, gastrointestinal infections and diagnosis and treatment of polyps, the bile duct stones, etc. The endoscopy is a minimally invasive procedure but it is not free from the unpleasant sensations and sometimes severe pain. The endoscopic procedure can be performed as hospitalization or outpatient examination. Staying in hospital and endoscopy can be a very unpleasant experience and a strong stress, that may cause the withdrawal of a child in the development up to the so-called "several stages of development". Children under 18 years old should be anesthetized and operated by trained personnel, in specialized pediatric centers possessing a recovery room, post-operative intensive care and intensive care unit. Children who do not cooperate due to age, stage of development, certain diseases of the CNS, lack of understanding of the situation, fear of the unknown, separation from parents or guardians, previous bad experiences, rebellion and negativism, etc. often than adults require general anesthesia for gastrointestinal endoscopic examinations and the installation of PEG. The presence of parents during the staying in the hospital, preparing for the endoscopic surgery and during the induction of anesthesia and immediately after regaining consciousness helps to alleviate stress and its associated complications. The child is accompanied by both parents and favorite items or toys such as "teddy bear Bordus". Qualifying children for anesthesia is based on medical interview with the parents and child, child's physical examination and full observation. To achieve the best results, avoid critical situations and complications children should be adequately prepared for anesthesia and endoscopy.

2. Preparation of children for anesthesia — Anesthetist visit

Before to a planned endoscopic examination and anesthesia, physical examination should be performed and detailed medical history from patient's parents or legal guardians should be obtained. In addition, the current documentation and results of laboratory tests should be analyzed. Physical examination is aimed at an accurate assessment of the work of the lungs, heart, presence of the heart rate and accurate looking into and assessment of the throat, nasal patency, breathing circuit and possible prediction of difficult intubation. The anesthetic examination of the child before anesthesia is always done in the presence of the parent, guardian or "other party" for example, anesthetic nurses or nurses from the gastroenterology unit. Such situation creates the so-called "triangle" where the anesthesiologist must meet the requirements of both the child and the parent or guardian. This allows to mutual awareness, good contact, to reduce stress to a minimum, gives the opportunity to parents to ask questions and obtain all necessary information needed to make an informed and voluntary decision to consent to anesthesia for endoscopy.

If necessary, the specialist consultation may be ordered for a more specific evaluation of patient's condition and the degree of anesthetic risk according to ASA scale. The decisive influence to the risk of anesthetic have the procedure, the presence of congenital malformations, underlying conditions, concomitant diseases, the history of diseases, infections and their consequences, the perinatal asphyxia, etc. Anesthesia and endoscopy are procedures not required the performance of unnecessary laboratory tests, which should be reduced to a minimum, unless the child's serious condition, results of the consultations, the physical examination, the interview determine the need to perform specific analysis that allows for the safe conduct of the planned procedures. During the preparatory stage because of the period of interruption of oral feeding for several hours and / or cleansing of the colon it is important to put on attention to adequate hydration, glucose levels or levels of electrolytes.

A decision about anesthesia is made by an anesthesiologist on the basis of examination and evaluation of the anesthetic risk in the relation to the mode in which the endoscopic procedure is performed. The course of an anesthetic visit is noted in the anesthetic examination record. After obtaining sufficient information, parents or legal guardians give their informed consent to anesthetic procedure. During the visit, the pharmacological premedication before anesthesia is ordered.

In children with asthma a chronic therapy should not be terminated on the day of anesthesia and surgery, they should receive all regular medications. Children with diabetes should be operated as first, additionally during the procedure 0.9% NaCl should be given because anesthesia and surgery causes hyperglycemia. In the case of hyperglycemia or prolonged surgery the child may receive continuous infusion of regular insulin with glucose. During the treatment it is required to control the levels of glucose, electrolytes and acid - base balance.

Procedures associated with endoscopy should be so created to reduce to a minimum staying of a child in the hospital. Complications of anesthesia in the form of cough, spasms of the larynx and bronchi or respiratory disorders may occur up to several weeks after infection. In cases of children after infection, the planned surgery should be postponed for about two weeks. After vaccination, anesthesia should be postponed for a week (occurrence of reactions after vaccination).

3. Informed parental consent for anesthesia

Informed consent of parents or legal guardians is to provide information about the purpose, types, course, possible consequences and complications of anesthesia in endoscopy.

After reviewing the written information, presented above problems connected with anesthesia, awakening and post-operative care, parents or guardians have the right to ask questions to obtain additional information, resolve doubts, understand and gain trust to anesthetic and used methods. When all doubts are dispelled, the parents or guardians express informed consent for anesthesia.

4. Preparation of children for anesthesia — Premedication

It is difficult to predict how a child will react in a situation of forced during disconnection from parents, and anesthesia. Even apparently brave child may panic at some time. Oral administration of benzodiazepines, ketamine (nasal) and in some cases, atropine at 30 to 45 minutes before examination causes sedation, easier introduction of anesthesia and reduces the amount of anesthetic agents but extends waking after anesthesia and requires special care and supervision in the form of monitoring of vital signs. Premedication in children is administered orally, nasally or less frequent rectally. Sedatives can have form of lotions, syrups, tablets, drops. Depending on the age and ability to cooperate, to achieve the desired result, the appropriate form of the drug can be applied. Midazolam, according to various authors, is used at doses from 0.2 to 06 mg / kg body-weight. To prevent postoperative nausea and vomiting brain serotonin receptors agonist drug is used - ondansetron at a dose of 0.05 to 0.1 mg / kg., generally only in patients with postoperative vomiting in an interview.

Preparation of children and their parents or legal guardians for anesthesia requires from both anesthesiologist and gastroenterologist meeting and discussion in order to explain the nature and necessity of the forthcoming procedures and to resolve any doubts. Premedication is aimed at decreasing the level of patient's anxiety and sedation while waiting for the procedure, on the way to the endoscopy laboratory and directly before and during induction of anesthesia. Premedication in children comprises three elements, two of them are not formal and do not have material form: the constant presence of the parent or guardian near the child, staff's interest and support (showed by an anesthesiologist and gastroenterologist) and appropriate doses of pharmacological agents. Pharmacological agents used for premedication include sedatives and soporifics, antiemetics and antacids. From 120 to 60 minutes before the scheduled surgery, to neutralize and reduce the volume of gastric juice ranitidine or omeprazole is used in doses of: ranitidine from 2 to 4 mg / kg, omeprazole from 0.5 to 3.5 mg / kg.

The advantage of pharmacological premedication is a calm, caring, willingness to cooperate of the child and also decreased need for anesthetics and analgesics necessary during anesthesia. These, outlined above undoubted advantages are reduced by a noticeable disadvantage of premedication which is prolongation of the time to awakening after an anesthesia. Premedication is applied ½ to ¾ h before a planned procedure. After premedication, the patient may show various reactions, e.g. agitation, lack of reaction, sedation or excessive sedation including anesthesia.

After the sedative injection may occur agitation and uncontrolled response of the patient (fighter) or anesthesia with all effects that may affect the unconscious patient. During sedation staff must have the monitoring equipment used in resuscitation. This can be illustrated on the six levels Ramsay sedation scale.

1	excited, frightened, impaired consciousness (fighter), inadequate reaction
2	calm, cooperates
3	drowsy, cooperating, responsive to verbal commands
4	deep sedation, does not respond to voice, observed the response to pain
5	anesthesia, sluggish ,vestigial reaction to pain
6	deep coma, no reaction to pain

Table 1. Ramsay sedation scale.

Due to the inability to predict the effect of the dose of a substance used as the premedication, which depends on the patient's individual reaction to the administered pharmacological agent, after its administration the patient must be supervised by anesthetic staff, and staff members should be provided with functional equipment for monitoring, intubation and with possibility of application of LMA, maintaining artificial respiration, oxygen therapy and cardiopulmonary resuscitation.

5. Withholding oral fluids and food

Withholding the intake of food and beverages should be considered individually due to the child's age, the eating habits and time of feeding. In the smallest children period of withholding food to the anesthesia should be equal to the gastric emptying time. Its the most common expression is a crying baby demanding food.

Every 2 to 3 hours the newborns' and infants' stomach is empty. Gastric emptying time depends also on the type of food. Gastric emptying after eating takes from 6 to 8 hours, after the liquid such as milk from 4 to 6 hours and after ingestion of a water or tea for about 2 hours. Regularly every 3 hours breastfed baby empties the stomach in such intervals. It should be noted that the bad general condition of the child, trauma, pain, anxiety can have unpredictably affect to the gastric emptying time. Chewing gum causes salivation and increased secretion in the stomach which increases stomach contents and growth pH.

Before anesthesia and endoscopy patient should be long enough in the fasting state for anesthetic reasons and gastrological indications. For the gastroenterologist empty stomach or intestine are necessary to correctly perform the examination. However, during anesthesia may occur regurgitation of gastric contents or vomiting. Sedation and general anesthesia causes weakness or total abolition of reflexes such as coughing and swallowing which may cause aspiration into the respiratory tract and related severe complications in the form of acute respiratory and / or chemical pneumonia. Withholding food and / or beverages intake depends on the child's age and type of diet. Solid foods should be withheld about 6 to 8 hours before the test, liquid foods about 4 hours, and water or tea can be given about 4 to 2 hours before the anesthesia and endoscopy. In infants fed naturally every signal of hunger and willingness of food intake is a kind of signal "to be fasting." It should also be remembered that withholding food does not guarantee an empty stomach. During the endoscopic examination almost always in the stomach contents can be found some air and colorless or yellow-tinged liquid secretions.

6. Indications for general anesthesia during endoscopic examination in children

Children who cooperate with the medical staff and understand the need for examination, the technique and the course, and who do not show anxiety before and during endoscopy, may be examined after premedication (in sedation). Children who do not cooperate with the staff, insertion of PEG and colonoscopy should be indications for general anesthesia. Anesthesia is intended to protect psyche, reduce fear and its consequences, and relieve pain. The experience of the child and parents, the conviction of the necessity of anesthesia or the total negation of anesthesia during endoscopic should be taken into account.

7. Equipment and special conditions in the endoscopic laboratory for children

The equipment of endoscopy laboratory comprises the general anesthesia apparatus, monitor of anesthesia parameters and vital functions of the patient, high-performance suction device, resuscitation equipment, equipment for difficult intubation, laryngeal masks, and available quick telephone connection with the operating theatre and more experienced colleague or superior. After anesthesia, children should wake up in the recovery room, and if a serious situation or a severe, life-threatening complications occur, intensive therapy (IT) must be available.

8. Vital functions monitoring

During sedation and general anesthesia in children, a continuous presence of anesthetic staff is required as well as adequate monitoring of patient's vital functions, airway patency, chest movements, hemoglobin saturation (SaO_2), ECG, arterial blood pressure, and in some cases in very young children, also body temperature. Staff should also pay attention to the color of skin, respiratory murmur over the lung fields which is a sign of normal alveolar ventilation.

9. Mode of anesthesia and endoscopy

Outpatient surgery refers to patients who have been admitted and examined in one day of staying in hospital. This mode is particularly relevant to children because of the short stay in the hospital and less harmful effect on the psyche. Proceedings under a one day requires proper organization, proper co-operation between all involved i.e. the gastroenterologist, the anesthesiologist, the patient, the family of the patient, family doctor. In this mode, the most important is qualification. First, the parental consent is required, then the patient's condition, appropriate treatment within 24 hours after surgery and anesthesia. In general, to the mode of one day are eligible patients from the risk of anesthesia ASA I and II (exceptionally III if the patient's condition is stable and shortened stay in hospital is beneficial for medical indications - stable diabetes, asthma, patients during chemotherapy). Patients qualified for the one day mode should be older than 6 months. Withholding the intake of food and beverages in children has the same rules as in the mode of hospitalization. Patients who require neutralization of acidic gastric juice should be anesthetized and operated in sufficient time for safe and full action of antacids in the stomach acid content. Shall also be required closer monitoring in the postoperative period.

Criteria for discharge of patients in one day mode: the circulatory and respiratory stability, full wake-up and orientation, the patient can intake food, no pain, no nausea and no vomiting, the patient is able to move themselves, the patient was observed after anesthesia at least 1 hour. Transport to home should be done after the removal of the intravenous cannula, the provision of written and oral information, the order of pain relief treatment, own transport with a 24-hour care and supervision of an informed person. The family must be informed about the possibility of telephone consultations if needed. Driving time to the hospital should not be longer than 1 hour. If one or more of the above criteria are not met, the patient should stay in hospital overnight.

10. Induction and maintaining anesthesia

Induction of anesthesia in children for endoscopy is sometimes a challenge for the pediatric anesthesiologist. If the child has catheter previously introduced into a vein, the induction of anesthesia can be started by giving intravenous anesthetics this way. However, in the absence of such catheter or in the case when the child's peripheral venous are destroyed by the past infusion due to chronic disease, long, unsuccessful searching of a vein can cause severe stress and mental trauma for both the child and for accompanying persons. The fear of the introduction of the intravenous catheter makes the inhaled induction the method of choice. Parent or guardian is present during induction of anesthesia. Inhalation of the anesthetic gas mixture through a face mask is painless, fast and efficient. Inhalation anesthesia is carried out with semi-closed system with a circular system of pipes for children or adults, and a built-in absorber of carbon dioxide. During inhalation anesthesia spontaneously breathing may be complicated by hypoventilation caused by respiratory depression due to high concentration of anesthetic, laryngospasm and bronchospasm which is caused by respiratory hypersensitivity to irritant effects of inhaled anesthetics and airway disorders of pharynx caused by a reduction in pharyngeal and tongue muscles tone. During inhaled induction of anesthesia should be done close monitoring of the movements of the chest, breath sounds, respiratory additional phenomena in the form of wheezing, rales or rhonchi, skin color, saturation of hemoglobin, heart rate. For inhalational induction in children only sevoflurane is suitable because of the least irritating effect on the respiratory mucosa. The safest method of introduction of anesthesia using sevoflurane is administered to breathe increasing concentrations of the anesthetic with the precise monitoring of the concentration of this gas in the breathing mixture.

Intravenous anesthesia can be performed in children after obtaining venous access. However, this treatment causes a strong stress not only for medical reasons. Often, parents who at that moment when they are unable to cope with the resistance of the child irresponsible scare the child: "if you don't eat dinner you will be injected and get a drip".

Intravenous access is accompanied by sharp, severe pain. Application of proper cream to the puncture site may be helpful and it is good to introduce a catheter into a vein in this place. It is known that for various reasons: age, obesity, previous long-term therapy, oncology treatment, etc. cause significant difficulties in obtaining intravenous access. In addition, it should be noted that the cream can stop the pain, but the stress of a view of the needle will not stop. In such a case, when the child and the parents show excessive anxiety sedative medications must be given. However, sedation raises another problem specific to effects of this drug - there is currently no method to predict the potential effects of the administered drug. Best represents it the Ramsay Sedation Scale (see above). If a child comes to anesthesia with access to the vein, it is very important to carefully check and make sure that the catheter is located in the vein. Paravenous administration of the drug does not give the intended result, may result in overdose or can cause pain, burning, necrosis with defects of adjacent tissue and other complications. In the intravenous induction in children most often is used thiopental at a dose of 4 to 8 mg / kg, but must be remembered that the concentration of this drug in the solution can not exceed 2%. Higher concentrations in the paravenous injection can cause damage to the surrounding tissues and necrosis followed by scarring. Another drug used for intravenous induction is propofol at a dose of 2 to 3.5 mg / kg, which lowers the blood pressure (positively works during intubation and implantation of laryngeal mask what prevent a sudden stroke of blood pressure). During intravenous anesthesia without tracheal intubation in spontaneously breathing planned dose should be administered slowly (in fractions) to prevent apnea. Induction of anesthesia should be rapid without unpleasant sensations. Anesthesia should result in the elimination of consciousness and pain, should be as short as possible and should stop immediately after endoscopy, waking should be quick and pleasant. On the one hand the patient should have ensured an adequate level of anesthesia, on the other hand analgesia should not cause respiratory and circulatory depression. Because essentially to this type of examination or procedure the tracheal intubation is not performed, the best care is required to maintain the airway patency and providing the stable alveolar ventilation and the gas exchange. During anesthesia, patients should be placed in the recovery position to provide adequate protection against aspiration in case of regurgitation or vomiting.

It is very important to perform induction very slowly in divided doses due to an individual sensitivity, in order to avoid respiratory disorders and provide adequate level of anesthesia. Analgesics seem to be indispensable due to a low pain threshold during endoscope insertion through the pharynx. A good analgesic agent seems to be fentanyl at a dose of 1 to 2 micrograms/kg b.w., administered in divided doses. The administration of rectal enemas with anesthetics is absolutely contraindicated for colonoscopy and in other cases can not be reliable as to the timing and strength of action - in assuming that the induction of anesthesia and awakening should be quick, pleasant and should not cause stressful situations this method is difficult and unpredictable.

During anesthesia, ECG, hemoglobin saturation and arterial blood pressure should be monitored. Oxygen therapy is important because it prevents desaturation. An equipment for ventilation and tracheal intubation should be kept handy, and in the case of difficult intubation a laryngeal mask and alternative intubation methods should be available (bijou probe, bronchofiberoscope, etc.) or immediate contact and help from an experienced colleague should be possible. It is impossible to predict all possible events, but in unclear cases proceedings should be adapted to the situation - preparation of adequate scenarios and discussing them with a gastroenterologist and intensive therapy staff, preparation of necessary equipment or earlier intubation of the patient.

During anesthesia for gastroscopy, colonoscopy, and especially for PEG insertion, a close cooperation between the members of gastroenterological and an aesthetic teams is necessary.

11. Oxygen therapy

During general intravenous anesthesia with preserved patient's own respiration, changes of ventilation and desaturation may occur due to respiratory centre depression. Each time it is necessary to ensure adequate oxygenation, sufficient breathing and maintain a clear airway. In the case of a decrease in ventilation, the respiratory support should be immediately start using an AMBU bag, face mask, tracheal intubation or laryngeal mask (LMA). If airway disorders caused by collapsing of the language occur it is necessary to use the oral airway (Guedel pattern airway). To passive oxygen therapy during upper gastrointestinal endoscopy, a facial mask for oxygen therapy may considerably hinder endoscopic examination. Use of oxygen masks in children is difficult, especially while waking up, when children poorly tolerate this device. The simplest method of oxygen therapy is insufflation using a thin catheter covered with 2% xylocaine gel, inserted in the nasal passage at depth of 3 to 4 cm; oxygen is administered via this catheter, at flow of 0.5 to 1 liter. The catheter may be fixed with an adhesive tape, and small oxygen flow does not irritate the nasal mucosa or cause needless discomfort. This method can be regarded as an extremely effective and also very economical.

12. Transport of the child after anesthesia

Preparation of the child for transport after anesthesia and endoscopy should be very careful. The level of anesthesia, respiratory efficiency (frequency and depth of breathing), and possibility to maintain airway patency should be evaluated. During transport, oxygen insufflations should be maintained, and ECG and SaO_2 should be monitored. The child should be placed in the recovery position in order to prevent the tongue from blocking patient's airway; in the case of regurgitation or vomiting, it prevents aspiration and related complications. During transport, an anesthesiologist and anesthetic nurse are present, and a resuscitation set is available.

13. Waking up the patient after anesthesia — Observation in the recovery room

During the postoperative period should be pay attention to the efficiency of ventilation, proper hemoglobin saturation, the evacuation of carbon dioxide, effective analgesic (paracetamol, diclofenac, ketonal) and in case of stimulation, confusion, short-term complement of sedation.

After anesthesia all children should be observed in the recovery room until they are fully conscious. In contrast to the adults, in children more common are critical situations what is mostly due to the immaturity of tissues and organs, anatomical and physiological differences that cause disturbances of the lung ventilation and an incorrect oxygenation.

While staying in the recovery room, patient's vital functions are monitored, and observation is carried out by an experienced anesthetic nurse. An anesthetist should be present or available if a critical condition or complications occur.

Statistically, in patients staying in the recovery room, critical situations or complications occur in 7%, i.e. in every 15 patients. Patients leave the recovery room after the complete return of consciousness, after examination performed by an anesthesiologist, which is noted in the patient record (time of discharge, patient's condition, doctor's signature and stamp).

Adequate preparation, anesthesia, transport and observation in the recovery room should guarantee that critical situations possible during anesthesia will not result in reversible or irreversible complications associated with anesthesia.

Author details

Ludwik Grzegorz Stołtny[1], Urszula Grzybowska–Chlebowczyk[2], Halina Woś[2] and

Anna Agata Stołtny[3]

1 Department of Anesthesiology and Intensive Care Upper-Sielsian Child Health Care Centre in Katowice, Poland

2 The Department of Peadiatrics Medical University of Silesia, Gastroenterology Unit, Upper-Sielsian Child Health Care Centre in Katowice, Poland

3 Department of Pediatric Surgery Upper-Sielsian Child Health Care Centre in Katowice, Poland

References

[1] Gregory GA; Pediatric Anesthesia. Fourth edition. Churchil Livingstone. (2002).

[2] Aschl G; Kirchgatterer A; Allinger S; Hinterreiter M; Huebner D; Kranewitter W; Stadler B; Wimmer L; Knoflach P; Indikationen und Komplikationen der perkutanen endoskopischen GastrostomieWiener Klinische Wochenschrifft (2003). Feb 28; 115(3-4): 115- 120.

[3] Gauderer, M W, Ponsky, J L, & Izant, R. J Jr. Gastrostomy without laparotomy: a percutaneous endoscopic technique. Journal of Pediatric Surgery. (1980). , 15, 872-875.

[4] Gozal D; Goldin E; Shafran-Tikva S; Tal D; Wengrower DLeigh syndrome: anesthetic management in complicated endoscopic procedures. Pediatric Anaesthesia (2006). , 16(1), 38-42.

[5] Wengrower D; Gozal D; Gozal Y; Meiri Ch; Golan I; Granot E; Goldin EComplicated endoscopic pediatric procedures using deep sedation and general anesthesia are safe in the endoscopy suite. Scandinavian Journal of Gastroenterology. (2004). , 39(3), 283-286.

[6] Fortunato, J. E, & Cuffari, C. Outcomes of Percutaneous Endoscopic Gastrostomy in Children. Current Gastroenterology Report (2011). , 13, 293-299.

[7] Allman, K. G, & Wilson, I. H. Oxford Handbook of Anaesthesia. Second edition. Red. Mayzner-Zawadzka E. Polish edition. Medipage (2009).

Chapter 2

Cardiorespiratory Complications During Moderate and Deep Sedation for Gastrointestinal Endoscopic Procedures

Somchai Amornyotin

Additional information is available at the end of the chapter

http://dx.doi.org/10.5772/52737

1. Introduction

Gastrointestinal endoscopic (GIE) procedures are now performed routinely because of their minimal invasiveness and their diagnostic and therapeutic capabilities. These procedures have been shown to cause various effects on cardiorespiratory systems, which can increase the risks of the procedure in patients with underlying cardiorespiratory diseases [1]. Additionally, the complications attributed to moderate and deep sedation levels are more often associated with cardiovascular and respiratory systems. Most predictors of cardiorespiratory-related complications are patient-centered factors and do not vary significantly from procedure to procedure although the procedure is complex [2].

The exact incidence of cardiorespiratory complications associated with GIE procedure is not precisely known, but probably is quite low. Risk factors for cardiorespiratory complications are age > 60 years, high American Society of Anesthesiologists (ASA) physical status, the use of supplemental oxygen, inpatient status, and the involvement of a trainee in the procedure [3,4]. Sedation-related complications during GIE procedures are commonly transient and mild degree. The risk for these complications while providing any level of sedation or general anesthesia is greatest when caring for the patients already medically compromised. The significant unwanted complications can generally be prevented by careful preprocedure assessment and preparation, appropriate monitoring and support as well as postprocedure management.

Before undertaking any GIE procedure, endoscopists should be obtained the informed consent from the patient, are familiar with the latest guidelines on sedation, aware of any medical, surgical and drug history elicited in the pre-admission process as well as the risk factors should be identified in both out-patients and in-patients. Additionally, the physicians must be prepared to manage these complications. Safety and monitoring should be part of a quality assurance program for endoscopy units. This article will review the cardiovascular and respiratory complications during moderate and deep sedation for gastrointestinal endoscopic procedures and also address their appropriate management.

2. Cardiovascular consideration

The autonomic nervous system (ANS) plays an important role in maintaining normal hemodynamics and an adequate coronary blood flow. The sympathetic nervous system regulates the heart rate and rhythm, increases the excitability of myocardium. The parasympathetic nervous system regulates the heart rate and rhythm, which when stimulated can lead to sinus bradycardia [1]. The cardiorespiratory complications account for about 50% of the potentially serious morbidity and about 50% of all the procedure-related deaths associated with GIE procedure. In many cases these complications are a direct or indirect consequence of elderly or risk patients being given unnecessarily high doses of sedative and analgesic drugs [5].

2.1. Hypotension

A significant decline in blood pressure from baseline should alert the clinicians. Hypotension is defined as the systolic blood pressure lest than 90 mmHg is due to a fall in either cardiac output or total peripheral resistance lowering the patient's mean arterial pressure.

Episodes of hypotension in clinical practice are most commonly associated with vasovagal events and are generally transient. However, they may become prolonged in the presence of central nervous system depressants [6]. Blood pressure is a reflection of cardiac output and total peripheral resistance and a fall in either or both will lower the patient's mean arterial pressure. In general, a systolic blood pressure of 90 mmHg should sustain mean arterial blood pressure sufficiently to perfuse tissues in the recumbent patient. Blood pressure lower than this combined with evidence of inadequate perfusion requires intervention.

The evaluation of tissue perfusion is the most significant component of cardiovascular assessment. Hypotension encountered during sedation is usually attributed to either vasovagal episodes or the use of sedative and anesthetic agents that depress sympathetic outflow to the cardiovascular system. Benzodiazepines such as midazolam and diazepam, have a mild vasodilator effect and usually produce a slight fall in arterial blood pressure even in normal sedative doses. The combination use of a benzodiazepine and an opioid can profoundly drop blood pressure. Propofol has been shown to be safe and effective for sedation during ERCP, endoscopic ultrasonography (EUS) and small bowel enteroscopy, because these procedures require more time and patient cooperation [7-11].

The cardiovascular effects of propofol include decreases in cardiac output, systemic vascular resistance, and arterial pressure. A fall in heart rate and/or cardiac stroke volume will also lower blood pressure. Additionally, more profound falls in blood pressure is occurred in a hypovolemic patient. Propofol also has been proven to reduce postprocedural hypoxemic events, which may be of significance in critically ill elderly patients [12] and sick pediatric patients [13].

Prevention of this complication is to be relevant medical and drug history before the procedure, particular detail required regarding current antihypertensive, anti-anginal and anti-arrhythmic therapy and the use of systemic corticosteroids. Additionally, blood pressure and heart rate should be recorded before, during and after endoscopic procedure.

2.2. Hypertension

Blood pressure continuously fluctuates due to the cyclic nature of the pumping action of the heart. The highest pressure occurs during ventricular contraction. The lowest pressure occurs during ventricular relaxation [14]. Generally, hypertension is defined as the systolic blood press is greater than 160 mmHg. Sudden elevations of systolic blood pressure ≥ 180 mmHg or diastolic blood pressure ≥ 110 mmHg are generally regarded as an acute hypertensive episode [5]. The causes of hypertension are the background systemic hypertension, anxiety or pain, and a reflex pressor response from intubation of the esophagus. Generally, asymptomatic patients and the patients without acute end-organ symptoms should not receive antihypertensive agents in the endoscopy unit.

2.3. Cardiac arrhythmias

Autonomic control of heart rate will respond to demands placed on the patient and may be initiated via several baroreceptor-mediated reflexes [12]. Electrocardiogram (ECG) is also a useful monitor for heart rate and a better assessment of heart rhythm. Continuous ECG monitoring is recommended for high risk patient with relevant cardiac history. Cardiac arrhythmias are frequently observed during GIE procedures. Fortunately, most of them are not clinically significant.

In the healthy patients, a heart rate up to 120 beats/min will usually allow adequate filling. Sinus tachycardia can be caused by patient's anxiety or related to pain, compensatory mechanism in patients who are hypotensive as a result of either dehydration or blood loss, and following intravenous anticholinergic drugs such as buscopan.

Heart rate < 50 beats/min in healthy patients may allow for more time in diastole, but ventricular filling becomes maximized [14]. Sinus bradycardia is most frequently seen in the patients who are taking beta blockers. It can also be induced by vagal stimulation, which occurs at the time of intubation of the esophagus or the stretching of the sigmoid mesentery during colonoscopy or flexible sigmoidoscopy.

2.4. Myocardial ischemia/infarction

Myocardial infarction occurs either during or in the few days after endoscopic procedures with or without sedation. A proportion of these are undoubtedly causally related to the endoscopic procedure. The causes of angina or myocardial Infarction are two factors; increased myocardial oxygen demand and reduced myocardial perfusion [6].

Increased myocardial oxygen demand is due to an increase in the mean arterial blood pressure and heart rate. This can cause angina in the patients with ischemic heart disease or occult symptomless myocardial ischemia. Additionally, marked hypertension and/or tachycardia increase myocardial oxygen consumption. In the other way, hypotension and/or bradycardia reduce myocardial perfusion. Stress-induced myocardial ischemia can occur even in the patients with or without clinically significant coronary disease [15]. This myocardial ischemia is related to the activation of the sympathetic nervous system, resulting in hemodynamic changes causing an increase in cardiac demand.

Prevention or minimization of myocardial ischemia/infarction during GIE procedure

1. Pre-oxygenation in risk patients and give continuous supplemental oxygen

2. Give patients on their normal anti-hypertensive and/or anti-anginal therapy right up to the time of the endoscopy

3. Angina developing during an endoscopy is usually best managed by giving sublingual nitroglycerine, oxygen supplementation and discontinuing the examination

4. If angina or myocardial infarction is suspected during or following an endoscopy, arrange an electrocardiogram to exclude an myocardial infarction

3. Respiratory considerations

Airway management is the most important aspect of patient care and examination of the patient's airway is an essential component of the preoperative assessment. Mallampati class correlates with increased difficulty in airway management. High oxygen concentration is indicated for patients who are spontaneously breathing, regardless of their level of consciousness during medical urgencies and emergencies. The equipment required to provide supplemental oxygen includes a 100% oxygen source, a regulator, tubing, and either a nasal cannula or mask. Every office should be equipped with a portable E-cylinder of oxygen.

3.1. Respiratory depression

Higher dose of benzodiazepine and/or opioid is also the greater the percentage benzodiazepine and/or opioid receptor occupancy in the central nervous system the greater is the degree of depression of consciousness. Intravenous benzodiazepines such as midazolam and diazepam can cause respiratory depression. Intravenous opioids such as pethidine and fentanyl occupy opioid receptor sites within the brain and brainstem and can similarly cause respiratory depression [6]. Drug induced hypoventilation may cause both hypoxemia and CO_2 retention.

Pulse oximetry is a very useful indicator of oxygenation but not ventilation. However when supplemental oxygen is used, the fall in SpO_2 may be significantly delayed for between 30-90 seconds. So that continuous capnography monitoring is recommended in the patients being sedated with propofol [16]. As for over-sedation, loss of verbal contact due to reduced conscious level may be the first sign of impending respiratory depression. Reduction in

SpO_2 on pulse oximetry is a good indicator but it can be a late sign of respiratory depression. Increased $PaCO_2$ is the most sensitive early warning of respiratory depression [17].

Management of oversedation is to stimulate the patient to wake up and take deep breaths both verbally and/or light shaking. If the patients are not responding then benzodiazepine antagonist such as flumazenil and/or opioid antagonist such as naloxone may be required. The airway may need to be protected with chin lift, jaw thrust, and, if necessary, airway or laryngeal mask [6].

3.2. Airway obstruction

Although, obstruction may result in hypoventilation and hypoxia. Airway obstruction must be distinguished from respiratory depression. Hypoxia is common in patients undergoing upper GIE procedure with or without sedation. Sedation significantly increases the incidence of desaturation and hypoxia. Supplementary nasal oxygen at 3 litres/min in sedated patients abolishes desaturation and hypoxia. Upper airway obstruction may be attributed to anatomical structures or foreign body [18]. Independent predictors of airway modifications include male sex, American Society of Anesthesiologists class of III or higher, and increased body mass index [19].

Laryngospasm is a reflex closure or spasm of the glottic muscles including the false and true vocal cords. It is more likely during deep sedation. Laryngospasm occurs more frequently in adults who are smokers. Bronchospasm is a lower airway obstruction due to contraction or spasm of the bronchial smooth muscle. It may be a result of an anaphylactoid reaction or a consequence of a hyper-reactive airway in the asthmatic patients [18]. Management of laryngospasm and bronchospasm depends on the severity and the causes of them.

3.3. Hypoxia

Hypoxia may be a consequence of respiratory depression or airway obstruction. The incidence of hypoxia is up to 1.5% to 70%, which make it the most common cardiorespiratory adverse event during the endoscopy [20]. Hypoxemia can lead to many complications, depending on the severity of hypoxemic attack. The use of supplemental oxygen during GIE procedure is routinely used by many endoscopists. However, oxygen supplementation will delay the detection of apnea and hypoxia [4]. Additionally, in patients given supplemental oxygen, saturation may be maintained in the progression of hypercapnia.

Multivariable logistic regressions revealed that independent risk factors for hypoxemia include high body mass index, hypertension, diabetes, gastrointestinal diseases, heart diseases and the procedures that combined esophagogastroduodenoscopy (EGD) and colonoscopy [21]. Hypoxemia occurs typically within 5 min of medication administration or endoscope intubation and only one third of all apnea and abnormal ventilation events eventually lead to hypoxemia [20].

3.4. Pulmonary aspiration

Aspiration of gastric contents into the lungs during GIE procedure is relatively common. It may cause pneumonia and may result in death. Risk factors for aspiration are the elderly patients, over-sedated patients, the patients with gastrointestinal bleeding, gastric stasis, gastric outlet obstruction, patients with hepatic encephalopathy, and the patients who have full stomach. Aspiration can also occur when a local anesthetic spray is used in combination with intravenous sedation [6].

Aspiration may be suspected when a patient starts coughing violently either during or soon after an endoscopic procedure and cyanosis may occur. Although the higher incidence of pulmonary aspiration because of the better sensitivity of 2-[^{18}F] fluoro-2-deoxy-D-glucose positron tomography. However, the low incidence of clinical events needed intervention may still reflect the safety of sedation used for gastrointestinal endoscopy [22]. Treatments of pulmonary aspiration include suction of fluids from oral cavity and throat, increasing the rate of supplemental oxygen, encouraging the patient to cough, chest film, antibiotics and physiotherapy.

4. Patients requiring anesthesiologists support for GIE procedures

Generally, GIE procedures can be performed by using topical anesthesia, intravenous sedation and general anesthesia [23-25]. The topical anesthesia and intravenous sedation techniques can be effectively done by non-anesthetic personnel. However, non-anesthetic personnel should be sedated the patients only in mild and moderate (conscious) sedation levels [26].

Elective cases – Indications include:

1. Hypotension (systolic blood pressure < 90 mmHg) due to a fall in cardiac output or total peripheral resistance
2. Patients with severe cardiac and/or pulmonary abnormalities
3. Patients with severe learning difficulties
4. Patients with history of failed sedation
5. Patients who may prove difficult to sedate such as alcoholic or drug addicted patients
6. Patients with poor venous access
7. Phobic or uncooperative patients such as children, dementia patients and psychiatric patients
8. Patient being sedated with intravenous propofol

Emergency cases- with high risk of aspiration and requiring endotracheal tube with general anesthesia include:

1. Patients with depressed levels of consciousness
2. Patients associated with encephalopathy
3. Patients suspected bleeding varices

4. Patients with severe cardiac and/or pulmonary abnormalities
5. Patients unlikely to cooperate during endoscopy procedure

5. Postprocedural period

Most of cardiorespiratory adverse events occur during the GIE procedure. Standard monitoring including non-invasive blood pressure, heart rate, pulse oxymetry and electrocardiogram is also routinely used in the postprocedural period. Postprocedural nausea/vomiting and pain need to be rescued especially in the ambulatory patients. Fortunately, a lower incidence of procedural nausea/vomiting and pain after the GIE procedure is observed even in the therapeutic endoscopy [27]. Opioid and cyclo-oxygenase-2-inhibitor can be safely and effectively used for procedural pain in the GIE patients [28].

My previous study showed that periodic objective evaluation of home-readiness revealed that the majority of patients would achieve a satisfactory score on or before 1 hour after the GIE procedure [29]. So that, the patients underwent GIE procedures should be admitted in the recovery room unit at least 30-60 min before discharge. The time to home-readiness by objective evaluation correlated with the type of procedure. Most delay after satisfactory home-readiness scores were reached, were due to non-medical reasons.

Sedation-related cardiorespiratory complications also occur immediately after the GIE procedure. The types of complications in the postprocedural period are similar as in the intraprocedural period. The patients who receive benzodiazepine and/or opioid antagonists should to be closely observed in the recovery room unit longer than the other patients.

6. Summary

Although the serious adverse events are rare for the GIE procedural sedation. However, the cardiorespiratory-related complications are common. These complications may be severe if the physicians do not detect and treat the patients earlier. An adequate preprocedural history should be obtained and physical examination performed on all patients. Particular attention should be paid to the patient's physical status and cardiorespiratory system. Appropriate preprocedural assessment and optimization of the patients undergoing moderate or deep sedation are essential to minimize complications. Periodical assessment of the level of sedation and continuous monitoring of cardiovascular and respiratory systems provides timely information. Pulse oxymetry and oxygen supplementation are recommended for the reduction of hypoxemia. Capnography monitoring is considered in the patients undergoing prolonged endoscopic procedures who are at risk of deep sedation. Additionally, the standardized discharge criteria should be used to determine the patient's readiness for discharge. Lastly, the physicians should remember that the risk for un-intended deeper level of sedation may be more common after the stimulation of the endoscopic procedure has been removed.

Author details

Somchai Amornyotin*

Department of Anesthesiology and Siriraj GI Endoscopy Center, Faculty of Medicine Siriraj Hospital, Mahidol University, Bangkok, Thailand

References

[1] Ross C, Frishman WH, Peterson SJ, Lebovics E. Cardiovascular considerations in patients undergoing gastrointestinal endoscopy. Cardiology in Review 2008; 16(2): 76-81.

[2] Romagnuolo J, Cotton PB, Eisen G, Vargo J, Petersen BT. Identifying and reporting risk factors for adverse events in endoscopy. Part I: cardiopulmonary events. Gastrointestinal Endoscopy 2011; 73(3): 579-585.

[3] Vargo JJ. Risks of sedation and analgesia. Techniques in Gastrointestinal Endoscopy 2007; 9: 218-224.

[4] Sharma VK, Nguyen CC, Crowell MD, et al. A national study of cardiopulmonary unplanned events after GI endoscopy. Gastrointestinal Endoscopy 2007; 66(1): 27-34.

[5] Becker DE, Haas DA. Recognition and management of complications during moderate and deep sedation. Part 2: Cardiovascular considerations. Anesthesia Progress 2011; 58(3): 126-138.

[6] British Society of Gastroenterology. Guidelines in Gastroenterology: Complications of gastrointestinal endoscopy. http://www.bsg.org.uk/pdf_word_docs/complications.pdf

[7] Amornyotin S, Chalayonnawin W, Kongphlay S. Propofol-based sedation does not increase rate of complication during percutaneous endosopic gastrostomy procedure. Gastroenterology Research and Practice 2011; Article ID 134819; 6 pages, doi: 10.1155/2011/134819.

[8] Amornyotin S, Kachintorn U, Chalayonnawin W, Kongphlay S. Propofol-based deep sedation for endoscopic retrograde cholangiopancreatography procedure in sick elderly patients in a developing country. Therapeutics and Clinical Risk Management 2011; 7: 251-255.

[9] Amornyotin S, Kachintorn U, Kongphlay S. Anesthetic management for small bowel enteroscopy in a World Gastroenterology Organizing Endoscopy Training Center. World Journal of Gastrointestinal Endoscopy 2012; 4(5): 189-193.

[10] Amornyotin S, Leelakusolvong S, Chalayonnawin W, Kongphlay S. Age-dependent safety analysis of propofol-based deep sedation for ERCP and EUS procedures at an

Endoscopy Training Center in a developing country. Clinical and Experimental Gastroenterology 2012; 5: 123-128.

[11] Amornyotin S, Prakanrattana U, Chalayonnavin W, Kongphlay S, Kachintorn U. Propofol based sedation does not increase perforation rate during colonoscopic procedure. Gastroenterology Insights 2010; 2(e4): 13-16.

[12] Riphaus A, Stergiou N, Wehrmann T. Sedation with propofol for routine ERCP in high-risk octogenarians: a randomized, controlled study. American Journal of Gastroenterology 2005; 100(9): 1957-1963.

[13] Amornyotin S, Kongphlay S. Esophagogastroduodenoscopy procedure in sick pediatric patients: a comparison between deep sedation and general anesthesia technique. Journal of Anesthesia and Clinical Research 2012; 3: 185. doi: 10.4712/2155-6148.1000185.

[14] Casabianca AB, Becker DE. Cardiovascular monitoring: physiological and technical considerations. Anesthesia Progress 2009; 56(1): 53-61.

[15] Lacy CR, Contrada RJ, Robbins ML, et al. Coronary vasoconstriction induced by mental stress (simulated public speaking). American Journal of Cardiology 1995; 75(7): 503-505.

[16] Pino RM. The nature of anesthesia and procedural sedation outside of the operating room. Current Opinion in Anesthesiology 2007; 20(4): 347-351.

[17] Cacho G, Pérez-Calle JL, Barbado A, et al. Capnography is superior to pulse oximetry for the detection of respiratory depression during colonoscopy. Revista Espanola de Enfermedades Digestivas 2010; 102(2): 86-89.

[18] Becker DE, Haas DA. Recognition and management of complications during moderate and deep sedation. Part 1: Respiratory considerations. Anesthesia Progress 2011; 58(2): 82-92.

[19] Cote GA, Hovis RM, Ansstas MA, et al. Incidence of sedation-related complications with propofol use during advanced endoscopic procedure. Clinical Gastroenterology and Hepatology 2010; 8(2): 137-142.

[20] Qadeer MA, Lopez AR, Dumot JA, Vargo JJ. Hypoxemia during moderate sedation for gastrointestinal endoscopy: causes and associations. Digestion 2011; 84(1): 37-45.

[21] Long Y, Liu HH, Yu C, et al. Pre-existing diseases of patients increase susceptibility to hypoxemia during gastrointestinal endoscopy. PLoS ONE 7(5): e37614, doi:10.1371/journal.pone.0037614.

[22] Hsieh TC, Wu YC, Ding HJ, et al. Clinically unrecognized pulmonary aspiration during gastrointestinal endoscopy with sedation: a potential pitfall interfering the performance of 18F-FDG PET for cancer screening. European Journal of Radiology 2011, doi: 10.1016/j.ejrad.2010.10.030.

[23] Amornyotin S, Srikureja W, Chalayonnavin W, et al. Topical viscous lidocaine solution versus lidocaine spray for pharyngeal anesthesia in unsedated esophagogastroduodenoscopy. Endoscopy 2009; 41(7): 581-586.

[24] Amornyotin S, Lertakayamanee N, Wongyingsinn M, et al. The effectiveness of intravenous sedation in diagnostic upper gastrointestinal endoscopy. Journal of Medical Association of Thailand 2007; 90(2): 301-306.

[25] Amornyotin S, Pranootnarabhal T, Chalayonnavin W, Kongphlay S. Anesthesia for gastrointestinal endoscopy from 2005-2006 in Siriraj Hospital: a prospective study. Thai Journal of Anesthesiology 2007; 33(2): 93-101.

[26] American Society of Anesthesiologists. Practice guidelines for sedation and analgesia by non-anesthesiologists. An update report by the American Society of Anesthesiologists Task Force on sedation and analgesia by non-anesthesiologists. Anesthesiology 2002; 96(4): 1004-1017.

[27] Amornyotin S, Phasurin T, Wongnuch P. Pain score within twenty-four hours post-endoscopic retrograde cholangiopancreatography: a comparison between diagnostic and therapeutic procedures. Gastroenterology Insights 2009; 1: e(7): 20-23.

[28] Amornyotin S, Chalayonnawin W, Kongphlay S. A randomized controlled trial of preprocedure administration of parecoxib for therapeutic endoscopic retrograde cholangiopancreatography. Journal of Pain Research 2012; 5: 251-256.

[29] Amornyotin S, Chalayonnawin V, Kongphlay S. Recovery pattern and home-readiness after gastrointestinal endoscopy. Journal of Medical Association of Thailand 2007; 90(11): 2352-2358.

Chapter 3

Pre–Endoscopy Screening of *Helicobacter pylori* Infection: Implication and Advantages

Maria Teresa Mascellino, Alessandra Oliva and
Barbara Porowska

Additional information is available at the end of the chapter

http://dx.doi.org/10.5772/52734

1. Introduction

Over the last 30 years, upper gastrointestinal endoscopy has become the investigation of choice for patients with symptoms referable to upper gastrointestinal tract. Owing to the increasing number of patients who should be undergone endoscopy with a consequent high cost and a marked workload and medical expenses for the hospitals, it has been recommended that pre-endoscopy screening strategies might identify patients at low risk of having major pathology. These patients could avoid prompt endoscopy and might safely undergo different management.

Considering that *Helicobacter pylori* (*Hp*) is the most frequent aetiologic agent in these pathologies, several invasive and non-invasive diagnostic tests have been taken into account for the diagnosis of *Hp* in the individual patient. The non-invasive tests obviate the need for endoscopy and can be surely more accepted by the subjects.

It has been proposed [1,2,3] that younger patients with symptoms of dyspepsia with non-alarming symptoms could be screened non-invasively for the infection in order to reduce endoscopy procedure. In addition, non-invasive tests are suitable, other than for pre-endoscopy screening of younger dyspeptics, also for use in research and for epidemiological surveys as well as for confirming successful eradication after treatment and for screening asymptomatic population.

The pre-endoscopy screening is based on different methodologies (such as serological markers, molecular markers, etc.) that will be discussed in the present chapter.

2. Serological markers

Serological testing has been recommended for initial pre-endoscopy or pre-treatment screening in dyspeptic patients. Serology is cheap and convenient and thus should be preferred in situations where the additional information yielded by an endoscopy is not needed.

Patients are prone to undergo this analysis because it only requires a simple peripheral blood collection for the investigation of anti-Hp IgG, IgM and IgA antibodies. The presence of even high levels of immunoglobulines does not appear to influence eradication of the bacteria from the stomach: the microorganism in fact is rarely eliminated and when it is not treated adequately, the infection generally persists in the rest of an individual's life [4].

For these reasons, the use of serological tests are very commonly used for clinically diagnosis of Hp-related infections. In general, the serum levels of anti-*H. pylori* IgG antibodies increase in the presence of infection and can be used as a marker. On the other hand, even if anti-Hp IgA antibodies are less appropriate for this purpose [5], serological findings of anti-Hp IgA in symptomatic patients might have significant clinical value for the diagnosis of infection, especially if the patient is seronegative for IgG. The disadvantage for serology is that past or current infections are not distinguished owing to the fact that past infections may lead to false positive, so that this test cannot be used for determining therapy success after treatment even if successful eradication can follow a substantial drop in antibody title, using repeat serology after a delay post-treatment. [6]

2.1. Serology as diagnostic tool

Serological testing is recommended for initial pre-endoscopy or pre-treatment screening in dyspeptic patients. The systemic response typically comprises a transient rise in IgM followed by a rise in specific IgA and IgG maintained throughout infection.

The consideration that patients with IgG antibodies to Hp have a greater risk of peptic ulcer disease as a cause of their dyspepsia, has led to screen dyspeptic patients under the age of 45 years using Hp serology. Three strategies are proposed after serology screening:

1. endoscopy of Hp seropositive patients and treatment of seronegative patients symptomatically;
2. treatment of seropositive patients for Hp and endoscopy of seronegative patients
3. eradication of infection from Hp seropositive patients, treatment of seronegative patients symptomatically and endoscopy for those with recurrent dyspepsia.

The attitude in both gastroenterologists and general practitioners with interest in gastroenterology towards the current pattern of use of pre-endoscopic Hp serology screening of young dyspeptics has been evaluated [7].

The most popular strategy among general practitioners is that of eradicating infection from seropositives and treating seronegatives symptomatically. In contrast, the most popular strategy among gastroenterologists is that of endoscoping seropositives and treating seronegatives symptomatically.

There is then wide variation in attitudes and practice between these two groups: general practitioners like more serological tests and strongly prefer eradicating infection in seropositives before addressing to endoscopy (even for cost consideration). On the contrary, the majority of gastroenterologists would endoscope seropositives before treating the infection.

In any case, it is recommended that non-invasive Hp testing should be used in place of endoscopy with all those testing positive being given anti-Hp therapy and those testing negative being treated symptomatically. The above strategy of "test and treat" used in clinical practice may include some inconveniences: expense morbidity from drug side effects and introduction of antibiotic resistance both in Hp and in other pathogens [8].

An important serological tool for the pre-endoscopy screening in patients at risk of carcinoma includes the quantitative determination of the different subclasses of IgG. In fact, a selective reduction of anti-Hp IgG subclass antibody is proven to occur in gastric carcinoma [9]. Cell-mediated immunity influences the outcome of infection including the development of gastric carcinoma (CG). The T-cell response comprises a secreted cytokine profile which influences the B-cell response including the production of the different IgG subclass antibody. In the adenocarcinoma, a fall in IgG level is demonstrated resulting to be particularly predictive of cancer [10]. This is thought to reflect premalignant gastric atrophy with loss of colonization and antigens stimulus [11]. A diminuished IgG antibodies response due to low immunogenicity of Hp-LPS or to the loss of Hp in some subjects evolving to GC, could reflect the premalignant phase of gastric atrophy. Significantly lower IgG2 levels are found in subjects with gastric carcinoma compared with those with reflux oesophagitis, chronic gastritis, gastric ulcer and peptic ulcer whereas IgG1 antibody remains at similar levels (Figure1). The levels of IgG 3 and IgG 4 are not affected and in most subjects are undetectable. The decreasing of IgG 2 subclass level, noticed in patients with adenocarcinoma and not in other Hp-related pathologies, depends on both the switching of mucosal cytokine secretion and the different kinetics of IgG response to gastric colonization by B-lymphocyte that can be influenced by cytokine profiles in secreting different antibody patterns.

Consequently, the patients showing low levels of IgG especially of subclass IgG 2 (below an established cut-off value) can be considered subjects at high risk of developing pre-malignant disease, gastric atrophy and adenocarcinoma [9]. These data show that above certain levels of antibody, irrespective of age, the risk of cancer is low and that primary endoscopy could be restricted to those with antibodies values below this level. In this way, the endoscopy could be avoided, as initial investigation, in 42% of dyspeptic subjects [9].

The value of this test as a predictive diagnostic tool in the pre-endoscopy screening strategy is crucial.

In conclusion, the screening strategy based on Hp serological status, determined with the enzyme-linked immunoadsorbent assay (ELISA) and Western blotting (WB), in patients with uncomplicated, simple dyspepsia up to 55 years of age, is able to identify 95%-100% of patients with significant gastroduodenal lesions while potentially saving 47% of endoscopies [12].

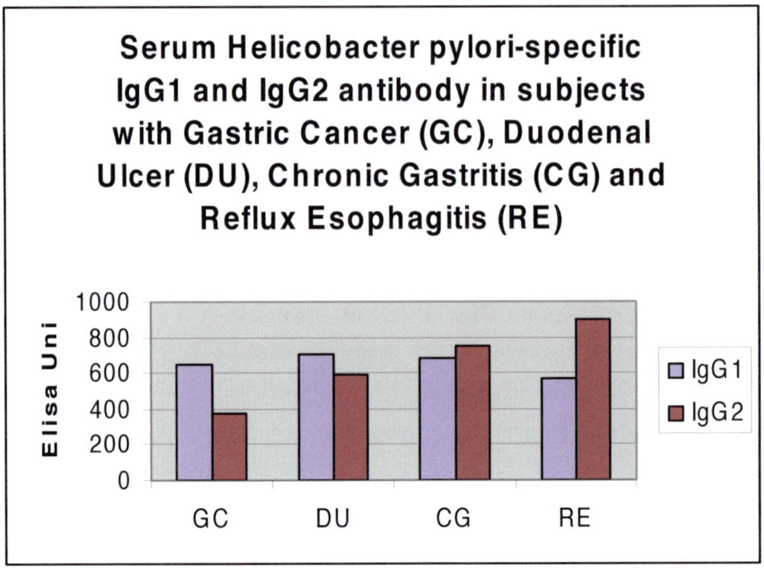

Figure 1. Serum Helicobacter pylori-specific IgG1 and IgG2 antibody in subjects with Gastric Cancer (GC), Duodenal Ulcer (DU), Chronic Gastritis (CG) and Reflux Esophagitis (RE)

2.2. Sensitivity and specificity of serological test

The concentration of serum IgG is reported to have sensitivity of 64%, specificity of 83.7 %, PPV (Positive Predictive Value) of 82%, NPV (Negative Predictive Value) of 66% and accuracy of 73.1% for the diagnosis of Hp infection [4]. For the same purpose, serum IgA has the following values: 72.0%, 65.9%, 72.0%, 64.4% and 69.8% respectively [4]. If the serological tests are considered together (when both test are positive or negative), some of these values could increase: the accuracy could be 80%, sensitivity 86.6%, specificity 74.2%, PPV 74.2 % and NPV 86.6%. In synthesis, the serological tests are efficient in the diagnosis of the presence or absence of Hp infection and when used simultaneously, they are more efficient in accuracy, sensitivity and negative predictive value than when used alone. (Table 1)

	Sensitivity (%)	Specificity (%)	PPV (%)	NPV (%)	Accuracy (%)
IgG alone	64	83.7	82	66	73.1
IgA alone	72	65.9	72	67.4	69.8
IgG + IgA (both positive or negative)	86.6	74.2	74.2	86.6	80

Modified from A. Locatelli et al. (2004)

Table 1. Sensitivity, Specificity, Positive Predictive Value (PPV), Negative Predictive Value(NPV), Accuracy of IgG and IgA detection in serum.

The detection of Hp IgA and IgG antibodies in serum is useful in distinguishing between infected and uninfected patients whereas the concentration of antibodies in duodenal fluid is not suitable at this purpose [13]

2.3. Advantages and disadvantages

Screening strategies, based on the serology used as marker of virulence, surely results to be very useful as reported above. The main advantage of serology is that it is a non-invasive and simple method for diagnosing *Hp* infections and for screening individuals at high risk to develop malignant disease. Furthermore, it reduces endoscopies taking also into account the patient's compliance. A drawback of using serology as predictive diagnostic marker of disease is that it could miss a proportion (even if irrelevant) of severe pathologies and underlying malignancy. However, in western countries, this is rare in patients less than 55 years of age presenting with dyspepsia in the absence of sinister symptoms [14].

3. Molecular markers

Knowing in advance if a *Hp* strain in a specific patient is virulent or not is vital for the approach that the clinician should have towards the infected individuals. In other words, the presence of virulence determinants (such as CagA, VacA, Hsp60 proteins) can address the gastroenterologists to a correct and suitable therapy. For this aim, strain typing could be generally useful in pre-endoscopy screening; for example endoscopy might be unnecessary in young dyspeptic patients without severe symptoms who are infected with non- virulent strains. It would be better not only to treat young dyspeptic patients infected with virulent strains without performing an endoscopy but also to treat patients likely to develop ulcers or gastric malignancy before those conditions arise.

In consequence of this, it would seem preferable to screen for and treat only strains which are known to cause disease. For this purpose, the serology towards the virulence determinants can be used instead of invasive endoscopy.

3.1. Vac–A and Cag–A

VacA serology is uncommon because there are some uncertainties about its interpretation owing to the mosaicism of antigens and to the variety of existing subtypes which are correlated to the different diseases (for example vacA s1 strains are more commonly associated with ulcer than vacA s1b strains or vacA s2). In this situation, the vacA genotype should be determined but that requires a gastric biopsy so vacA genotyping cannot be used in non-invasive screening strategies.CagA serology is more reliable than VacA serology due to the strong immunogenicity and the less variability of CagA protein respect to VacA.

CagA seropositivity reflects the presence of cagA gene together with the cag PAI (pathogenicity island). Some problems linked to CagA serology could occur. First of all, the infection with CagA+ strains is common so that treating CagA seropositive subjects might result in unnecessary treatment even if it has been demonstrated [15] that people with CagA seropositive infection are at higher risk of ulcers or more severe pathologies than CagA-negative subjects.

A second problem concerns the fact that avoiding treatment for CagA-negative patients would lead to miss some infected individual patients who later develop malignancy.

Third the presence of CagA-negative strains may be rare in some populations depending on geographical area. Further, it would be advisable to know, in CagA-negative subjects, if their risk of developing more severe disease such as carcinoma is higher than in uninfected people. If any significant risk is confirmed between CagA-negative infected and uninfected individuals, the treatment of CagA-negative patients would be strongly recommended.

In synthesis, if there is evidence that treatment of CagA-positive patients reduces the possibility of subsequent *Hp*-related malignancy, CagA serology can be considered a viable test for selecting strains to treat [16, 17].The *Hp* infectious status is determined serologically using a commercially available enzyme-linked immunosorbent assay ELISA with a sensitivity and specificity of 96% and confirmed by Western blotting (WB).

3.2. Hsp60 (Heath schock protein 60)

Antibodies to Hsp60 have been suggested as markers of chronic inflammation so the detection of anti-Hsp60 covers a crucial role as serological marker of strain-virulence and may therefore be good predictors for the risk of vascular diseases as well as it has been reported for Chlamydia species [18]. High levels of anti-Hsp60 antibodies may constitute a marker and/or a concomitant pathogenic factor of these pathologies.

Lenzi C et al, 2006 [19] found an increased prevalence of CagA-positive Hp infection as well as increased levels of antibodies to Hsp60 in patients with CHD (Coronary Heart Disease) compared with controls. The accurate definition of this new risk factor may lead to novel strategies for the prevention of ischemic heart disease since simple procedures such as the detection of anti-Hsp60 may be a good predictor of ischemic illness.

Wick et al [20] demonstrated that the association between high levels of anti-Hsps60 antibodies and atherosclerotic vascular disease is due to an autoimmune reaction to endothelial cells that express high levels of Hsps in response to different stimuli such as free radicals, local infections, cytokines etc.

Antibodies to Hsp60 are determined by ELISA test using a commercially available human hsp60 (Sigma Che. Co., Milan, Italy) (19).

4. Multiplex PCR assay (Molecular screening)

The molecular markers of virulence, listed above, can be easily detected, other than by the evidence of antibodies towards them through the serology, also by multiplex assays based on PCR. Multiplex PCR assay is an advancement, compared to uniplex or single locus PCR, because it is suited to diagnose and specifically identify virulence *Hp* strains and their main virulence genes cagA, cagE, cagT, vacA, hrgA. This method is able to genotype *Hp* isolates based on the main virulence genes analysis of cagA alleles as well as vacA is performed by polymerase chain reaction (PCR). The methodology for performing Multiplex PCR is reported by Tiwari *et al.* 2007 [17]. Briefly, samples in sterile phosphate bufferd saline after being vortexed, are boiled, cooled in ice and centrifuged. The supernatant is transferred to another tube where 1 μl of the template for amplification is added. Multiplex PCR is carried out in 25-μl volumes using DNA, *Taq* polymerase, oligonucleotide primers of all the selected genes, deoxynucleotide triphosphate and $MgCl_2$ in standard PCR buffer for 35 cycles.

PCR products are electrophoresed in agarose gel with ethidium bromide in a Tris-borate-EDTA buffer. Gel is visualized under UV transilluminator. Polymerase chain reaction products of each target genes are sequenced directly after purification.

The PCR products were inspected by eletrophoresis on 2% agarose gels. Reference strain *H. pylori* ATCC 49503 is used as a positive control whereas water for cell culture grade was used as negative control. [21].

This method results very useful in distinguishing five potential virulence genes also including the two subtypes of vacA signal region (s1 and s2). This new strategy, which not only predicts mere presence or absence of *Hp* infection but also gives information about its genetic heterogeneity, is highly recommended especially because it is a fast and reliable alternative to others methods and also can be employed even in highly contaminated samples. Different genotypes are reported to be correlated to various infection kind by Tiwari *et al.* 2007 [17].

In this study, they report the distribution of the above genes in the different pathologies (Table 2).

	Gastric carcinoma	Duodenal ulcer	Pre-pyloric ulcer	Peptic ulcer	GERD*	NUD**
	%	%	%	%	%	%
vacA s1	85	64	100	100	50	50
vacA s2	14	35	/	/	50	50
cagA	100	78	100	50	100	66
cagE	100	85	100	100	100	83
cagT	100	92	100	100	100	83
hrgA	100	100	100	100	100	100

Modified from S.K. Tiwari et al. (2007)

GERD* : Gastric oesophageal reflux disease; NUD**: Non-ulcer disease

Table 2. Distribution of major virulence genes of *Helicobacter pylori* in various diseases.

An important finding of this study is that hrgA gene results to have 100% prevalence among all disease groups irrespective of clinical category. This result differs from that obtained by Ando 2002 [22] who reported a more marked presence of hrgA in patients with cancer than in those with other pathologies. These discordant data can depend on different geographical areas considered in the two researches and on the need of examining a more large number of subjects. Higher prevalence of the genotype cagT +, hrgA +, cagA +, cagE + and vacAs1 + is found among patients with pre-pyloric ulcer (100%) and gastric carcinoma (85.7%) followed by duodenal ulcer subjects (60.7%). Overall, this genotype is present in 67% of the total subjects analysed with higher occurrence among those with ulceration and gastric carcinoma than among those with GERD (gastric oesophageal reflux disease) and NUD (non-ulcer disease). The genotype cagT +, hrgA +, cagA-, cagE + and vacAs2 subtype is least prevalent. The vacAs1 subtype is more correlated with the presence of cagA than the vacAs2 subtype and only 2.44% CagA-negative strains possess the vacAs1 allele. Then with reference to the clinical status, vacAs1 is prominent in patients with pre-pyloric ulcer (100%), gastric carcinoma (85%) and duodenal ulcer (64%).However, this study has been performed using gastric tissues (biopsies). Consequently it is an invasive method and cannot be used as a pre-endoscopy screening. The same authors in a previous attempt, had reported saliva as one of the effective non-invasive specimen not only for the detection of *Hp* infection but also for genotyping the strain infecting [23]. The 16S rRNA gene of *Hp* is a highly specific target for amplification, able to confirm *Hp* infection. Positive amplification of *Hp* specific DNA may be considered as a direct evidence of the presence of the pathogen. Non-invasive methods for the rapid diagnosis of *Hp* in salivary secretion of patients with various gastric diseases using 16S rRNA PCR analysis result to be very useful in pre-endoscopy screening thus showing comparable results with those obtained when biopsies are used (Table 3).Consequently saliva of infected persons serves as a reliable non-invasive alternative to detect the presence of *Hp* infection compared to currently diagnostic invasive tests. Tiwari *et al* [24] in another research also report salivary secretion as a sample suitable for detecting cag PAI (pathogenicity island) of infecting *Hp* correlating this with the disease status of the patients. Hence, analysis of complete cag PAI of *H. pylori* isolated from saliva would be of immense importance in standardizing saliva as a reliable non-invasive diagnostic specimen and also to evaluate the type of *Hp* infection. cagE and cagT are found in a larger proportion of the ulcer group than in the non-ulcer group [24,25].

	Symptomatic subjects		**Asymptomatic subjects**	
	(80)		(20)	
	N°	%	N°	%
Stomach biopsy	72	(90)	10	(50)
Saliva	70	(87.5)	12	(60)

Modified from S.K. Tiwari et al. (2005)

Table 3. Detection of *H. pylori* in biopsies and in salivary secretions by multiplex PCR.

5. Multiplex bead array assay and pre–endoscopy screening

A number of new methodologies and assays have been defined during the last years in order to have reliable, rapid, precise and cost-effective results for the management of many diseases. Furthermore, these methods include the use of non-invasive specimens such as serum and plasma being then a useful tool for pre-endoscopy screening. Multiplex bead array assays (MBAA) and Luminex X-map constitute an advancement in detecting contemporaneously bio-markers in plasma and serum. They result comparable to ELISA method and in addition have the advantage of revealing, independently and quantitatively, a large number of analytes using an automated 96-well plate format. These methods also permit the molecular study of genetic variables involved in virulence mechanisms of important bacterial strains.

The clinical applications of MBAA are reported in Table 4.

Application	Available kits*
Autoimmune	ASCA (h), β-2 Microglobulin (h,m) Centomere B (h)
Cancer markers	α-Fetoprotein (h), Cancer antigen 125 (h), Carcinoe
Cytokine	Aβ40 (h), Aβ42 (h), BDNF (h) DR-5 (h), EGF (h,m)
Gene expression	1L6R (h), ACTB (h), BAD (h), BAK1 (BAK) (h), BCL
Genotyping	FlexMAP (G), Mitochondrial DNA Screening (h)

* (h)= human, (m)= mouse

Modified from F.M. Elshai et al. (2006)

Table 4. Principal clinical applications of MBBA.

The most important application of this test is the quantitative detection of cytokines. The measurement of soluble cytokines and other analytes plays a pivotal role in Hp-related infections. In fact, in Hp diseases, a number of pro-inflammatory cytokines such as tumor necrosis factor-α (TNF- α), interleukin-1β (IL-1β), IL-6, IL-8, IL-2, IL-24 etc, is on the basis of the host immune response and of the immunopathology of this microorganism. Practically multiplex assays rely upon the determination of soluble analytes in serum or plasma through the utilization of specific beads for each ligand with subsequent detection of the captured ligand by a second "reporter" antibody. Positive reaction is detected by the fluorescences where ELISA method uses enzyme amplification of a colorimetric substrate.

Protein microarray kits that use capture antibodies in a multiplex fashion similar to MBAA, are relatively new but they are not accepted as a "gold standard" for clinical use and may be of limited sensitivity [26].

Problems for the MBAA technique can arise for the multiplex nature of the test that can lead to cross-reactions and to anomalies in quantifying some analytes. Interferences can also occur in anti-cytokine antibodies which may cross-react whit other cytokines and other interfering substances. Kits have been optimized to eliminate or minimize any artefact from multiplexing. Nevertheless the problem of interferences can exist.

Test ELISA has been considered as a "gold-standard" for the determination of the analytes in plasma and serum but MBAA test is comparable to it [27]. Even if these two tests have been correlated in many studies [26, 27], it can be difficult to evaluate the results because various investigators use different methods of comparison between MBAA and ELISA. Most of published studies [28,29] have shown good correlation and reproducibility between these two methodologies for the majority of cytokines tested even if the degree of correlation has varied widely. MBAA test has proven to be easy to perform, reliable, time saving and cost-effective so that its use in the clinical practice and in the research area is suggested. (27)

6. Luminex X–MAP technology

Among various MBAA tests that generally incorporate an automatic software able to evaluate the cytokine levels in the samples (plasma and serum), significantly reducing the complexity of the assay and requiring less user interaction, Luminex X-MAP technology plays an important role. It uses digital signal processing capable of classifying polystyrene beads (microspheres) dyed with distinct proportion of red and near-infrared fluorophores.

A spectral address for each bead population can be defined by these proportions. In this case, different detection reaction can be carried out simultaneously on various bead populations. Some recent applications with Luminex-based fluorescent microspheres include cytokine quantitation [30] and polymorphism genotyping [31]. In conclusion we can say that it is possible to measure, with these new methodologies, the level of important cytokines involved in *Hp* immunopathology. These results can make us know, through non-invasive methods, the pattern of cytokines involved in the infection which accounts for the disease status and the strain virulence.

7. Conclusions

The non-invasive tests as diagnostic tool in *Hp* infections of patients with various gastrointestinal disorders, are strongly important because they make the endoscopy unnecessary in different situations. The pre-endoscopy screening may be performed principally through serological markers (detection of different kinds of immunoglobulines) or through molecular markers (presence of CagA or Hsp60).

For CagA detection, serology has proved to be useful, being CagA protein a factor with good antigenic properties, easy and realiable to perform and prone to reveal the presence of Cag pathogenicity island [12]. Hsp60 is also a good antigen so that its detection can be performed through the appearance of specific antibodies against it.[32]

Strain typing could also be useful in pre-endoscopy screening: in fact the invasive gastroscopy could be avoided in young populations with non-ulcer dyspepsia and with non-alarming symptoms. It might be even better to treat patients infected with virulent strains without performing an endoscopy. For these problems, the fact to know in advance if a *Hp* strain is virulent or not, could allow us to treat only isolates with proved aptitude to cause disease.

What we would suggest concerns the rapid and easy detection of virulent strains avoiding both invasive techniques and the consequences of a long-lasting untreated infection. The best approach for this is the new development of multiplex PCR assay considered an advancement over other PCR-based methods which could contribute to gain insights at the genotypic variability exhibited by this pathogen. Multiplex PCR assay by which the presence of various markers can be detected in a single reaction constitutes an important tool [17].

Other new methods such as new multiplex assays (Multiplex Bead Array Assays-MBAA) and Luminex-X map technology, constitute a considerable advancement for genotyping *Hp* thus using non-invasive samples as serum, plasma and salivary secretions [26, 27].

Further problems that should be more deeply examined concern the possible link that may exist between strains with more combinations of virulence determinants and antibiotic resistance that is known to be a crucial drawback in the disease treatment.

Author details

Maria Teresa Mascellino[1*], Alessandra Oliva[1] and Barbara Porowska[2]

*Address all correspondence to: mariateresa.mascellino@uniroma1.it

1 Department of Public Health and Infectious Diseases, Sapienza University, Rome, Italy

2 Department of General and Specialistic Surgery, "Paride Stefanini", Sapienza University, Rome, Italy

References

[1] Censini S., Lange C., Xiang Z.Y. et al. CagA pathogenicity island of *Helicobacter pylori,* encoder type I-specific and disease associated virulence factors. *Proc Natl Acad Sci* USA, 1996;93: 14648-14653.

[2] Center for Disease Control. Universal precaution for prevention of transmission of human himmunodeficiency virus, hepatitis B virus and other bloodborne pathogens in healt-care settings.*United States Morbid Mortal Weekly Rep* 1988;37:377-382, 387-388.

[3] Corrado E., Novo S.. Role of inflammation and infection in vascular disease. *Acta Chir Belg 2005; 105 :567-579.*

[4] Locatelli A., Catalani W.R., Gomes Junior C.R., Battistin C., Paula Silva, Waisberg J.. Detection of Anti-Helicobacter pylori antibodies in serum and duodenal fluid in peptic gastroduodenal disease. *World J Gastroentreol* 2004; 10:2997-3000.

[5] Andersen L.P., Kiilerick S., Pedersen G., Thoreson A.C., Jorgensen F., Rath J., Larsen N.E., Borup O., Krogefelt K., Scheibel J., Rune S.. An analysis of seven different methods to diagnose Helicobacter pylori infections. *Scand J Gastroenterol* 1998; 33: 24-30.

[6] Kosunen T.U., Hook J., Rautelin H.I., Myllyla G.. Age dependent increase of *Campylobacter pylori* antibodies in blood donors. *Scand J Gastroenterol* 1989;24: 110-114.

[7] Lim A.G. , Martin R.M., Monteleone M., Walker A.C., Gould S.R.. *Helicobacter pylori* serology and the managment of young dydpeptics: a UK survey of gastroenterologists and general practitioners with an interest in gastroenterology. *Aliment Pharmacol Ther* 1997; 11: 299-303.

[8] Atherton J.C. *H. pylori* virulence factors. *British Medical Bulletin* 1998; 54: 105-120.

[9] Ren Z., Borody T., Pang G., Chen Li L., Dunkley M., Clancy R. Selective reduction of Anti-*Helicobacter pylori* IgG Subclass Antibody in Gastric Carcinoma. *Journal of Gastroenterology and Hepatology.* 2005; 20:1338-1345.

[10] Tulinius H., Ogmundsdottir H.M., Kristinsson K.G. *et al. Helicobacter pylori* antibodies and gastric cancer in Iceland: the decline in IgG antibody level is a risk factor. *APMIS* 2001; 109:835-841.

[11] Correa P. Human gastric carcinogenesis:a multistep and multifactorial process- first American Cancer Society Award Lecture on cancer epidemiology and prevention. *Cancer Res* 1992; 52:6735-6740.

[12] Bodger K., Wyatt J.L., Heatley R.V. Serologic screening before endoscopy: the value of *Helicabacter pylori* serology, serum recognition of the CagA and VacA proteins, and serum pepsinogen I. *Scand J Gastroenterol* 1999; 34:856-863.

[13] Mc Nulty C.A., Nair P., Watson B.E., Uff J.S., Valori R.M. A comparison of six commercial kits for *Helicobacter pylori* detection. *Commun Dis Public Health* 1999;1: 59-63.

[14] Mc Coll K. Should non-invasive *Helicobacter pylori* testing replace endoscopy in investigation of dydpepsia? *Helicobacter* 2000;5: 11-31.

[15] Blaser M.J., Pèrez-Pèrez G.I., Kleanthas H. *et al.* Infection with *Helicobacter pylori* strains possessing *cagA* is associated with an increate risk of developing adenocarcinoma of the stomach. *Cancer Res* 1995;55: 2111-2115.

[16] Rhead J.L., Letley P.D., Mohammad M., Hussein N., Mohagheghi M.A., Hosseini M.E., Atherton J.C.. A new *Helicobacter pylori* Vacuolating Cytotoxin Determinant, the Intermediate Region, Is Associated With Gastric Cancer. *Gastroenterology* 2007; 133.926-936.

[17] Tiwari S.K., Khan A.A., Manoj G., Ahmed S., Abid Z., Habeeb A., Habibullah C.M.. A simple multiplex PCR assay for diagnosing virulent *Helicobacter pylori* infection in

human gastric biopsy specimens from subjects with gastric carcinoma and other gasto-duodenal diseases. *Journal of Applied Microbiology* 2007;103: 2353-2360.

[18] Mascellino M.T., Ciardi M.R., Oliva A., Cecinato F., Borghese L. *Chlamydia trachomatis* detection in a population of asymptomatic and symptomatic women: correlation with the presence of serological markers for this infection. *New Microbiologica* 2008;31: 249-256.

[19] Lenzi C., Palazzuoli A., Giordano N., Alegente G., Gonnelli C., Campagna M.S., Cantucci A., Sozzi M., Papakostas P., Rollo F., Nuti R., Figura N. *H pylori* infections and systemic antibodies to CagA and heat shock protein 60 in patients with coronary heart disease. *World J Gastroenterol* 2006;48: 7815-7820.

[20] Wick G., Knoflach M., Henderson B., Bernhard D. Heat shock proteins and stress in atherosclerosis. *Autoimm Rev* 2004;3: 30-31.

[21] Lozniewski A., Muhale F., Hatier R. *et al.* Human embryonic gastric xenografts in nude mice: a new model of *Helicobacter pylori* infection. *Infect. Immun* 1999;67: 1798–1805.

[22] Ando T., Wassenaar M., Peek R.M., Aras R.A., Tschumi A.I., van Doorn L.J., Kusugami K., Blaser M.J. A *Helicobacter pylori* restriction endonuclease replacing gene, *hrgA*, is associated with gastric cancer in Asian strains. *Cancer Res* 2002;62: 2385-2389.

[23] Tiwari S.K., Khan A.A., Ahmed K.S., Ahmed I., Kauser F., Hussain M.A., Alì S.M., Alvì, Habeeb A., Abid Z., Ahmed N., Habibullah C.H. Rapid diagnosis of *Helicobacter pylori* infection in dyspeptic patients using salivary secretion: a non-invasive approach. *Singapore Med J* 2005;5:224-228.

[24] Tiwari SK, Sharma V, Sharma VK, Gopi M, Saikant R, Nandan A, Bardia A, Gunisetty S, Katikala P, Habeeb MA, Khan AA, HabibullahCM Phylogenetic analysis, based on EPIYA repeats in the cagA gene of Indian Helicobacter pylori, and the implications of sequence variation in tyrosine phosphorylation motifs on determining the clinical outcome. *Genet Mol Biol.* 2011 ;34(2):280-285.

[25] Tiwari SK, Manoj G, Sharma V, Sivaram G, Saikant R, Bardia A, Sharma VK, Abid Z, Khan AA, Habeeb MA, Habibullah CM, Kumar BS, Nandan A.Relevance of Helicobacter pylori genotypes in gastric pathology and its association with plasma malondialdehyde and nitric oxide levels. *Inflammopharmacology*. 2010 Apr;18(2):59-64. Epub 2010 Feb 9.

[26] Copeland S., Siddiqui J. and Remick D. Direct comparison of traditional ELISAs and membrane protein arrays for detection and quantification of human cytokines.*J Immunol Methods* 2004;284:99-106.

[27] Elshal M.F. and Mc Cay J.P. Multiplex bead array assays: Performance evaluation And comparison of sensitivity to ELISA. *Science Direct* 2006;4: 317-323.

[28] Dubois A., Berg D.E., Incecik E.T., Fiala N., Heman-Ackah L.M., Perez-Perez G.I., Blaser M.J. Transient and persistent infections of non-human primates with *Helicobacter pylori:* implications for human disease. *Infect Immun* 1996;64: 2885-2891.

[29] Hildesheim A., Ryan R.L., Rineart E., Nayak S., Wallace D., Castle P.E., Niwa S. and Kopp W. Simultaneous measurement of several cytokines using small volumes of biospecimens. *Cancer Epidemiol Biomarkers Prev* 2002;11:1477-1484.

[30] de Sager W., Velthuis H.T.E., Prakren J., Kuis W., Rijkers G.T. Simultaneous detection of 15 human cytokines in a single sample of stimulated peripheral blood mononuclear cells.*Clin Diagn Lab Immunol* 2003;1: 133-139.

[31] Keyes K., Mann L., Cox K., Treadway P., Iverson P., Chen Y.F., Teicher B.A.. Circulating angiogenic growth factor levels in mice bearing human tumors using Luminex Multiplex technology *Cancer Chemother Pharmcol* 2003;4:321-327.

[32] Kusters J.G., Van Vliet A.H.M., Kuipers E.J. Pathogenesis of *Helicobacter pylori* Infection. *Clinical Microbiology Reviews* 2006; 19(3): 449-490.

Chapter 4

Diagnostic Endoscopy

Akash Nabh, Muhammed Sherid, Charles Spurr and Subbaramia Sridhar

Additional information is available at the end of the chapter

http://dx.doi.org/10.5772/ 52826

1. Introduction

Gastrointestinal (GI) endoscopy is defined as the direct visualization of the digestive tract, with or without therapy. Endoscopic technology has rapidly advanced over the past 40 years and has become an integral part of clinical gastroenterology. The utilization of endoscopy for both diagnostic evaluation and screening has markedly increased over the last two decades. Many innovations have expandedthe indications for endoscopy. Successful endoscopy relies upon the ability to recognize abnormalities and diagnose disease. It is imperative for the endoscopist to detect GI lesions in its early stage to ensure that the patient can receive less invasive treatment and have better prognosis. To make a correct diagnosis of early neoplasm in the GI tract, we first need to detect any lesions with subtle morphologic change.

In this chapter we describe various GI conditions and the role of various endoscopic methods in their diagnosis.

2. Esophagogastroduodenoscopy (EGD)

EGD is performed by passing a flexible scope through mouth to the esophagus, stomach and duodenum. This procedure is the best method to examine upper gastrointestinal mucosa can be performed under conscious sedation in most patients.

The indications for EGD are persistent upper abdominal symtoms despite trial of therapy, upper abdominal symptoms with suspected organic disease (anorexia, weight loss etc.), dysphagia, odynophagia, recurrent or persistent gastroesophageal reflux disease (GERD), persistent vomiting, familial adenomatous polyposis (FAP),GI bleeding, portal hypertension to treat and document esophageal varices, management of achalasia/ esophageal strictures/

stenotic lesions, removal of foreign bodies, placement of feeding tubes, palliative stenting, surveillance of malignancy in Barrett's esophagus, and banding of esophageal varices [1].

Contraindications of EGD are medical instability, patient incooperation and suspected perforation.

Complications of diagnostic EGD are cardiopulmonary events, perforation (0.03%),and bleeding (<0.1%)[2].

2.1. Esophagus

2.1.1. Eosinophilic esophagitis

Eosinophilic esophagitis is a chronic inflammatory disease of the esophagus,usually associated with allergic syndromes.It is increasingly diagnosed in patients presenting with episodic dysphagia and occurs predominantly in males.Endoscopically it is characterized by longitudinal furrows (linear furrowing), widespread white spots,diffuse mucosal nodularity,and multiple rings which fail to disappear with insufflation with air (feline esophagus).Mucosal fragility is frequent. Esophageal mucosa may bleed or become fissured with the scope passage,particularly in the case of a small-caliber or felinized esophagus[3,4].

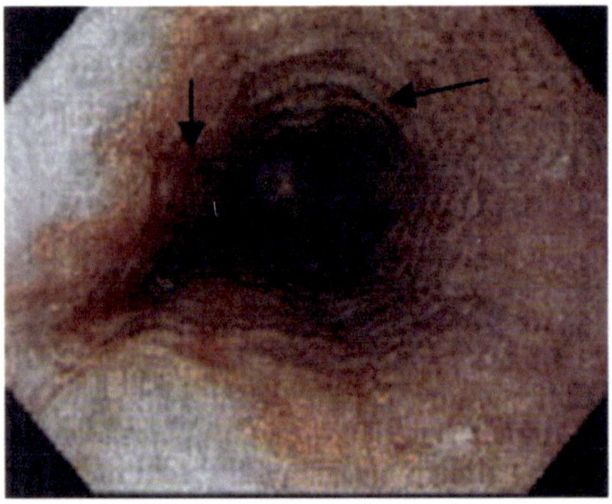

Figure 1. Eosinophilic esophagitis with linear furrowing and rings(pointed by arrows)

2.1.2. Pill-induced esophagitis

Prolonged contact with certain medications can irritate the esophageal mucosa causing esophageal ulcer and esophagitis. Medication-induced esophagitis presents with sudden onset of odynophagia and retrosternal pain. A clinical diagnosis may be made by history without the requirement for confirmatory endoscopy [5](19). The common culprit medications arenon-steroidal anti-inflammatory drugs (NSAIDS), tetracyclines, bisphosphonates, potassium chloride, and iron supplements. Endoscopyallows diagnostic confirmation and is a more sensitive procedurethan barium swallow [5,6].

Endoscopically, pill-induced esophageal injury presents as a discrete ulcer with relatively normal surrounding mucosa. Exudative inflammation with esophageal thickening and stricture formation are also seen.

The most common sites of injury are the proximal esophagus near the compression from the aortic arch and the distal esophagus in patients with left atrial enlargement.It can also occur in motility disorders which allow prolonged contact of medications with the esophageal wall [5].

2.1.3. *Reflux esophagitis and Gastroesophageal reflux disease (GERD)*

GERDis defined as the backward passage of stomach contents through the lower esophageal sphincter. The symptoms of GERD include heart burn, chest pain, water brash and odynophagia.

Endoscopy at initial presentation should be considered in patients who have alarm symptoms suggestive of complicated disease or those at risk for Barrett's esophagus.These alarm symptoms are failure to respond to appropriate antisecretory medical therapy, dysphagia, upper GI bleeding,anemia, odynophagia, and weight loss [7].

The severity of esophageal erosions is predictive of a patient's response to therapy and of the likelihood of relapse after therapy. Therefore it is important to grade the severity of erosive reflux esophagitis.Two grading systems which are commonly usedare Savary-Miller endoscopic classification and Los-Angeles grading [7].

The Savary-Miller endoscopic classification system is used widely but usage and interpretation are very variable. The "MUSE" (Metaplasia, Ulceration, Stricturing, and Erosions) classification provides clear definitions of the relevant endoscopic features, and it is based on a standardized report form, which allows the endoscopist to make a clear record of esophagitis severity.

Grade I: One or more supravestibular, non-confluent reddish spots, with or without exudates

Grade II: Erosive and exudative lesions in distal esophagus thatmay be confluent, but not circumferential

Grade III: Circumferential erosions in the distal esophagus, covered by hemorrhagic and pseudomembranous exudates

Grade IV: Chronic complications such as deep ulcers, stenosis, or scarring with Barrett's metaplasia

The "L.A." (Los Angeles) classification describes four grades of esophagitis severity (A to D), based on the extent of esophageal lesions known as "mucosal breaks," but it does not record the presence or severity of other GERD lesions.

Grade A: One or more mucosal breaks each ≤5 mm in length

Grade B: At least one mucosal break >5 mm long, but not continuous between the tops of adjacent mucosal folds.

Grade C: At least one mucosal break that is continuous between the tops of adjacent mucosal folds, but which is not circumferential

Grade D: Mucosal break that involves at leastthree-fourths of the luminal circumference.

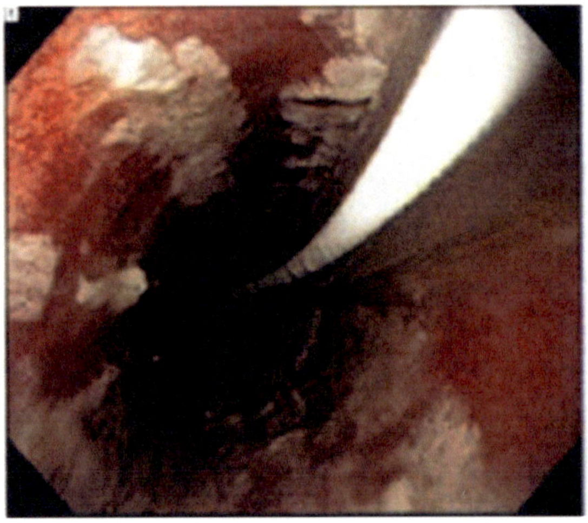

Figure 2. LA grade D esophagitis

Chronic GERD can cause esophageal stricture and Barrett's esophagus(which are described in later sections)

2.1.4. Barrett's Esophagus

Barrett's esophagus is a condition in which metaplastic columnar epithelium that predisposes to cancer development replaces the stratified squamous epithelium that normally lines the distal esophagus. Barrett's esophagus is well recognized as a complication of GERD. Patients with GERD who develop Barrett esophagus tend to have a combination of clinical features, including hiatal hernia, reduced lower esophageal sphincter (LES) pressures or delayed esophageal acid clearance time. The annual incidence of esophageal cancer in a population of patients with Barrett's esophagus is approximately 0.5% per year.

Endoscopically,the typical appearance of Barrett's esophagus is a salmon pink mucosa which extends down and joins the gastric mucosa.

The American Gastroenterologic Association (AGA) suggests endoscopic screening for Barrett's esophagus in patients with multiple risk factors associated withesophageal adenocarcinoma "age 50 years or older,male sex, white race, chronic GERD, hiatal hernia,elevated body mass index, and intra-abdominal distributionof body fat". Once identified, patients with Barrett esophagus should undergo periodic surveillance endoscopy to identify dysplasia.It is recommended that endoscopic evaluation be performedtaking 4-quadrant biopsies every 2 cm with biopsy sampling of any mucosal irregularities. Four-quadrant biopsy specimens be obtainedevery 1 cm in patients with known or suspecteddysplasia.If there is no dysplasia surveillance endoscopy is recommended every 3-5 years.With low grade dysplasia, 6-12 month surveillance intervals are recommended. High grade dysplasia requires endoscopic biopsy every 3 months if eradication therapy is not performed.The AGA recommends endoscopic eradication therapywith radiofrequency ablation, photodynamic therapy or endoscopic mucosal resection rather than surveillance for treatment of patients with high-grade dysplasia with Barrett's esophagus[8].

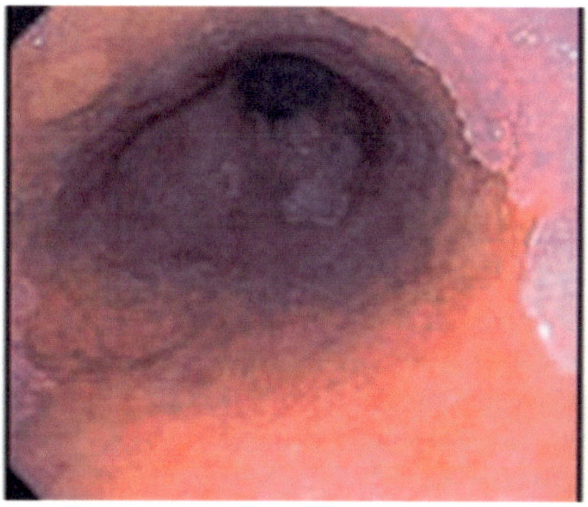

Figure 3. Long segment Barrett's esophagus

2.1.5. Esophagitis related to infections

Candida

Candida species colonize in 20 % of healthy adults.The risk factors are AIDS, cancer, antibiotic or steroid therapy.The causative organism is almost always C. albicans. Candida esophagitis usually present as odynophagia or dysphagia.The diagnosis is based on the endoscopic picture, microscopic examination and culture of the mucosal brushings, and histological examination of the esophageal mucosa. About two-third of patients have signs of oral thrush (thus its absence does not exclude esophageal involvement).EGD with brushings orbiopsy is currently the most sensitive and specific method of diagnosis.Endoscopy demonstrates patchy, whitish plaques covering a friable, erythematous mucosa.When the infection is severe, ulceration may be present as well [9]. Confirmatory biopsy shows the presence of yeasts and pseudohyphae invading mucosal cells, and the culture reveals Candida.

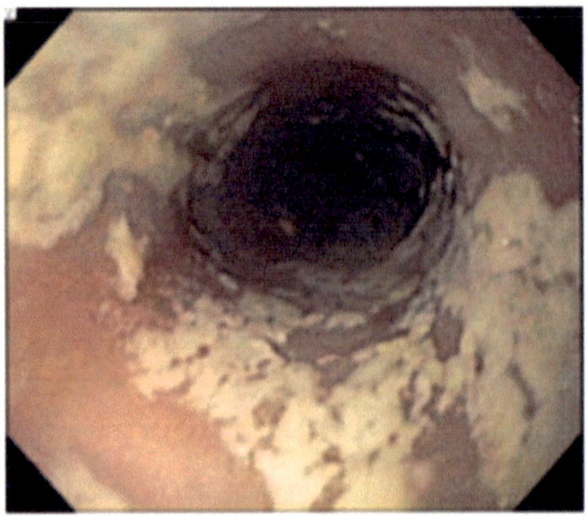

Figure 4. Pale plaques with erythematous mucosa – esophageal candidiasis

Herpes simplex virus

HSV-1 infection of the esophagus is usually seen in immunocompromisedconditions such asorgan or bone marrow transplantation. Less commonly in HIV patients and occasionally immunecompetent patients acquire HSV-1 infection. Endoscopically, there are well circumscribed ulcers with raised margins and a punched out" appearance,distinguishing them from the ulcers seen in CMV infection.Exudates, plaques, or diffuse erosive esophagitis and vesicles can also be seen. Biopsies should be taken from the edge or margin of the ulcer where viral cytopathic effects are most likely to be present [10].

Cytomegalovirus

The most common cause of esophagitis in patients with advanced AIDS is Candida, whereas the most common viral cause is CMV. CMV esophagitis is seen in post-transplantation, long-term renal dialysis, human immunodeficiency virus (HIV) infection, and AIDS and other debilitating diseases. Endoscopically,extensive ulceration of the esophagus is hallmark of CMV esophagitis.It may present as asolitary ulcer or multiple ulcers.Most ulcers are noted in the distal esophagus [11]. The multiple biopsy specimens should be taken from the base of the ulcer.

2.1.6. Esophageal diverticulum

The formation of diverticula occurs due pulsion from increased intraluminal pressure resulting in pushing of esophageal mucosa andsubmucosa through the focal weakness of mucosal wall. The risk factors are esophageal dysmotility or stricture which contribute to intraluminal pressure[12].Esophageal diverticula are rare but can occur in any part of the esophagus.If it occurs in the upper esophagus above the upper esophageal sphincter through a weak spot (Killian's triangle)form above the upper esophageal sphincter in the midline posteriorly at the pharyngoesophageal junction, it is called Zenker's diverticulum. When it occurs in the distal esophagus just abovethe lower esophageal sphincter, it is called epiphrenic diverticula. Endoscopically appear round with a wide neck.

Endoscopy does not play important role in the diagnosis but the endoscopistshould be aware and cautious about their presence as perforation can occur with endoscopy especially when side viewing scopes are used. Esophageal diverticula are well seen on barium x-ray examination, which is the best modalityfor diagnosis.

2.1.7. Esophageal rings and webs

Esophageal webs are thin membrane like structure containing mucosa and submucosa which can occur anywhere in the esophagus.The patients are asymptomatic or have only intermittent dysphagia. It is frequently discovered incidentally during radiographic studies for other reasons. However, esophageal webs have been described in Plummer-Vinson syndrome which present as iron deficiency anemia, glossitis and koilonychia. Endoscopically, the webs are seen with difficulty due to proximal location.They are covered with squamous mucosa [13,14].

Esophageal rings are thin, fragile structures that partially or completely obstruct the esophageal lumen.They present with dysphagia if the lumen is <13 mm. They are usually seen in the distal esophagus. If the ring occurs at squamocolumnar junction covered with squamous mucosa above and columnar epithelium below, it is called Schatzki ring or Type B ring. If the ring occurs about 1.5 cm proximal to the squamocolumnar junction, it is called Type A ring. Endoscopy is less sensitive than the barium esophagram in detecting esophageal rings [13,14].

Endoscopically, an esophageal ring appears as a thin membrane with a concentric smooth contour that projects into the lumen.

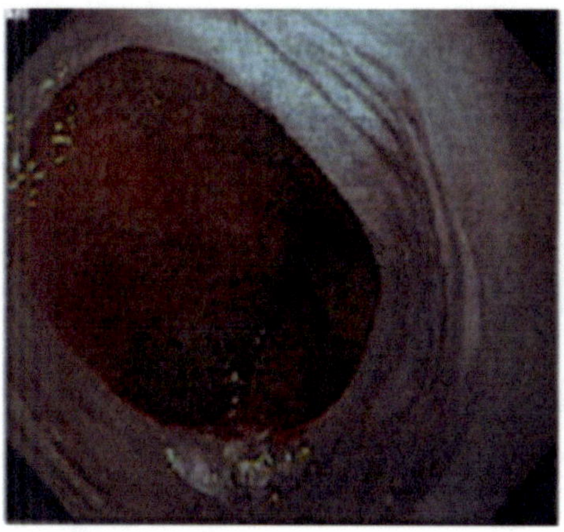

Figure 4. Schatzki ring

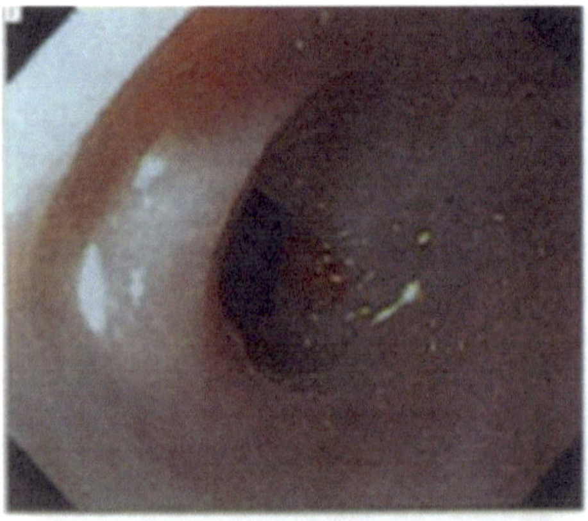

Figure 5. Esophageal web

2.1.8. Stricture

The esophageal stricture is narrowing of esophagus which can be benign or malignant.The symptoms of esophageal stricture are usually insidious but progressive with dysphagia to solids followed by dysphagia to liquids. Dysphagia corresponds to the caliber of the stricture; dysphagia to solids is usually present when the esophageal lumen is narrowed to 13 mm or less. The causes of esophageal stricture formation are GERD, long-term use of a nasogastric (NG) tube, complication of sclerotherapy for varices, infectious esophagitis, post surgical resection for esophageal or laryngeal cancer, caustic ingestion, pill esophagitis, and radiation exposure [15].

Endoscopy is helpful as it allows direct visualization, tissue sampling to rule out malignancy, and dilation of the narrowed part of the esophagus.

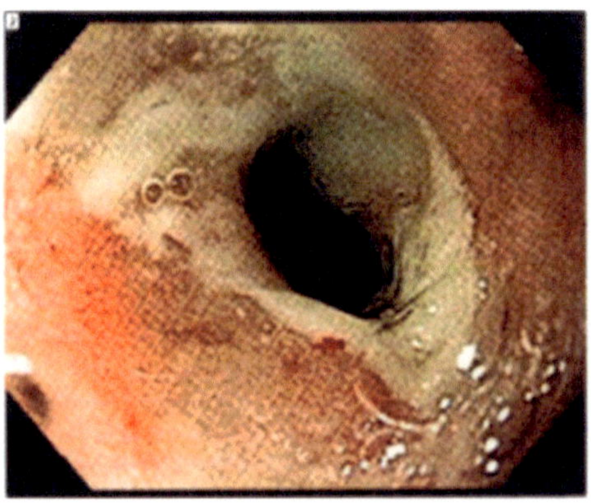

Figure 6. Esophageal stricture

http://dx.doi.org/10.5772/ 52826

2.1.9. Hiatus hernia

Hiatus hernia refers to herniation of elements of the abdominal cavity most commonly stomach,into the mediastinum, through the esophageal hiatus of the diaphragm.Endoscopic and radiographic studies have shown a significant relation between GERD and hiatal hernia [16]. The main types of hiatal hernia are sliding type and para-esophageal type.

Sliding hiatal hernia accounts for more than 95 % of cases. It is characterized by widening of the muscular hiatal tunnel and circumferential laxity of the phrenoesophageal membrane, allowing a portion of the gastric cardia to herniate upward. Hiatal hernias that are larger than 2 cm in axial span can be diagnosed easily by barium swallow radiography, endoscopy, or esophageal manometry. Smaller hernias are more difficult to define. Endoscopically, the squamocolumnar junction appears 2-3 cm above the diaphragmatic hiatus. On endoscopic retroflexed view appears as pouch like area just below mucosal junction and above the diaphragm [17].

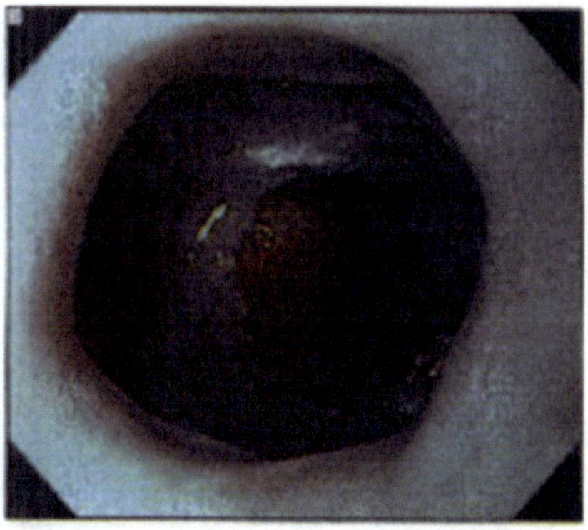

Figure 7. Sliding hiatal hernia visible in the esophagus

Para-esophageal herniasaccount for about 5 % of all hiatal hernias.Anatomically,the pouch of stomach herniatesinto the chest adjacent to the esophagus.Most complications of a para-esophageal hernia are related to mechanical problems caused by the hernia. Para-esophageal hernias are best diagnosed with a barium swallow, although their presence is usually suggested by endoscopy.Endoscopically, they can cause difficulty in locating the main gastric lumen.

Cameron lesions are erosions or ulcers occurring in the sac of a hiatal hernia. They have been described in up to 5.2 % of patients with a hiatal hernia who undergo upper endoscopy. They are usually an incidental finding but rarely cause acute or chronic upper gastrointestinal bleeding and iron deficiency anemia[18].

2.1.10. Motility disorders of the esophagus

Motility disordersin the esophagus present as dysphagia. Evaluation of esophageal motility disorders often begins with endoscopy.The diagnosis can be made with endoscopy alone, however some cases require manometry or barium swallowing study for confirmation.

Endoscopy typically reveals a dilated esophagus in achalasia that often contains residual material. A''popping''effect with difficulty in passing the endoscope through the gastro-esophageal junction may be noted.The esophageal mucosa usually appears normal. Endoscopy is also essentialin achalasia to exclude malignancy.

Endoscopic findings in spastic disorders of the esophagus such as nutcracker esophagus and diffuse esophageal spasm are often normal; however, it may reveal sacculations, diverticula, and chaotic contractile activity along the mid or distal esophagus.Endoscopyis usually performed to exclude structuralesophageal obstruction.

In scleroderma, endoscopic findings usually relate to a hypotensive lower esophageal sphincter [12].

2.1.11. Other benign lesions of the esophagus

The prevalence of benign esophageal tumors is 0.5%. The majority of these benign tumors are asymptomatic which diagnose incidentally. Dysphagia is the most common presenting symptomin patients with symptomatic benign esophageal tumors which occurs with large sized tumors. Other symptoms include regurgitation, vomiting and retrosternal discomfort [19].

Leiomyomas

Leimyomas are the most common benign tumors of the esophagus. They arise from smooth muscle cells. Dysphagia can occur only with large sized tumors. Endoscopically, they appear as submucosal masses with smooth margins and normal overlying mucosa.

Esophageal Cyst

Esophageal cysts are second most common benign tumors. Cysts are usually located in the upper esophagus and are lined by ciliated columnar epithelium. Endoscopically, they appear as protruding mass in the lumen. Surgical resection is required as they can cause complication line obstruction or hemorrhage.

Fibrovascular polyps

Fibrovascular polyps are thin, solitary polyps which usually occur in upper esophagus. They present with symptomatic dysphagia. Over 75 % are 7cm or larger. They have large mucosal folds or large pedicles containing blood vessel.

Squamous cell papilloma

Squamous cell papilloma is usually solitarysessile, warty lesion less than 1.5cm occurring most commonly in lower third of the esophagus.Histologically they are finger like projections of hyperplastic squamous tissue. Etiology of these lesions is felt to be due to human papillomavirus (HPV) infection.

Inlet patch

Inlet patch is isolated area in the esophagus resembling gastric mucosa usually found in the proximal esophagus.It can be associated with Barrett's esophagus and esophagitis in about 20% cases. Histologically, oxyntic type gastric mucosa is most commonly seen [20].

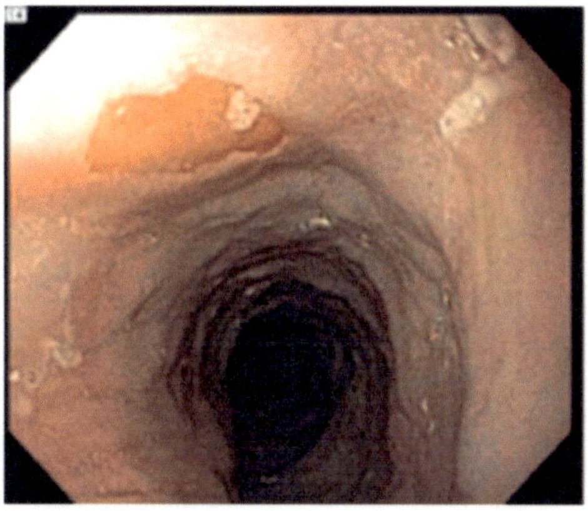

Figure 8. Inlet patch in the esopghagus

Glycogen acanthosis

Glycogen acanthosis presents as elevated gray-white plaques in the esophagus that range in diameter from 1 to15 mm. They are seen in 20–40% of endoscopic procedures and are more prominent in the lower third of the esophagus. Histologically, the epithelium is thickened by the proliferation of large squamous cells filled with glycogen. Glycogen acanthosishas been associated with Cowden's syndrome and celiac disease.

2.1.12. Foreign bodies of the esophagus

Ingestion of foreign bodies occursmost commonly among those with psychiatric disorders, mental retardation, prisoners, and alcoholics.Thepresence of esophageal stricture or ring predispose to impaction of foreign body or food bolus in the esophagus. Fortunately, most pass through the gastrointestinal tract harmlessly. However, 10–20% will require non-operative intervention. Endoscopic extraction is themainstay of non-operative interventions which usually attempt after radiographic localization. Foreign bodies at the level of the hypopharynx or cricopharyngeus muscle are best treated with rigid laryngoscopy using a grasping clamp.In all other cases esophagoscopy is the method of choice [21].

2.1.13. Esophageal Varices

Varices are dilated veins which develop in the esophagus and stomach due to portal hypertension. Severe upper GI bleeding from varicesas a result of portal hypertension develops in about 30-40%of cirrhotic patients. Mortality of the first variceal bleed is 25-35%. Endoscopic grading of size and stigmata is very important in predicting the risk of hemorrhage.Endoscopic stigmata which are associated with risk of variceal hemorrhage are red wale markings, white nipple sign, cherry red and hematocystic spots andvariceallarge size [22]. It is recommended that all the patients with cirrhosis have a screening test to determine presence of varices, so that preventive treatments can be recommended to prevent bleeding [23].

Endoscopically, esophageal varices are graded according to their size, as follows [24]:

Small (Grade 1): Small straight varices

Medium (Grade 2): Enlarged tortuous varices occupying less than one third of the lumen

Large (Grade 3): Large coil-shaped varices occupying more than one third of the lumen.

Upper endoscopy plays vital role in diagnosis, management, screening and surveillance of esophageal varices.

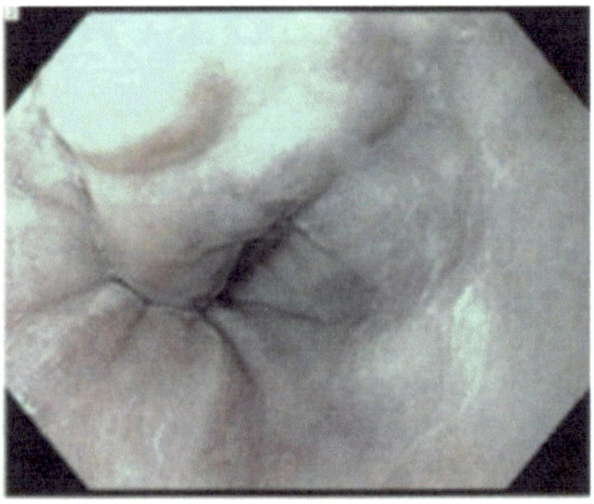

Figure 9. Grade 2 esophageal varices

2.1.14. Mallory Weiss Tear

Mallory Weiss tear is a mucosal lacerationat the level of gastroesophageal junction or gastric cardia usually caused by forceful emesis or retching. Most tears occur with in 2 cm of the cardia side of the gastroesophageal junction on the lesser curvature. The majority of patients present with gastrointestinal bleeding. Endoscopy is the diagnostic test of choice which also helps in allowing visualization of any active bleeding. Usually,a single tear is noted and the most common location is the right posterior aspect of the cardia. Between 2 and 6 O'clock position with patient in left lateral decubitus position. If endoscopy is delayed, a healing tear may be seen with grayish or erythematous granulation tissue [25].

http://dx.doi.org/10.5772/ 52826

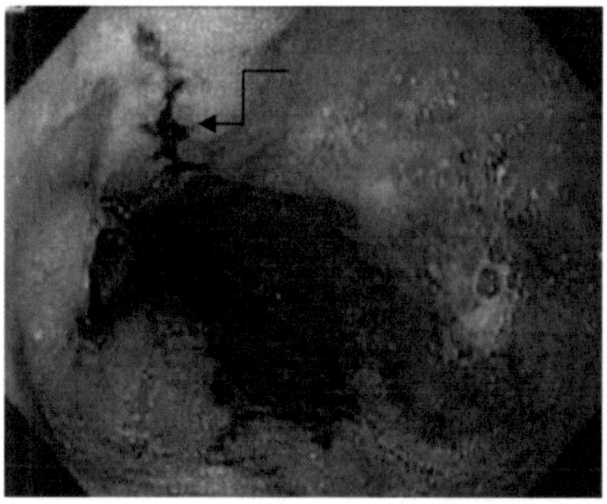

Figure 10. Mallory Weiss Tear at GE junction (pointed by the arrow)

2.1.15. Esophageal neoplasm

Carcinoma of the esophagus presents with dysphagia to solid food usually which progresses gradually to both solids and liquids.There are two main types of esophageal carcinoma: squamous cell type and adenocarcinoma.

Squamous cell carcinoma presents as three typical forms

polypoid mass (most common),

mass with central depressed ulceration,and

diffuse infiltrating form associated with malignant stricture.

Adenocarcinoma usually appears as an infiltrative lesion, with a narrowed lumen with or without associatedmass. It often has a nodular appearance with friable and eroded mucosa; stricture may occur.

Endoscopic visualization with multiple biopsies to increase diagnostic yield must be performed to confirm the diagnosis. Chromoendoscopy using Lugol's iodine (discussed later) is helpful to direct the biopsies and identify the disease extent. Endoscopic ultrasound along with PET /CT further defines the extent of the disease.

2.2. Stomach and duodenum

2.2.1. Peptic ulcer disease

Endoscopy is the most accurate diagnostic test for peptic ulcer disease (PUD) which could be benign or malignant ulcers.

Benign Ulcer

Benign ulcers have smooth, regular, rounded edges, with a flat, smooth ulcer base often filled with exudates.The ulcer base is white covered by fibrinous granulation tissue.In the event of recent bleeding, stigmata of recent bleeding can be seen in the ulcer base.

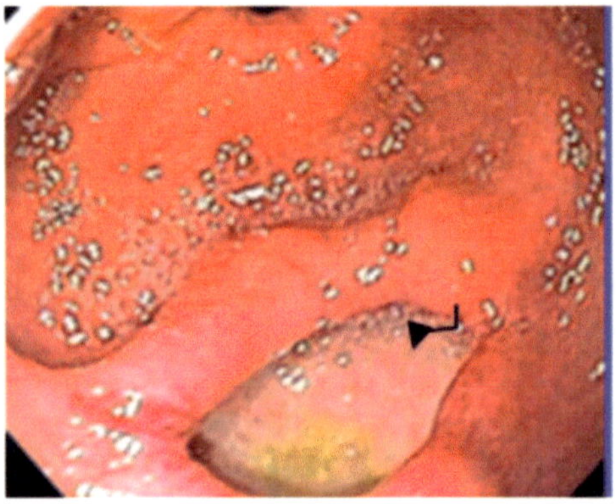

Figure 11. Large cratered clean based gastric ulcer

Malignant ulcer

An ulcerated mass with nodular looking folds and irregular overhanging, nodularmargin is suggestive of malignant ulcer. The chance of malignancy is greater in large gastric ulcers.In about 20 % of cases, endoscopic appearance cannot distinguish benign from the malignant ulcer. 4-6 biopsies of the ulcer margin are shown to detect the vast majority of cancers. Multiple endoscopic biopsies of even benign-appearing gastric ulcerations should be performed due to the risk they may harbor malignancy [26].

Refractory ulcers

Refractory ulcers have been defined as those that fail to heal despite 8 to 12 weeks of antisecretory therapy.I n patients with refractory PUD, surveillance endoscopy should be considered until healing is documented or until the etiology is defined (eg. NSAID use, highgastrin states, ischemia).

Bleeding ulcers

Endoscopy is an effective tool in the diagnosis, prognostication, and management of ulcer bleeding. Randomized studies have shown early endoscopic interventions (within 24 hours of admission) reduce blood transfusionr equirements, shorten intensive care unit and hospital stays, decrease need for surgery, and lowermortality rate [27]. Patients who are hemodynamically stable with endoscopy revealing ulcers without high-risk stigmata may be safely discharged home after endoscopy. Patients with endoscopic stigmata indicating a high risk of rebleeding which includes adherent clots, visible vessels, and active arterial bleeding should all undergo endoscopic therapy to achieve hemostasis and reduce the risk of rebleeding. Recurrent bleeding may occur in as many as 10% of patients despite endoscopic therapy and the use of high-dose proton pump inhibitors. In patients who rebleed after initial endoscopic therapy, repeat endoscopic therapy is suggested before considering surgicalor radiologic intervention [28].

2.2.2. Gastric outlet obstruction

Gastric outlet obstruction may occur as a result of PUD with inflammation and scarring of the pylorus or duodenum. Patients typically present with loss of appetite, epigastric pain, bloating, nausea, vomiting, and weight loss. Endoscopy is important in confirming the diagnosis and differentiating benign from malignant obstruction. Active ulcers may be noted in association with gastric outlet obstruction in as many as one third of patients undergoing endoscopy for this condition [29]. Biopsies to excludem alignancy should be considered.

2.2.3. Gastritis and gastropathy

Gastritis is an inflammatory process while gastropathy demonstrates minimal to no inflammation.

Gastritis

Gastritis is a term that covers entities that induceacute inflammatory changes in the gastric mucosa. The inflammation may involve the entire stomach or a region of the stomach. Acute gastritis is classified as erosive or non-erosive. Erosive gastritis appears as superficial, deep or hemorrhagic erosions. Non erosive gastritis generally caused by Helicobacter pylori.

Vascular gastropathy

Vascular gastropathies are abnormalities in the gastric tissue that involve mucosal vessels with or without inflammation. The two most important vascular gastropathies are gastric antral vascular ectasias(GAVE) and portal hypertensive gastropathy (PHG).

GAVE is characterized by longitudinal columns of vascular ectasias that cross the antrum and converge on the pylorus.The columns have the appearance of the outside of a watermelon. Thus, this disorder commonly being referred as" water melon stomach" [30]. Histpathological exam shows minimal inflammation in the lamina propria, but there is prominent fibromuscular hyperplasia with dilated muscular capillaries. It is common in females and is associated collagen vascular disease and liver disease. It can lead to iron deficiency anemia and the patient may become transfusion dependent. GAVE can be treated with endoscopic therapy using argon plasma coagulation.

Portal hypertensive gastropathy (PHG) or (congestive gastropathy) is a rare cause of significant upper GI bleeding in patients with portal hypertension. PHG characteristically appears as a fine white reticular pattern separating areas of pinkish mucosa on endoscopy, giving the gastric mucosa a "snakeskin" appearance. The vascular abnormalities involve deeper submucosal vessels that are dilated, irregular and tortuous. Patients with severe PHG may develop iron deficiency anemia due to active oozing requiring blood transfusions. Since deeper vessels are involved endoscopic treatment is not effective. Treatment is aimed at

1. decreasing portal pressure with beta blockers,

2. portal decompression withtransjugular intrahepatic portosystemic shunt (TIPS), or

3. liver transplantation.

Hypertrophic Gastropathy

Gastric mucosal hypertrophy refers to giant gastric folds. Diffuse mucosal hypertrophy may be described as hyperplastic or nonhyperplastic.In hyperplastic gastropathy gastric epithelial cells which compose the oxyntic glands may become hyperplastic and give rise to giant mucosal folds. The conditions include: Ménétrier's disease, hyperplastic hypersecretorygastropathy, and Zollinger-Ellison syndrome. In nonhyperplasticgastropathy - gastric mucosa may contain other cell types which result in enlargement of the gastric folds. These conditions include infiltrative diseases, infections, and malignancy.

Endoscopy with mucosal biopsy is required to distinguish between acute, chronic active and chronic gastritis and gastropathy. All gross abnormalities should be biopsied withmultiple biopsies of both the corpus and the antrum to establish the diagnosis of Helicobacter pylori or autoimmune gastritis.Biopsies of the duodenum may also be helpful for diagnosing some forms of chronic gastritis such as Crohn's disease in patients with granulomatous gastritis and celiac disease in patients with lymphocytic gastritis [31].

2.2.4. Dieulafoy's lesions

Dieulafoy's lesion is a rare but important cause of upper GI bleeding. Arterial bleeding from an aberrant vessel isvisualized without an associated ulcer or mass lesion.The lesion can be easily missed on endoscopy in the absence of active bleeding. It may look like a raised nipple or visible vessel without an associated ulcer. Endoscopy is the diagnostic modality of choice for a Dieulafoy's lesion during acute bleeding [32].

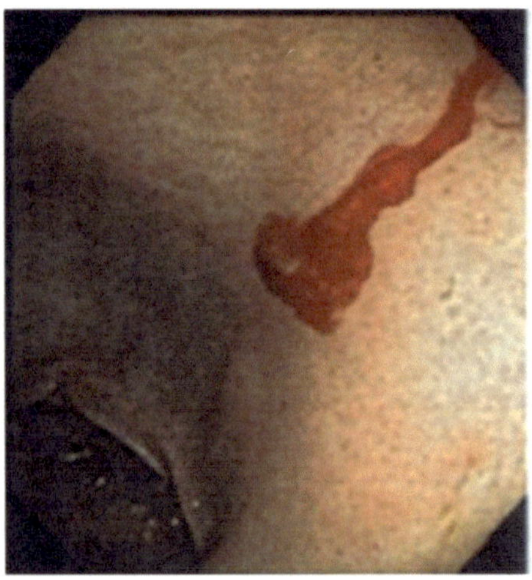

Figure 12. Actively bleeding dieulafoy's lesion

2.2.5. Gastric polyps

Gastric polyps are usually found incidentally when upper GI endoscopy performed for an unrelated indication. They are important since some types of polyps have malignant potential [33]. Adenomatous gastric polyps are at increased risk for malignant transformation and should be resected completely. Hyperplastic polyps have a rare malignant potential. Endoscopic polyp appearance cannot differentiate histologic subtypes, therefore biopsy or polypectomy is recommended when a polyp is encountered. When multiple gastric polyps are encountered, a biopsy of the largest polyps should be performed or they should be excised. Surveillance endoscopy 1 year after removing adenomatous gastric polyps is reasonable to assess recurrence at the prior excision site, new or previously missed polyps, and/or supervening early carcinoma. If the results of this examination are negative, repeat surveillance endoscopy should be repeated no more frequently than at 3- to 5-year intervals. Follow-up after resection of polyps with high-grade dysplasia and early gastric cancer should be individualized. No surveillance endoscopy is necessary after adequate sampling or removal of non-dysplastic gastric polyps [34].

The various types of gastric polyps are briefly described below.

Fundic Gland Polyps

Fundic gland polyps are the most common type of polyps detected by endoscopy. These lesions are typically less than 5 mm in size, sessile and smooth in appearance. They are located in body and fundus. Fundic gland polyps are commonly seen in patients who take proton pump inhibitors (PPIs) on a long-term basis. They have an extremely low malignant potential. The PPI-related lesions may regress in 3 months, once use of the PPI is discontinued. A polyp associated with familial polyposis carries a defined 30% to 50% risk of developing dysplasia. When multiple fundic gland polyps are evident in younger patients, evaluation for familial polyposis should be considered.Biopsy of fundic polyps is done to exclude dysplasia [35].

Hyperplastic polyps

Hyperplastic polyps are caused by an inflamed or atrophic gastric mucosa. They have a smooth, dome-shaped appearance. Hyperplastic polyps can be large in size, and patients may present with chronic blood loss or even gastric obstruction. Elimination of the underlying cause, such as H pylori infection, typically results in polyp regression. The risk of malignancy is higher if polyps exceed 2 cm in size. For this reason, large polyps must be completely excised.

Adenomatous Polyps

Adenomatous polyps occur sporadically or in association with familial polyposis. Thesepolyps are circumscribed, pedunculated, or sessile. They are associated with chronic atrophic gastric metaplasia and have a defined cancer risk. Complete removal should be performed.

Polyposis Syndromes

Polyposis syndromes are characterized by multiple polyps.They include juvenile polyposis, Cronkite-Canada syndrome, Peutz-Jeghers syndrome, and Cowden's disease. Hamartomatouspolyps may be present in all of these syndromes. Adenomatous polyps may be found in familial polyposis.

Gastrointestinal Stromal Tumor

Gastrointestinal stromal tumors (GISTs) make up 1% to 3 % of gastric neoplasms and occur more frequently in men than in women. GISTs are typically located in the fundus. Biopsy is typically normal. Endoscopic ultrasonography-guided biopsy with fine-needle aspiration provides the best tissue sample for diagnosis. GISTs are categorized as having malignant potential ranging from low risk to high risk on the basis of polyp size and level of mitotic activity. All GISTs should be regarded as having neoplastic potential. Surgical resection is recommended for lesions larger than 2 cm. Endoscopic resection is an option for smaller GISTs [35].

Pancreatic Heterotopia

Pancreatic heterotopia may present assubmucosal nodular involvement (single or multiple) at the esophagogastric junction or as asubmucosal nodular lesion located in the antrum and prepyloric area.There is a characteristic nodule with a central dimple is seen endoscopically. Histological features resemble normal pancreatic tissue.Pancreatic heterotopia is a benign and asymptomatic condition.

2.2.6. Gastric neoplasm

Esophagogastroduodenoscopy has a diagnostic accuracy of 95% in diagnosing gastric cancer. Early gastric cancers may appear as a subtle polypoid protrusion, superficial plaque, mucosal discoloration, depression, or ulcer [33]. Improved detection of abnormal lesions may be possible with chromoendoscopy, narrow band imaging and magnification endoscop y(discussed later). Endoscopy is also the primary method for obtaining a tissue diagnosis of suspected lesions. Biopsy of any ulcerated lesion should include at least 6 specimens taken from around the lesion because of variable malignant transformation.The early use of upper endoscopy in patients presenting with gastrointestinal complaints may be associated with a higher rate of detection of early gastric cancers. During endoscopy, any suspicious-appearing gastric ulceration should be biopsied. The diagnosis of anaggressive form of diffuse-type called "linitisplastica", can be difficult endoscopically. Because these tumors infiltrate the submucosa and muscularispropria, superficial mucosal biopsies may be falsely negative.

In selected cases, endoscopic ultrasound may be helpful in assessing depth of penetration of the tumor in the layers of the stomach or involvement of adjacent structures.

3. Push enteroscopy

The evaluation of small intestine is difficult due to its length, intraperitoneal location and tortuousity. Recent developments of push enteroscopy, balloon assisted endoscopy, and capsule endoscopy have made endoscopic examination of the entire small bowel examination practical. Methods used to evaluate the small bowel include push enteroscopy, single balloon, double balloon enteroscopy and wireless capsule endoscopy [36].

Push enteroscopy using the enteroscope or pediatric or adult colonoscope allows evaluation of small bowel 70-150 cm beyond ligament of Treitz. The disadvantage is looping of scope resulting in patient discomfort. It helps in diagnosis and therapeutics in small bowel lesions in the proximal small bowel [36].

4. Deep small bowel enteroscopy

Diagnostic indications for deep small bowel enteroscopy include obscure gastrointestinal bleeding, tattooing of suspected small bowel malignancies or abnormal findings on other imaging studies and wireless capsule endoscopy, suspected nonsteroidal anti-inflammatory drug-induced small bowel injury, suspected or established small bowel Crohn's disease, refractory celiac disease,detection of polyps in patients with polyposis syndromes such as familial adenomatous polyposis or Peutz-Jeghers syndrome, examination of the gastric remnant in patients who have undergone Roux-en-Y gastric bypass and removal of foreign bodies like retained wireless capsule [37,38].

Deep small bowel enteroscopy can be performed with balloon-assisted or spiral enteroscopy. Single and double balloon techniques are described. These techniques allow deeper access to the small bowel than push enteroscopy.

Single balloon enteroscopy (SBE) uses the scope's flexible tip to anchor the scope to the bowel and intestinal tract is pleated over the overtube and shortened.On the other hand double balloon uses a second balloon to anchor the bowel instead of the scope tip.The working length of double balloon endoscope (DBE) is about 150-200 cm as a result 150-350 cm of small bowel can be visualized. The success rate of complete inspection of small intestine is 40-80%.Balloon-assisted enteroscopy (ie, DBE and SBE) which can be performed orally or per rectum, where as spiral enteroscopy can only be performed orally. The complications of double balloon enteroscopy are ileus, pancreatitis, perforation and prolonged duration of procedure [38].

Spiral enteroscopy is a diagnostic and therapeutic intervention of the small bowel. A small enteroscope is used with overtubethat has helical spirals on the surface. The overtube slides over the enteroscope.There are no major complications reported.The limitations are increased sedation requirement [36].

5. Wireless capsule endoscopy

Wireless capsule endoscopy is an ambulatory procedure which has become a first line test for visualizing the mucosa of the small intestine.The PillCam is a capsule comprise of a lens imager, battery and transmitter. The capsule moves from mouth to the anus with peristalsis taking two images per second at 1:8 magnification. The PillCam SB is FDA approved for visualization of the small bowel mucosa in adults and children aged >10 years(4).

The most common indications include evaluation of obscure GI bleeding including iron deficiency anemia, suspected Crohn's Disease, small intestinal tumors and surveillance in patients with polyposis syndromes, refractory malabsorptive syndromes (eg, Celiac disease)[39].

Contraindications suspected GI obstruction, gastroparesis, swallowing disorders, pregnancy, dementia, strictures or fistulas (based on the clinical picture or preprocedure testing), cardiac pacemakers or other implanted electro-medical devices.

5.1. Small intestine

5.1.1. Celiac disease

Celiac disease is a condition in which the immune system responds abnormally to a protein called gluten causing damage to the lining of the small intestine.It affects about 1% of the western population.Patients with celiac disease usually have positive IgA endomysial or-transglutaminase antibody.Patients with positive antibodies should undergo endoscopy with small bowel biopsy.

The duodenal mucosa may appear atrophic with loss of folds, contain visible fissures, have a nodular appearance or the folds may be scalloped. Multiple biopsies should be obtained in the second and third portion of the duodenum by upper GI endoscopy. Staining techniques and high resolution magnification endoscopy canalso help identify areas of villous atrophy for biopsy (discussed later) [40]. Videocapsule endoscopy shows good sensitivity and excellent specificity for the detection of villous atrophy in patients with suspected celiac disease [41]. The advantages of video capsule endoscopy (VCE) are that it is noninvasive, it images the entire length of the small bowel, and it is able to detect minute mucosal details. For these reasons VCE may be a useful tool for the diagnosis of Celiac disease [42].

5.1.2. Crohn's disease

Crohn's disease is characterized by transmural inflammation of the gastrointestinal tract. Crohn's disease may involve the entire gastrointestinal tract from mouth to the perianal area. It mostly affects distal small bowel and right colon and 20-30% have disease limited to the small bowel only. Thus colonoscopy with ileoscopyand biopsy is a very important test in the diagnosis of Crohn's disease. It can be diagnosed by upper endoscopy, enteroscopy, wireless capsule endoscopy or colonoscopy with terminal ileum intubation based on the location of GI tract involvement. Capsule endoscopy and double balloon enteroscopy have comparable yield. Therefore, capsule endoscopy may be part of an initial evaluation followed by double balloon enteroscopy if biopsy or intervention is needed [43]. Capsule retention is the main and only complication which is indefinite presence of capsule which occurs most commonly in patients of known Crohn's disease [39]. This can be avoided by the use of patency capsule (disintegration time-controlled capsule) in patients with high risk of capsule retention [44].

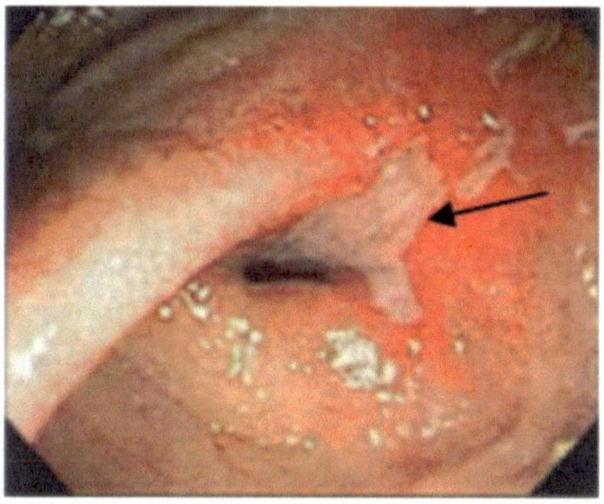

Figure 13. Crohn's disease ulcer in the colon (pointed with an arrow)

On enteroscopy,the findings inCrohn's Disease are linear ulcers,aphthous ulcers,round or irregular ulcers,pseudopolyps,cobble stoning, stricture or stenosis.

5.1.3. Tumors of small bowel

Tumors of the small bowel are relatively uncommon andaccount for approximately 3% of gastrointestinal neoplasms. As the symptoms are vague and conventional diagnostic tests are unsatisfactory.These tumors often present a clinical, radiological, and endoscopic challenge. Endoscopy is very accurate in diagnosing and identifying small bowel lesions[45]. Capsule endoscopy is helpful in the diagnosis of small bowel tumors[46]. Double balloon endoscopy is shown to have good diagnostic capabilities due to its ability to take biopsies[47]. However, isolated mass lesions can be missed on incomplete balloon endoscopy or capsule endoscopy[48]. The clinical conditions that predispose to small bowel neoplasms are Familial adematous polyposis, hereditary non-polyposis colorectal cancer (HNPCC), Peutz-Jegherssyndrome, celiac disease, and Crohn's disease[45].

Adenocarcinomas are the most common type of primary malignant small bowel tumors mostly occurring in duodenum.They appear as circumscribed,polypoid usually large and circumferentially involving the bowel wall.

Carcinoids mostly occur in the terminal ileum,less than 1 meter from IC valve. They are usually small and found incidentally.

GISTs appear as dome shaped submucosal with central ulceration, commonly seen in jejunum.

6. Colonoscopy

Colonoscopy is endoscopic visualization of colonic mucosa.A complete exam is possible in 95-99% of patients.The main indications to colonoscopy are screening and surveillance for colon polyps, pathological bowel wall thickening notedon imaging procedures,diarrhea, malabsorption, rectal bleeding,unexplained iron deficiency anemia, positive fecal occult blood test,suspected short strictures of the colon,rectal foreign bodies,weight loss and abdominal pain [49]. The contraindications of colonoscopy are peritonitis, perforation, fulminant colitis and recent surgical anastomosis.

Complications of colonoscopy are perforation (0.2% with diagnostic colonoscopy and 0.32% with polypectomy), hemorrhage (0.09% with diagnostic colonoscopy and 1.7% with polypectomy) and postpolypectomy coagulation syndrome(electrocoagulation injury inducing transmural burn in 0.5-1.2%,occurs 1-5 days of polypectomy, requires no surgical intervention) and sedation related complications [50]. Thus, polypectomy is the single greatest risk factor for complications of colonoscopy.

6.1. Colon

6.1.1. Screening colonoscopy

Screening for colorectal cancer with colonoscopy is the most common procedure performed by gastroenterologists in the US. Identification of premalignant polyps is primary goal.Some polyps are only hyperplastic with minimal malignant potential. Polyps of concern are called adenomas which are premalignant. Guidelines recommend colonoscopy every 10 years beginning at age 50 years. The follow up colonoscopy should be based on number, size and pathologic findings of the adenomatous polyps removed. Patients with 1-2 small (<1cm) tubular adenomas with only low grade dysplasia should get follow up after 5 years, whereas patients with 3 or more or advanced adenomatous lesions should get repeat colonoscopy in 3 years or before if colonoscopy was incomplete, preparation was poor or >10 polyps are removed.If surveillance colonoscopy is normal, follow up colonoscopy is recommend after 5 years. Patients with large,sessile adenomatous lesions which are removed in piecemeal should have repeat examination within 2-6 months to exclude and remove remnant polypoid tissue [51].

6.1.2. Colonic polyps

Colonic polyps are benign neoplasms that arise from the epithelial cells lining the colon. Colonic polyps are divided into 3 groups: hyperplastic polyps, adenomas, and polyposis syndromes [52].

Hyperplastic polyps

Hyperplastic polyps comprise about 90% of all polyps. They are rounded and sessile measuring few millimetersin size and cannot be distinguished from adenomas. Hyperplastic polyps most commonly occur in the rectosigmoid region.Theylack malignant potential especially if they are located in the rectosimoid area and if the size is few mm. Malignant potential is present only in the setting of very large polyps.

Polyps with architecture similar to hyperplastic polyps but the cytology is different with surface mitotic activity, higher nuclear /cytoplasmic ratio and serrated glandular pattern as a result they are termed as "serrated adenomas"[52]..

http://dx.doi.org/10.5772/ 52826

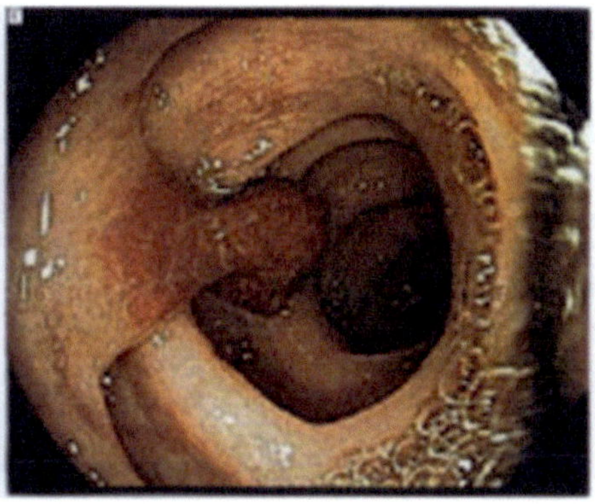

Figure 14. Stalked colon polyp

Adenomas

Adenomas can be seen throughout the colon.Most(70%) found in the left colon and are <1cm.Three histological subtypes are described: tubular, villous and tubulovillous.Tubular adenomas are the most common and can be found anywhere in the colon. Villous adenomas most commonly occur in the rectal area,larger than the other two types, and tend to be non-pedunculated, velvety, or cauliflower-like in appearance. They are more likely to harbor carcinoma in situ or invasive carcinomacompared toother adenomas.The risk of progression to carcinoma is related to both the size and the histology of the adenoma. Adenomas that are greater than 1 cm with villous component carry an increased cancer risk.

The shape or gross structure of the polyp is also clinically significant.Polyps with a stalk are called pedunculated. Those polyps without a stalk are called sessile. Sessile polyps are more concerning than large pedunculated polyps for two reasons. First, the pathway for migration of invasive cells from the tumor into submucosal and more distant structures is shorter. Second, complete endoscopic removal is more challenging and more difficult to accomplish. Premalignant flat lesions are now more readilydetected by new endoscopic imaging methods, such as narrow-band imaging or mucosal staining (described later). The colon polyps are removed with snare cautery, cold biopsy,hot biopsy or cold snaring [53].

6.1.3. Inherited syndromes

Familial adenomatous polyposis(FAP) is an autosomal dominant condition in whichat least 100 adenomatous polyp in the colon, most numerous in the distal colon. When left untreated these polyps develop into colon cancer by third to fifth decade [52].

Hereditary non-polyposis colorectal cancer (HNPCC)/Lynch syndrome is a misnomer as these patients have adenomas similar to general population. However, the adenomas appear at younger age and presents with early on set of colorectal cancer before the age 40, mostly in the right colon. There can be metachrnous or synchronous colorectal malignancies, associated with tumors of other organs especially endometrium, ovary and stomach.

Peutz-Jegherssyndrome is characterized by the presence of hemartomatous polyps occurring more frequently in the small bowel and colon. Melanin spots may be seen on lips and buccal mucosa.These polyps are not precancerous but patients are prone for tumors of breast, lung, ovary and pancreas.

Juvenile polyposis is a conditionpresenting with hamartomatous polyps in the colon, stomach and small bowel. These polyps may be precancerous andrequire close endoscopic surveillance.

6.1.4. Ischemic Colitis

Ischemic colitis is the most frequent form of mesenteric ischemia, presenting with sudden onset of abdominal pain followed by bloody diarrhea. Colonoscopy or sigmoidoscopy is often required to establish the diagnosis of ischemic colitis. The examination usually performed without bowel preparation (to avoid reducing blood flow from dehydrating cathartics), and with minimization of air insufflation (to avoid distention and perforation). Colonoscopy is more sensitive in detecting mucosal lesions allows biopsies, and does not interfere with subsequent angiography.

Colonoscopic findings in the acute setting frequently include pale mucosa with petechial bleeding withbluish hemorrhagic nodules may be seen representing submucosal bleeding [54]. Cyanotic mucosa and hemorrhagic ulcerations are seen later in the course [55]. Segmental distribution, abrupt transition between injured and non-injured mucosa and rectal sparing favor the diagnosis of ischemic colitis [54].

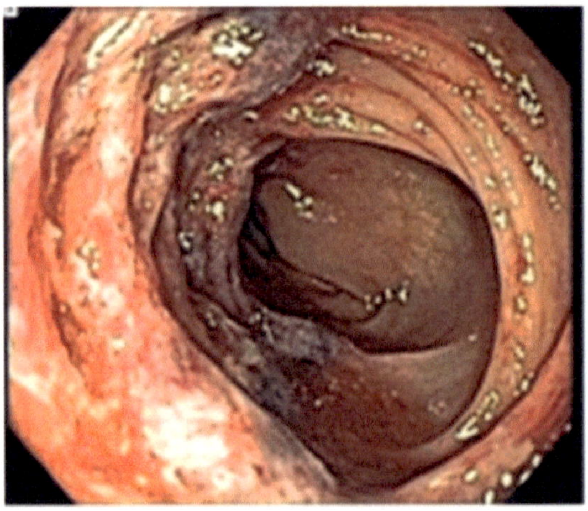

Figure 15. Ischemic colitis

6.1.5. Pseudomembranous colitis

Pseudomembranes are pathognomonic of pseudomembranous colitis (Clostridium difficile associated colitis) but are not found in all cases. Clostridium difficiletoxins cause cytoskeleton disruption causing shallow ulcerations which exude serum proteins and inflammatory cells forming pseudomembranes. Endoscopic findings include raised yellow or off-white plaques up to 2 cm in diameter scattered over the colorectal mucosa which cannot be removed by lavage. These lesions are discrete but may become confluent plaques in more advanced cases. The other colonic findings are edema, erythema, and inflammation with or without pseuodomembranes [56].

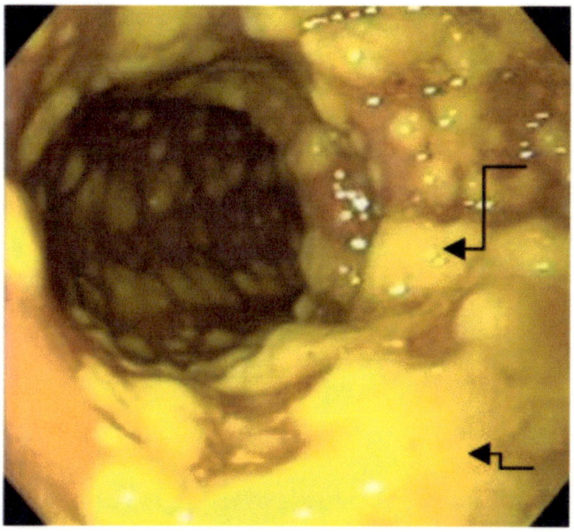

Figure 16. Pseudomembranous colitis- pseudomembranes(pointed by arrows)

6.1.6. Diverticular disease of colon

Diverticula are outpouching of mucosa through the muscle wall of the colon. Colonic diverticula are most frequent source of hematochezia followed by angiodysplasia and inflammatory bowel disease (IBD) [55]. Approximately 95% diverticulosis is noted in descending and sigmoid colon. The prevalence increases with age, from less than 5 % at age nearly two-third by age 80.The diverticular bleed presents as painless, acute hematochezia which is arterial in origin occurring at dome or neck of the diverticulum. About 60 % of diverticular bleeds occurs in left colon, however angiography study recognizes diverticular bleeding more often in the right colon. Bleeding stops spontaneously in 80% cases [55].

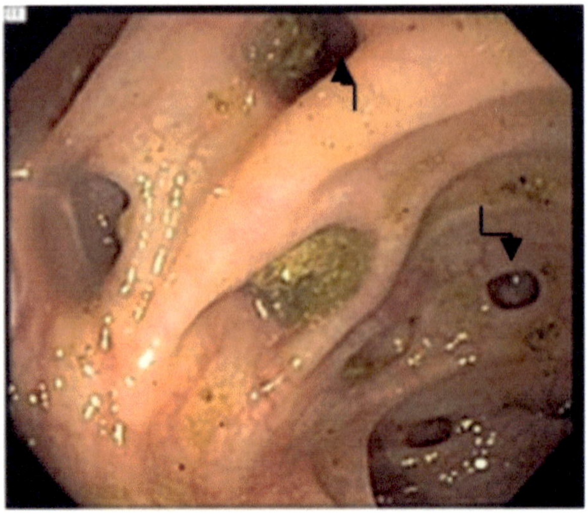

Figure 17. Diverticulosis of colon (pointed by the arrows)

6.1.7. Arteriovenous malformations or Angiodysplasia

Angiodysplasia are detected in about 3-12% cases of lower GI bleeding.Most patients are asymptomatic and overt bleeding occurs in presence of coagulopathy or platelet dysfunction.They are mainly found as multiple lesions in the right colon, appearing as red, circumferential lesions measuring from one millimeter to a few centimeter. The incidence increases with age.

Multiple telagiectasias in pale mucosa can also be seen in case of radiation induced proctopathy which occurs following radiation therapy for prostatic carcinoma [55].

6.1.8. Inflammatory bowel disease

Endoscopic findings in ulcerative colitis (UC) are mucosal erythema and edema with loss vascular pattern. Granularity of mucosa with friability, spontaneous bleeding and ulcers are also seen. Some of patients of UC have focal inflammation around the appendiceal orifice that is not contiguous with disease elsewhere in the colon which is known as "cecal patch".It is important to obtain adequate mucosal biopsies to help distinguish Crohn'sileocolitisfrom pan-ulcerative colitis with backwash ileitis (UC with distal ileum involvement).

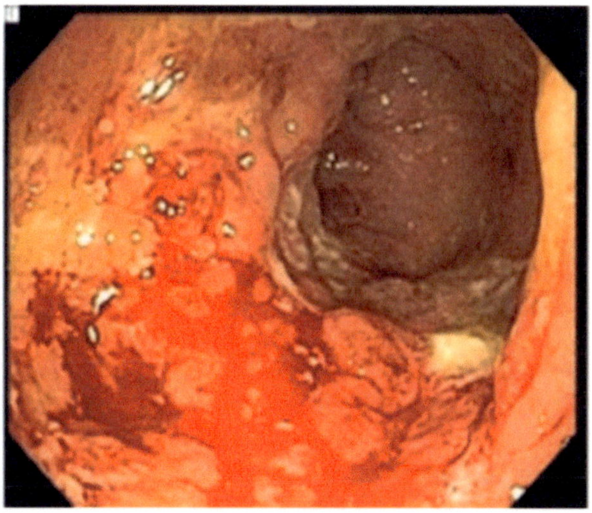

Figure 18. Ulcerative colitis- friable colon mucosa

Endoscopy in Crohns disease reveals aphthous ulcers, cobble stoning or skip lesions .A normal rectum supports the diagnosis of Crohn's disease, since UC always involves the rectum. The presence of normal vasculature adjacent to affected tissue is seen in Crohn's disease, while loss of vascularity and friability is more typical of UC [57].

6.1.9. Hemorrhoids

Hemorrhoids are clusters of veins, smooth muscle and connective tissue lined by the normal epithelium of the anal canal. They are categorized into internal and external hemorrhoids. These categories are anatomically separated by the dentate (pectinate) line. External hemorrhoids are hemorrhoids covered by squamous epithelium below the dentate line, where as internal hemorrhoids are lined with colonic columnar epithelium proximal to dentate line. Internal hemorrhoids are not supplied by somatic sensory nerves and therefore cannot cause pain.Internal hemorrhoids are classified in 4 degrees by the Goligher classification (Table 1). They are best viewed on retroflexed view on flexible endoscopy [58].

First degree	Bleeds but donot prolapse
Second degree	Prolapse but spontaneously reduce
Third degree	Prolapse but require manual reduction
Fourth degree	Unable to reduce

Table 1. Stains used in chromoendoscopy

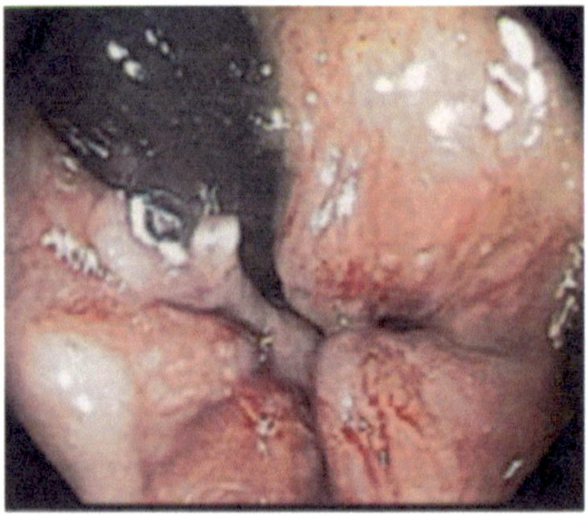

Figure 19. Internal hemorrhoids on retroflexed view

External hemorrhoidal veins are found circumferentially under the anoderm and are innervated by cutaneous nerves that supply the perianal area. Symptoms may occur anywhere around the circumference of the anus [58].

6.1.10. Melanosis coli

Deposition of pigment in the intestinal mucosa is commonly observed on endoscopy, especially within the colon. Electron microscopy has shown that this pigment is not melanin at all, but lipofuscin deposition in macrophages of colon mucosa. Herbal remedies or anthraquinone containing laxatives are often implicated. The pigment intensity is not uniform, being more intense in the cecum and proximal colon compared to the distal colon. Colorectal adenomas do not contain the melanin-like pigmentation. The association of adenomas with melanosis coli can be explained by the ease of detection of even tiny polyps as white spots within a dark-colored colonic mucosa [59]. The condition is benign requiring no treatment.

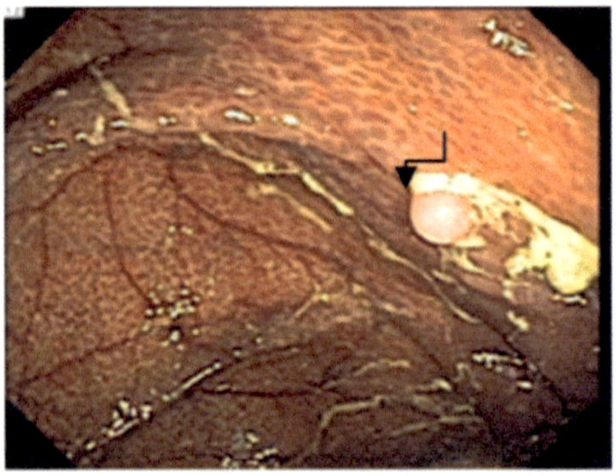

Figure 20. Melanosis coli – colon polyp noted (pointed by an arrow)

6.1.11. Solitary rectal ulcer syndrome

Solitary rectal ulcer syndrome (SRUS) is a rare disorder of defecation presenting as bleeding per rectum.The term SRUS is a misnomer, as 34% of the endoscopic findings are multiple lesions. Endoscopic findings include mucosal ulcerations, polypoid lesions or simply erythema. It is a rare and poorly understood disorder that occurs in people with chronic constipation [60]. Treatments for solitary rectal ulcer syndrome range from changing diet and fluid intake to surgery.

6.1.12. Stercoral ulcer

Stercoral ulceration is the loss ofbowel integrity from the pressure effects of inspissated feces. It usually occurs in constipated and bedridden patients. Because of associated diseases in the population at risk, perforation and hemorrhage are the principal complications resulting in a mortality exceeding 50%. Endoscopically, it appears as an isolated lesion in the rectosigmoid area [61].

6.1.13. Colorectal cancer

Colorectal cancer presents commonly as abdominal pain, hematochezia, change of bowel habits, anemia, or weight loss. Early diagnosis depends on routine screening. Colonoscopy is the single best diagnostic test in symptomatic individuals, since it can localize and biopsy lesions throughout the large bowel, detect synchronous neoplasms, and remove polyps. Air contrast barium enema (BE), supplemented with flexible sigmoidoscopy, is also used to evaluate symptomatic patients.

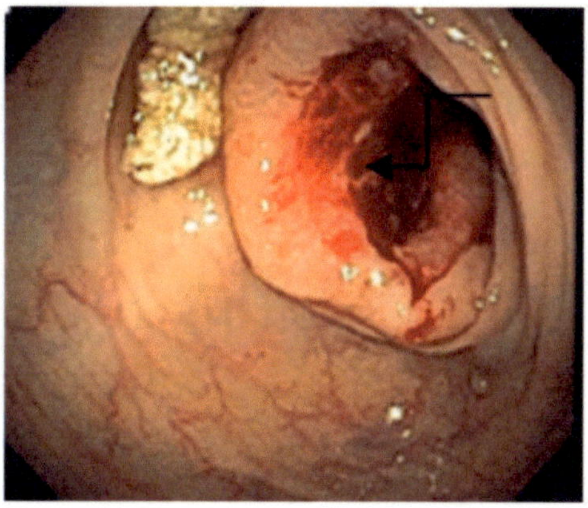

Figure 21. Colon cancer (pointed by an arrow)

Most colon cancers are adenocarcinomas which can be detected on colonoscopy and is undoubtedly the single best diagnostic test in symptomatic individuals since it can localize and biopsy lesions throughout the large bowel, detect synchronous neoplasms, and remove polyps.Endoscopically,lesions may appear as circular proliferating,exophytic or stenosing lesions and uncommonly as plaque like, flat discoid mass with slight depression or ulcer [52]. The likelihood of detection of colorectal cancer can be enhanced by novel methods like chromoendoscopy, narrow band imaging, confocal laser endomincroscopy and high resolution and high maginification endoscopy (described later).

7. Novel and adjunct methods with endoscopy

It is shown that certain flat adenomaswith subtle dysplastic and early neoplastic changes are missed with white light endoscopy as they as they are too small,flat or depressed to be detected. This has led to the development of techniques that compliment conventional endoscopic methods and help in detection of subtle GI lesions by enhancing the image by high magnification or high definition. Image enhanced endoscopy technology can either be dye based (Chromoendoscopy), equipment based (Narrow band imaging), or electronic based [62].

7.1. Chromoendoscopy

Chromoendoscopy involves the topical application of various stains or pigments to subtle GI lesions to improve tissue localization and characterization resulting in targeted biopsies of those lesions. The mucosa is pretreated with a mucolytic agent to remove excess mucus from the mucosal surface. Most commonly 10 % N-acetylcysteine is used. Targeted spraying via a spray catheter is performed for colon polyps and entire surface is stained inthe evaluation Barrett's esophagus. Glucagon is administered just before spraying to decrease contractions and uneven spraying.It is considered to be a safe and nontoxic procedure [63]. The table below describes various stains used in various conditions with their side effects (Table 2).

Stains	Conditions	Side effects
Methylene Blue	Esophagus: Barrett's mucosa/Post ablation to find Barrett's mucosa. Gastric: Intestinal metaplasia Colon:Chronic ulcerative colitis	Harmless , transient blue green discoloration of urine and feces
Toluidine blue	Esophagus: Squamous cell cancer	None reported
Lugol's solution	Esophagus: Squamous dysplasia and early squamous cell carcinoma,	Retrosternal burning and nausea which can be treated with application of 5% sodium thiosulfate which can neutralize residual iodine. Avoided in patients with Iodine hypersensitivity and hyperthyroidism
Indigo carmine	Colon : Colorectal neoplasia,chronic ulcerative colitis	None reported

Table 2. Stains used in chromoendoscopy

Chromoendoscopy has been shown to detected higher number of lesions per patient compared with narrow band imaging (NBI), autofluorescence, or white light colonoscopy [64]. It is an inexpensive, safe and relatively easy to perform but it is not standardized and is subject to observer interpretation.

7.2. Narrow band imaging

Conventional white light endoscopy uses full visible wavelength (red-green-blue) to produce an image. On the other hand narrow band imaging uses special filters which increase relative intensity of the blue band thus enhancing the image quality. NBI used along with magnifying endoscopy allows the analysis of thesurface architecture of the epithelium (pit pattern) and theanalysis of the vascular network resulting in better characterization of distinct types of gastrointestinal epithelia (e.g. intestinal metaplasia in Barret's esophagus),as well as the disorganization of the vascular pattern ininflammatory disorders and the irregular pit pattern in earlyneoplastic lesions of the esophagus, stomach and largebowel [65].

The NBI generates a darker field of view than white light and allows adequate inspection of the mucosal surface. The tip of the endoscope needs to be closer to the mucosa.The presence of bile and blood strongly absorb narrow band light thus obscuring the view under NBI. The NBI images are not yet standardized. There are no reported complications with NBI [66].

7.3. Confocal Laser Endomicroscopy

Canfocal Laser Endomicroscopy (CLE) is new imaging modality of GI endoscopy which allows in vivo imaging of the mucosal layer at cellular and subcellular resolution making in vivo histology possible during endoscopy. CLE is based on the principle of illuminating a tissue with a low-power laser and then detecting fluorescent light reflected from the tissue. To illuminate the tissue, an exogenousagent ??is applied topically or systemically. Most commonly used agent is intravenous fluorescein sodium which highlights the extracellular matrix enabling confocal imaging. The laser is focused at a specific depth and only light reflected back from that plane is refocused and able to pass through the pinhole confocal aperture. As a result, scattered light from above and below the plane of interest is not detected, increasing special resolution. The area being examined is scanned in the horizontal and vertical planes and an image is reconstructed. In this manner, microscopic imaging of biological tissue in vivo is possible due to the high lateral resolution of confocal imaging. It helps in differentiation of neoplastic from non-neoplastic polyps, for example, neoplastic lesion in patients with Barrett's esophagus [67], or ulcerative colitis, differentiation of benign from malignant biliary strictures.

Currently, there are two CLE systems used, probe based (confocal probe passes through the accessory channel of a standard video-endoscope) and integrated endoscopy (CLE integrated in the distal tip of endoscope).

More data is needed to support these modalities. In future, CLE will develop multicolor analysis of several layers with 3-dimensional reconstruction allowing deeper penetration depth [68].

7.4. High resolution and high magnification endoscopy

High-resolution imaging improves the ability to discriminate detail while magnification enlarges the image. Magnification endoscopy often utilizes a movable lens controlled by the endoscopist to vary the degree of magnification(100X as compared with 30X in standard endoscopy). Both high magnification and high-resolution endoscopes were designed to be used in conjunction with chromoendoscopy. High-resolution and high-magnification endoscopy may enhance the diagnosis and characterization of some mucosal lesions and may detect changes in vascular architecture of patients with early esophageal cancer. Magnification chromoendoscopy has been used to characterize Barrett's esophagus, early gastric cancer and villous atrophy [69]. The magnification endoscopy is simple, inexpensive, requiring no special light processors.The disadvantages are lack of standardization and prolongation of procedure time [70]. Whether high-resolution or high-magnification endoscopy will decrease the need for endoscopic biopsy or increase the diagnostic yield of endoscopic procedures has not yet been determined [71,72].

7.5. Autofluoresence imaging

Autofluorense imaging utilizes changes in concentrations of endogenous fluorophores, for example flavin adenine dinucleotide, collagenand nicotinamide adenine dinucleotide. The video-endoscopy adds green and red reflectance improving the image quality.The dysplastic tissue there is lack of fluorescence due to lack of collagen resulting in increased red and decreased green fluorescence.It has been shown useful in detection of dysplasia in Barrett's esophagus and early esophageal cancer but there is insufficient data to support its routine clinical use [62].

7.6. Endocytoscopy

Endocystoscopy is a new imaging method which provides combination which combines chrmoendoscopy with ultra-high magnification catheter which is passed through the working channel of the endoscope [73]. Unlike confocal endomicroscopy, it provides images in color but is limited to superficial layer. It has been shown to give accurate results which are almost comparable with histological results.The diagnosis based on endocytoscopic imaging is subject to interpretation,and there is no validated criteria regarding tissue diagnosis and differentiation for various GI conditions.

Author details

Akash Nabh[1*], Muhammed Sherid[2], Charles Spurr[1] and Subbaramia Sridhar[1]

*Address all correspondence to: anabh@georgiahealth.edu

1 Department of Gastroenterology and Hepatology, Georgia Health Sciences University, U. S. A.

2 Department of internal medicine, division of gastroenterology, Saint Francis Hosiptal, U. S. A.

References

[1] Cohen, J., Safdi, M. A., Deal, S. E., Baron, T. H., Chak, A., Hoffman, B., Jacobson, B. C., Mergener, K., Petersen, B. T., Petrini, J. L., Rex, D. K., Faigel, D. O., & Pike, I. M. (2006). ASGE/ACG Taskforce on Quality in Endoscopy. Quality indicators for esophagogastroduodenoscopy. *Am J Gastroenterol. Apr*, 101(4), 886-91.

[2] Eisen, G. M., Baron, T. H., Dominitz, J. A., Faigel, D. O., Goldstein, J. L., Johanson, . J. F., Mallery, J. S., Raddawi, H. M., Vargo, J. J. 2nd, Waring, .J. P., Fanelli, R. D., & Wheeler-Harbough, J. (2002). American Society for Gastrointestinal Endoscopy. Complications of upper GI endoscopy. *Gastrointest Endosc. Jun*, 55(7), 784-93.

[3] Croese, J., Fairley, S. K., Masson, J. W., Chong, A. K., Whitaker, D. A., Kanowski, P. A., & Walker, N. I. (2003). Clinical and endoscopicfeatures of eosinophilic esophagitis in adults. *Gastrointest Endosc. Oct*, 58(4), 516-22.

[4] Cantù, P., & Penagini, R. (2010). Eosinophilicoesophagitis: the essentials for daily-practice. *Scand J Gastroenterol. May*, 45(5), 528-32.

[5] Zografos, G. N., Georgiadou, D., Thomas, D., Kaltsas, G., & Digalakis, M. (2009). Drug-induced esophagitis. *Dis Esophagus Epub Apr 15*, 22(8), 633-7.

[6] Kikendall, J. W., Friedman, A. C., Oyewole, Fleischer. D., & Johnson, L. F. (1983). Pill-inducedesophagealinjury. Case reports and review of the medicalliterature. *Dig Dis Sci. Feb*, 28(2), 174-82.

[7] Lichtenstein, D. R., Cash, B. D., Davila, R., Baron, T. H., Adler, D. G., Anderson, M. A., Dominitz, J. A., Gan, S. I., Harrison, M. E., 3rd Ikenberry, S. O., Qureshi, W. A., Rajan, E., Shen, B., Zuckerman, M. J., Fanelli, R. D., & Van Guilder, T. (2007). Standards of Practice Committee. Role of endoscopy in the management of GERD. *Gastrointest Endosc. Aug*, 66(2), 219-24.

[8] Spechler, S. J., Sharma, P., Souza, R. F., Inadomi, J. M., & Shaheen, N. J. (2011). American Gastroenterological Association. American Gastroenterological Association medical position statement on the management of Barrett's esophagus. *Gastroenterology*, Mar, 140(3), 1084-91.

[9] Underwood, J. A., Williams, J. W., & Keate, R. F. (2003). Clinical findings and risk factors for Candida esophagitis in outpatients. *Dis Esophagus*, 16(2), 66-9.

[10] Canalejo, Castrillero. E., García, Durán. F., Cabello, N., & García, Martínez. J. (2010). Herpes esophagitis in healthy adults and adolescents: report of 3 cases and review of the literature. *Medicine (Baltimore).*, Jul, 89(4), 204-10.

[11] Wilcox, C. M., Straub, R. F., & Schwartz, D. A. (1994). Prospectiveendoscopiccharacterization of cytomegalovirusesophagitis in AIDS. *GastrointestEndosc.*, Jul-Aug;, 40(4), 481-4.

[12] Kopelman, Y., & Triadafilopoulos, G. (2011). Endoscopy in the diagnosis and management of motilitydisorders. Dig Dis Sci. Mar Epub Feb 1., 56(3), 635-54.

[13] Smith, M. S. (2010). Diagnosis and management of esophageal rings and webs. *GastroenterolHepatol (N Y).*, Nov, 6(11), 701-4.

[14] Tobin, R. W. (1998). Esophageal rings, webs, and diverticula. *J ClinGastroenterol*, Dec, 27(4), 285-95.

[15] Pregun, I., Hritz, I., Tulassay, Z., & Herszényi, L. (2009). Peptic esophageal stricture: medical treatment. Dig Dis Epub May 8., 27(1), 31-7.

[16] Wright, R. A., & Hurwitz, A. L. (1979). Relationship of hiatal hernia to endoscopicallyprovedreflux esophagitis. *Dig Dis Sci*, Apr, 24(4), 311-3.

[17] Kahrilas, P. J., Kim, H. C., & Pandolfino, J. E. (2008). Approaches to the diagnosis and grading of hiatal hernia. *Best Pract Res ClinGastroenterol*, 22(4), 601-16.

[18] Weston, A. P. (1996). Hiatal hernia with cameron ulcers and erosions. *GastrointestEndoscClin N Am*, Oct, 6(4), 671-9.

[19] Choong, . C. K., & Meyers, B. F. (2003). Benign esophageal tumors: introduction, incidence, classification, and clinical features. *SeminThoracCardiovasc Surg*, Jan, 15(1), 3-8.

[20] Tang, P., Mc Kinley, Sporrer. M., & Kahn, E. (2004). Inlet patch: prevalence, histologic type, and association with esophagitis, Barrett esophagus, and antritis. *Arch Pathol Lab Med*, Apr, 128(4), 444-7.

[21] Athanassiadi, K., Gerazounis, M., Metaxas, E., & Kalantzi, N. (2002). Management of esophageal foreign bodies: a retrospective review of 400 cases. *Eur J Cardiothorac Surg*, Apr, 21(4), 653-6.

[22] Jensen, D. M. (2002). Endoscopicscreening for varices in cirrhosis: findings, implications, and outcomes. *Gastroenterology*, May, 122(6), 1620-30.

[23] Merli, M., Nicolini, G., Angeloni, S., Rinaldi, V., De Santis, A., Merkel, C., Attili, A. F., & Riggio, O. (2003). Incidence and natural history of small esophageal varices in cirrhotic patients. *J Hepatol*, Mar, 38(3), 266-72.

[24] Reliability of endoscopy in the assessment of variceal features. (1987). The Italian Liver Cirrhosis Project. *J Hepatol*, Feb, 4(1), 93-8.

[25] Younes, Z., & Johnson, D. A. (1999). The spectrum of spontaneous and iatrogenic esophageal injury: perforations, Mallory-Weiss tears, and hematomas. *J ClinGastroenterol*, Dec, 29(4), 306-17.

[26] Graham, D. Y., Schwartz, J. T., Cain, G. D., & Gyorkey, F. (1982). Prospective evaluation of biopsy number in the diagnosis of esophageal and gastric carcinoma. *Gastroenterology*, Feb, 82(2), 228-31.

[27] Barkun, A., Bardou, M., & Marshall, J. K. (2003). NonvaricealUpper GI BleedingConsensus Conference Group. Consensusrecommendations for managingpatients with nonvaricealupper gastrointestinalbleeding. *Ann Intern Med*, Nov 18;, 139(10), 843-57.

[28] Banerjee, S., Cash, B. D., Dominitz, J. A., Baron, T. H., Anderson, M. A., Ben-Menachem, T., Fisher, L., Fukami, N., Harrison, M. E., Ikenberry, S. O., Khan, K., Krinsky, M. L., Maple, J., Fanelli, R. D., & Strohmeyer, L. (2010). ASGE Standards of Practice Committee. The role of endoscopy in the management of patients with peptic ulcer disease. *GastrointestEndosc.*, Apr, 71(4), 663-8.

[29] Di Sario, J. A., Fennerty, M. B., Tietze, C. C., Hutson, W. R., & Burt, R. W. (1994). Endoscopic balloon dilation for ulcer-induced gastric outlet obstruction. *Am J Gastroentero*, Jun, 89(6), 868-71.

[30] Primignani, M., Carpinelli, L., Preatoni, P., Battaglia, G., Carta, A., Prada, A., Cestari, R., Angeli, P., Gatta, A., Rossi, A., Spinzi, G., & De Franchis, R. (2000). Natural history of portal hypertensive gastropathy in patients with liver cirrhosis The New Italian Endoscopic Club for the study and treatment of esophageal varices (NIEC). *Gastroenterology*, Jul, 119(1), 181-7.

[31] Dixon, M. F., Genta, R. M., Yardley, J. H., & Correa, P. (1997). Histological classification of gastritis and Helicobacter pylori infection: an agreement at last? The International Workshop on the Histopathology of Gastritis. *Helicobacter*, Jul, 2(1), S17-24.

[32] Nagri, S., Anand, S., & Arya, Y. (2007). Clinical presentation and endoscopic management of Dieulafoy's lesions in an urban communityhospital. *World J Gastroenterol*, Aug 28, 13(32), 4333-5.

[33] Kajitani, T. (1981). The generalrules for the gastriccancerstudy in surgery and pathology. Part I. Clinical classification. *JpnJSurg.*, Mar, 11(2), 127-39.

[34] Hirota, W. K., Zuckerman, M. J., Adler, D. G., Davila, R. E., Egan, J., Leighton, J. A., Qureshi, W. A., Rajan, E., Fanelli, R., Wheeler-Harbaugh, J., Baron, T. H., & Faigel, DO. (2006). Standards of PracticeCommittee, AmericanSociety for Gastrointestinal Endoscopy. ASGEguideline: the role of endoscopy in the surveillance of premalignantconditions of the upper GI tract. *GastrointestEndosc*, Apr, 63(4), 570-80.

[35] Goddard, A. F., Badreldin, R., Pritchard, D. M., Walker, M. M., & Warren, B. (2010). British Society of Gastroenterology. The management of gastricpolyps. GutSep Epub Jul 30., 59(9), 1270-6.

[36] Voelkel, J. P., & Di Palma, J. A. (2010). Deep enteroscopy. *South Med J.*, Oct, 103(10), 1045-8.

[37] Westerhof, J., Weersma, R. K., & Koornstra, J. J. (2009). Investigatingobscuregastrointestinal bleeding: capsule endoscopy or double balloon enteroscopy? *Neth J Med.*, Jul-Aug, 67(7), 260-5.

[38] Yano, T., & Yamamoto, H. (2009). Current state of double balloon endoscopy: the latest approach to small intestinal diseases. *J GastroenterolHepatol.*, Feb, 24(2), 185-92.

[39] Eliakim, R. (2010). Videocapsuleendoscopy of the smallbowel. *CurrOpinGastroenterol*, Mar, 26(2), 129-33.

[40] Lo, A., Guelrud, M., Essenfeld, H., & Bonis, P. (2007). Classification of villousatrophy with enhancedmagnificationendoscopy in patients with celiac disease and tropicalsprue. *GastrointestEndosc*, Aug, 66(2), 377-82.

[41] Culliford, A., Daly, J., Diamond, B., Rubin, M., & Green, P. H. (2005). The value of wireless capsule endoscopy in patients with complicated celiac disease. *GastrointestEndosc*, Jul, 62(1), 55-61.

[42] Rondonotti, E., Spada, C., Cave, D., Pennazio, M., Riccioni De, Vitis. I., Schneider, D., Sprujevnik, T., Villa, F., Langelier, J., Arrigoni, A., Costamagna, G., & de Franchis, R. (2007). Video capsule enteroscopy in the diagnosis of celiac disease: a multicenter study. Am J GastroenterolAug Epub Apr 24., 102(8), 1624-31.

[43] Pasha, S. F., Leighton, J. A., Das, A., Harrison, Decker. G. A., Fleischer, D. E., & Sharma, V. K. (2008). Double-balloon enteroscopy and capsule endoscopy have comparable diagnostic yield in small-bowel disease: a meta-analysis. ClinGastroenterolHepatolJun Epub Mar 20., 6(6), 671-6.

[44] Signorelli, C., Rondonotti, E., Villa, F., Abbiati, C., Beccari, G., Avesani, E. C., Vecchi, M., & de Franchis, R. (2006). Use of the Given Patency System for the screening of patients at high risk for capsule retention. Dig Liver DisMay Epub Mar 9., 38(5), 326-30.

[45] Abu-Hamda, E. M., Hattab, E. M., & Lynch, P. M. (2003). Small bowel tumors. *CurrGastroenterol Rep*, Oct, 5(5), 386-93.

[46] Sîngeap, A. M., Trifan, A., Cojocariu, C., Sfarti, C., & Stanciu, C. (2010). Capsule endoscopy role in diagnosis of small bowel tumors]. [Article in Romanian, Abstract in English]. *Rev Med ChirSoc Med Nat Iasi*, Oct-Dec, 114(4), 988-92.

[47] Almeida, N., Figueiredo, P., Lopes, S., Gouveia, H., & Leitão, M. C. (2009). Double-balloon enteroscopy and small bowel tumors: a South-European single-center experience. Dig Dis SciJul Epub 2008 Oct 29., 54(7), 1520-4.

[48] Paski, S. C., & Semrad, C. E. (2009). Small boweltumors. *GastrointestEndoscClin N Am*, Jul, 19(3), 461-79.

[49] Jechart, G., & Messmann, H. (2008). Indications and techniques for lower intestinal endoscopy. *Best Pract Res ClinGastroenterol*, 22(5), 777-88.

[50] Fisher, D. A., Maple, J. T., Ben-Menachem, T., Cash, B. D., Decker, G. A., Early, D. S., Evans, J. A., Fanelli, R. D., Fukami, N., Hwang, J. H., Jain, R., Jue, T. L., Khan, K. M., Malpas, P. M., Sharaf, R. N., Shergill, A. K., & Dominitz, J. A. (2011). ASGE Standards of Practice Committee. Complications of colonoscopy. *GastrointestEndosc*, Oct, 74(4), 745-52.

[51] Davila, R. E., Rajan, E., Baron, T. H., Adler, D. G., Egan, J. V., Faigel, D. O., Gan, S. I., Hirota, W. K., Leighton, J. A., Lichtenstein, D., Qureshi, W. A., Shen, B., Zuckerman, M. J., Van Guilder, . T., & Fanelli, R. D. (2006). Standards of Practice Committee, American Society for Gastrointestinal Endoscopy. ASGE guideline: colorectal cancer screening and surveillance. *GastrointestEndosc*, Apr, 63(4), 546-57.

[52] Ponz de, Leon. M., & Di Gregorio, C. (2001). Pathology of colorectal cancer. *Dig Liver Dis*, May, 33(4), 372-88.

[53] Tappero, G., Gaia, E., De Giuli, P., Martini, S., Gubetta, L., & Emanuelli, G. (1992). Cold snare excision of small colorectal polyps. *GastrointestEndosc*, May-Jun, 38(3), 310-3.

[54] Barnert, J., & Messmann, H. (2009). Diagnosis and management of lower gastrointestinal bleeding. *Nat Rev GastroenterolHepatol*, Nov, 6(11), 637-46.

[55] Sherid, M., & Ehrenpreis, E. D. (2011). Types of colitis based on histology. *Dis Mon*, Sep, 57(9), 457-89.

[56] Hookman, P., & Barkin, J. S. (2009). Clostridium difficile associated infection, diarrhea and colitis. *World J Gastroenterol*, Apr 7;, 15(13), 1554-80.

[57] Waye, JD. (1977). The role of colonoscopy in the differential diagnosis of inflammatory bowel disease. *GastrointestEndosc*, Feb, 23(3), 150-4.

[58] Appalaneni, V., Fanelli, R. D., Sharaf, R. N., Anderson, M. A., Banerjee, S., Ben-Menachem, T., Decker, G. A., Fisher, L., Fukami, N., Harrison, M. E., Strohmeyer, L., Friis, C., Ikenberry, S. O., Jain, R., Jue, T. L., Khan, K. M., Krinsky, M. L., Malpas, P. M., Maple, J. T., & Dominitz, J. A. (2010). ASGE TECHNOLOGY COMMITTEE.The role of endoscopy in patients with anorectal disorders. *GastrointestEndosc.*, Dec, 72(6), 1117-23.

[59] Freeman, H. J. (2008). Melanosis" in the small and large intestine. *World J Gastroenterol*, Jul 21;, 14(27), 4296-9.

[60] Chong, V. H., & Jalihal, A. (2006). Solitary rectal ulcer syndrome: characteristics, outcomes and predictive profiles for persistent bleeding per rectum. *Singapore Med J*, Dec, 47(12), 1063-8.

[61] Maull, K. I., Kinning, W. K., & Kay, S. (1982). Stercoralulceration. *Am Surg*, Jan, 48(1), 20-4.

[62] Buchner, A. M., & Wallace, M. B. (2008). Future expectations in digestive endoscopy: competition with other novel imaging techniques. *Best Pract Res ClinGastroenterol*, 22(5), 971-87.

[63] Wong, ., Kee, Song. L. M., Adler, D. G., Chand, B., Conway, J. D., Croffie, J. M., Disario, J. A., Mishkin, D. S., Shah, R. J., Somogyi, L., Tierney, W. M., & Petersen, B. T. (2007). ASGE Technology Committee.Chromoendoscopy. GastrointestEndosc Oct; Epub Jul 23., 66(4), 639-49.

[64] Matsumoto, T., Esaki, M., Fujisawa, R., Nakamura, S., Yao, T., & Iida, M. (2009). Chromoendoscopy, narrow-band imaging colonoscopy, and autofluorescence colonoscopy for detection of diminutive colorectal neoplasia in familial adenomatous polyposis. *Dis Colon Rectum*, Jun, 52(6), 1160-5.

[65] Gheorghe, C. (2006). Narrow-bandimagingendoscopy for diagnosis of malignant and premalignantgastrointestinallesions. *J Gastrointestin Liver Dis*, Mar, 15(1), 77-82.

[66] Song, L. M., Adler, D. G., Conway, JD, Diehl, D. L., Farraye, F. A., Kantsevoy, S. V., Kwon, R., Mamula, P., Rodriguez, B., Shah, R. J., & Tierney, W. M. (2008). ASGE TECHNOLOGY COMMITTEE.Narrow band imaging and multiband imaging. *GastrointestEndosc*, Apr, 67(4), 581-9.

[67] Pohl, H., Rösch, T., Vieth, M., Koch, M., Becker, V., Anders, M., Khalifa, A. C., & Meining, A. (2008). Miniprobeconfocallaser microscopy for the detection of invisible-neoplasia in patients with Barrett's oesophagus. Gut Dec; Epub Aug 28., 57(12), 1648-53.

[68] Neumann, H., Kiesslich, R., Wallace, M. B., & Neurath, M. F. (2010). Confocal laser endomicroscopy: technical advances and clinical applications. GastroenterologyAug e1-2., 139(2), 388-92.

[69] Boeriu, A. M., Dobru, D. E., & Mocan, S. (2009). Magnifying endoscopy and chromoendoscopy of the upper gastrointestinal tract. *J Gastrointestin Liver Dis*, Mar, 18(1), 109-13.

[70] Sharma, P. (2005). Magnification endoscopy. *GastrointestEndosc*, Mar, 61(3), 435-43.

[71] Stevens, P. D., Lightdale, C. J., Green, P. H., Siegel, L. M., Garcia-Carrasquillo, R. J., & Rotterdam, H. (1994). Combinedmagnificationendoscopy with chromoendoscopy for the evaluation of Barrett's esophagus. *GastrointestEndosc*, Nov-Dec, 40(6), 747-9.

[72] Lee, C. T., Chang, C. Y., Lee, Y. C., Tai, C. M., Wang, W. L., Tseng, P. H., Hwang, J. C., Hwang, T. Z., Wang, C. C., & Lin, J. T. (2010). Narrow-band imaging with magnifying endoscopy for the screening of esophageal cancer in patients with primary head and neck cancers. *Endoscopy*, Aug, 42(8), 613-9.

[73] Kwon, R. S., Wong, Kee., Song, L. M., Adler, D. G., Conway, J. D., Diehl, D. L., Farraye, F. A., Kantsevoy, S. V., Kaul, V., Kethu, S. R., Mamula, P., Pedrosa, M. C., Rodriguez, S. A., & Tierney, W. M. (2009). ASGE Technology Committee. *Endocytoscopy.Endosc*, Oct, 70(4), 610-3.

Chapter 5

Capsule Endoscopy: A New Era of Gastrointestinal Endoscopy

Uday C Ghoshal

Additional information is available at the end of the chapter

http://dx.doi.org/10.5772/52732

1. Introduction

Background: Since the discovery of fiber-optic endoscopy to examine upper and lower gastrointestinal tract, diagnosis and therapy of gastrointestinal diseases were revolutionized. However, by these methods, of the small bowel, only the proximal duodenum and distal ileum could be examined. Hence, rest of the small bowel, which is more than four meters in length, remained like a black box. With the discovery of capsule endoscopy in 2000,[1] not only the small bowel became visible to the Gastroenterologist, but also it led to discovery of a new technology by which a swallowed capsule could take images of the gastrointestinal track and send these to a computer using radio-frequency transmitter. The value, safety and acceptability of this novel technology are further documented by the fact that within a year of its discovery (2001), it was approved by US Food and Drug Administration.[2] These led to an era of physiological endoscopy the scope of which is now increasing day by day to include colon and esophageal capsule endoscopy, steerable capsule and therapeutic capsule endoscopy.

Aims and Methods: The aims of this chapter are to, (a) review histotical aspects of this important development in medical science, (b) outline the principles of this technology, (c) review existing evidences on clinical impact of capsule endoscopy and its limitation, (d) project the future of capsule endoscopy. Literature was searched for studies on capsule endoscopy using various electronic search engines to review data on capsule endoscopy in relation to various gastrointestinal diseases.

2. Historical aspects of capsule endoscopy

In science, what is fiction today, may become reality tomorrow. This is amply documented once again by discovery of capsule endoscopy. Capsule endoscopy is a combination of the device that physicist G. Iddan had developed and that devised by Paul Swain.[2], [3] This was an attempt to reproduce the movie fiction filmed by R. Fleischer in 1966, based on a story by I. Asimov.[2] The first reported use of capsule endoscopy in ten human volunteers was published in 2000 by P. Swain in Nature.[1] The first model of capsule endoscopy was made available by Israeli Company Given Imaging by the name of M2A. Within a year of first publication, the capsule endoscopy was approved by US Food and Drug Administration.[4] Subsequently, it has been widely used throughout the World for diagnosis of small bowel diseases.

3. Small bowel capsule endoscopy: The method

Indications of capsule endoscopy: Indications of capsule endoscopy are summarized in Table 1. Capsule endoscopy is indicated in various small bowel diseases such as obscure gastrointestinal bleeding, celiac disease and other types of malabsorption syndrome, polyposis, Crohn disease etc. Colon capsule and esophageal capsules are used for esophageal and colonic diseases.[5]

Organ evaluated	Diseases or conditions
Small bowel	
	Obscure gastrointestinal bleeding (overt and occult)
	Chronic small bowel diarrhea including celiac disease
	Abnormal small bowel imaging
	Chronic abdominal pain with reasonable suspicion of organic cause in the small intestine
	Evaluation of Crohn disease and its extent
	Visualization of surgical anastomosis
	Suspected small bowel tumor
	Polyposis syndrome
	Portal hypertensive enteropathy and small intestinal varices
Esophagus	
	Barrett esophagus
	Esophageal varices
Colon	
	Colon polyps and colorectal cancer

Table 1. Indications for capsule endoscopy.

The capsule: Most capsules consist of a lens, 4 light emitting diodes, a color camera, 2 batteries, a radiofrequency transmitter and an antenna (Fig. 1).[4] The camera transmits multiple (usually 2/second) images by radiofrequency through sensor to a recorder. Currently, capsule endoscopy system is marketed by different suppliers, which somewhat differ in technology and in length and weight of capsule, number of cameras and antennas, frame rate per second and duration of battery life. Table 2 summarizes these variables.[5] Before patient swallows the capsule, 8 skin antennas are taped to the anterior abdominal wall (Fig. 1). The capsule, while moving inside gastrointestinal tract, takes images and sends these through radio-frequency transmitters and the sensor array that are fixed at different locations on the anterior abdominal wall (Fig. 1) to the data logger, which is hang on the patient. After study completion, the images are downloaded to a computer and seen as video images with software. The use of the real time viewer may shorten procedures, as the patient can be disconnected once the cecum is visualized.[6] Recently, softwares have been upgraded with additional capabilities to assist the reader, such as ability to localize the capsule, blood indicator, a multi-viewing feature and quick view modality.

	Pillcam SB2	Pillcam eso	Pillcam colon	Mirocam	Endocapsule	OMOM
Length in mm	26	26	26	24	26	27.9
Weight (g)	3.4	3.4	3.4	3.4	3.8	6
Number of cameras	1	2	2	1	1	1
Frame rate per second	2	18	4-35	3	2	2
Image sensor	CMOS	CMOS	CMOS	CCD	CCD	CCD
Battery life (h)	8	8	8	11	9	8
Antennas	8	3	8	9	8	14
Sleeping mode	No	No	Yes	No	No	No

Abbreviations used: CMOS: complementary metal oxide semiconductor, CCD: charge-coupled device.

Table 2. Comparison of various types of capsules used in capsule endoscopic examinations

Patient preparation: Initially, capsule endoscopy was done without any preparation. However, dark or opaque fluids, food, biliary secretions, air bubbles and mucus can cause incomplete visualization of small bowel mucosa. Slow gastric emptying and small bowel transit may also lead to incomplete examination of the small bowel in 17 to 25% of patients.[7], [8] Several subsequent studies demonstrated that various methods of bowel preparation using osmotic laxatives such as sodium phosphate, polyethylene glycol, and prokinetics such as erythromycin, metoclopramide, tegaserod, domperidone may improve image quality and completeness of examination of small bowel.[8]-[14] Sodium phosphate and polyethylene glycol, which may also shorten gastric and small intestinal transit time, were found to be superior to erythromycin for this purpose.[8], [15, 16] However, a meta-analysis demonstrated that improved visualization of small bowel mucosa during capsule endoscopy with bowel preparation is independent of any effect on transit time.[17] Oral simethicone, which may reduce intra-luminal air bubble, was associated with better mucosal visibility than placebo.[18, 19] Hence, such preparation to improve small bowel visualization and 12-h fasting before the procedure and ingestion only of clear liquids 2-h hours after capsule ingestion are recommended by most capsule endoscopists.

However, the best type of preparation, its dose and time of administration remain to be determined. Concerns have also been raised in relation to use of prokinetics that shorten small bowel transit as this may lead to shorter stay of the capsule at the site of lesions raising possibility of missing the lesions and some workers even suggested that bowel preparation may reduce patients' acceptability of the procedure.[20, 21] Some studies also suggested that keeping the patient in right lateral position may hasten passage of capsule from stomach to small intestine though there are studies to contradict this.[8], [22] It is important to note that typical gastic passage time of the capsule is one hour and small bowel passage time was four hours.[8]

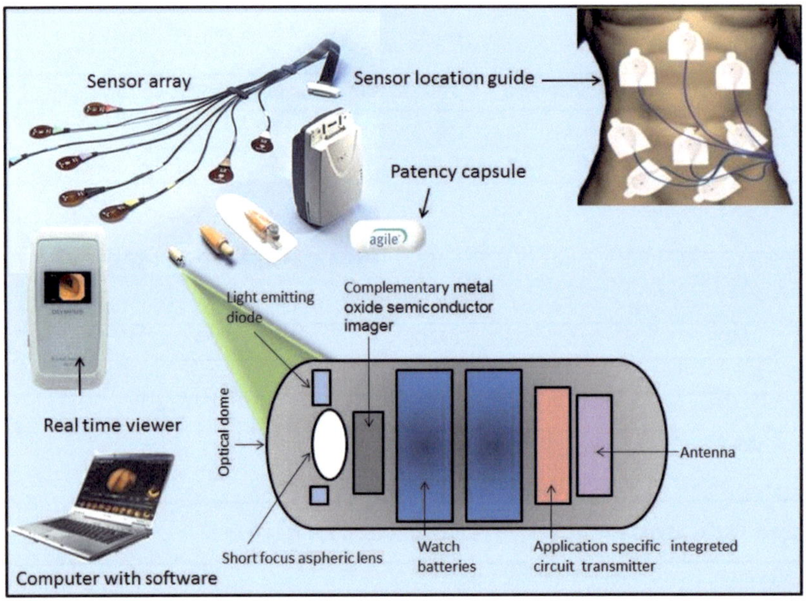

Figure 1. Components of capsule endoscopy system including schematic representation of parts of capsule and sensor location guide.

Clinical impact of capsule endoscopy: Several meta-analyses documented that small bowel capsule endoscopy is superior to other methods of small bowel evaluation such as barium small bowel series, CT enteroclysis, double balloon and single balloon endoscopy.[23], [24] Table 3 summarizes yield of capsule endoscopy in patients with obscure gastrointestinal bleeding in some series published during last decade. Capsule endoscopy detected lesions in small bowel in 45-89% patients with obscure gastrointestinal bleeding. Most series showed that lesions are detected more often in patients with obscure overt than occult gastrointestinal bleeding[25], [26] though a few series did contradict this observation.[27] It has also been shown that if capsule endoscopy is performed early after a bleeding episode, it detects lesion more frequently than if it is done late. In some studies, authors showed that second capsule endoscopy may pick-up some of the lesions missed by first study.[28], [29]

Other diseases of small bowel in which capsule endoscopy is indicated are summarized in Table 1. However, capsule endoscopy done in some of these conditions has limitations. For example, in celiac disease,[30] taking biopsy is very important to detect villous atrophy. However, in other conditions such as Crohn disease, small intestinal tumor, polyposis syndrome and portal hypertensive enteropathy and varices, capsule endoscopy is useful.[31]-[36] In endemic areas, hookworm infestation is not uncommonly detected in patients undergoing capsule endoscopy for obsure gastrointestinal bleeding.[27], [37], [38] Fig. 2 (A to F) and 3 (A to F) depict some of these findings on capsule endoscopy. Fig. 4 outlines a practical approach to use various small bowel endoscopic techniques in patients with obscure gastrointestinal bleeding.

Study	Location	Year	Number of patients	Indications	Overall diagnostic yield
Albert JG et. al.[55]	England	2008	285	OGIB	76.8%
Almeida N[56]	Australia	2009	15	Severe overt OGIB	73.3%
Apostolopoulos P[57]	Germany	2006	51	Occult OGIB	57%
Apostolopoulos P[58]	United States	2007	37	Acute mild-to-moderate OGIB	91.9%
Ghoshal UC[27]	India	2011	86	Occult and overt OGIB	74.4%
Ben Soussan E[59]	France	2004	35	OGIB overt (n=17) and occult (n=18)	45.7%
Bresci G[60]	Japan	2005	64	OGIB	62.5%
Calabrese C[61]	Italy	2011	346	OGIB	71%
Carey EJ[26]	Unites States	2007	260	OGIB overt (n=126) and occult (n=134)	53%
Carlo JT[62]	United States	2005	532	532 studies for OGIB	49.3%
Chao CC[63]	China	2005	35	OGIB	89%
Chong AK[64]	Australia	2003	47	OGIB	68%
De Leusse A[65]	Germany	2005	64	64 OGIB (overt 69% and occult 31%)	45%
Gupta R[25]	India	2006	154	OGIB (overt 74, occult 80)	51%
Enns R[66]	Canada	2004	167	167 studies, 88 overt, 79 occult)	50.8%
Estevez E[67]	England	2006	100	OGIB (overt 52, occult 48)	68%
Fireman Z[68]	England	2004	160	OGIB	57.7%
Fireman Z[69]	Israel	2004	293	OGIB	72%

Abbreviations used: OGIB: obscure gastrointestinal bleeding.

Table 3. Summary of some studies on small bowel capsule endoscopy

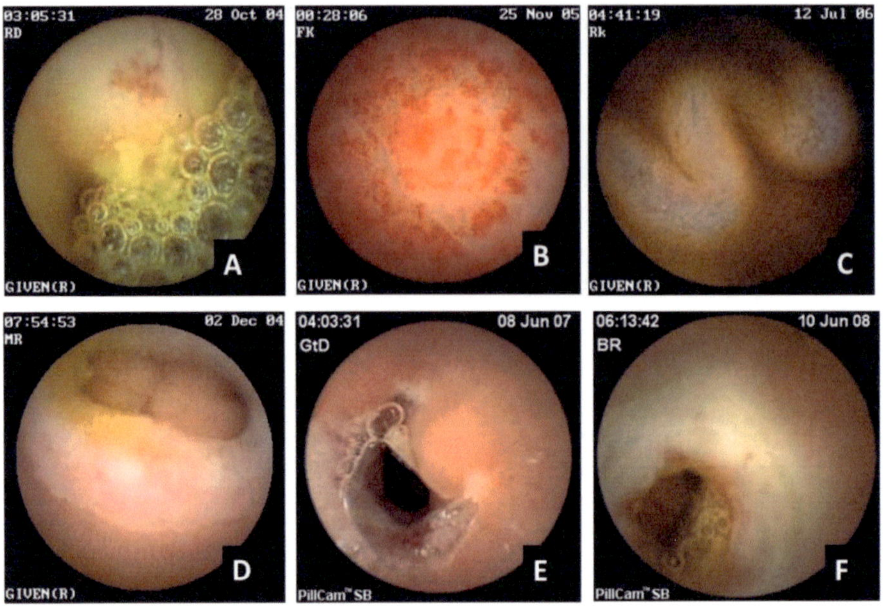

Figure 2. Representative pictures of capsule endoscopy in patients with small bowel angiodysplasia (A), portal hypertensive jejunopathy (B), varices (C), ileocecal ulceration in a patient with intestinal tuberculosis (D), small bowel stricture in a patient with intestinal tuberculosis (E) and in a patient with Crohn disease (F).

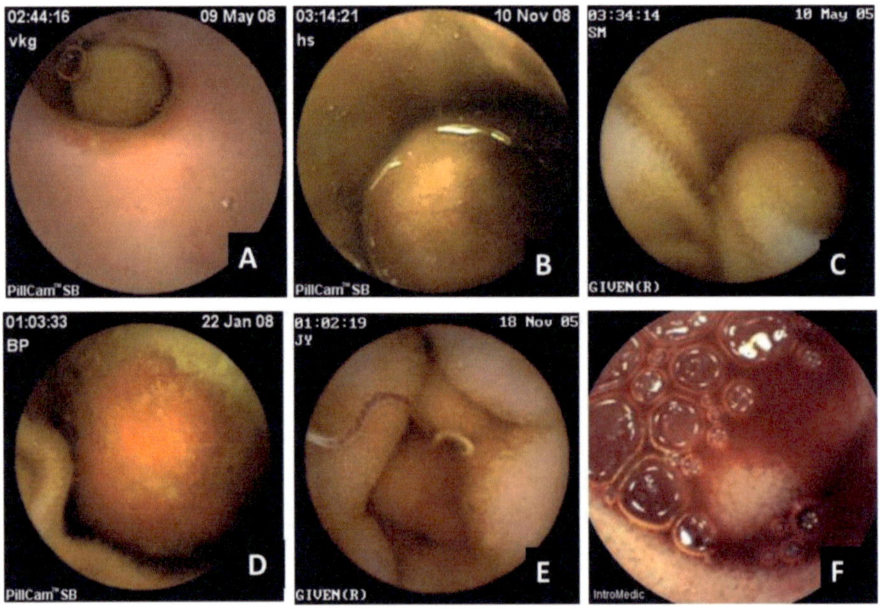

Figure 3. Representative pictures of capsule endoscopy in patients with intestinal stricture due to tuberculosis with enterolith (A), small bowel tumors (B, C, D), hookworm (E) and active bleeding without an identifiable causative lesion (F).

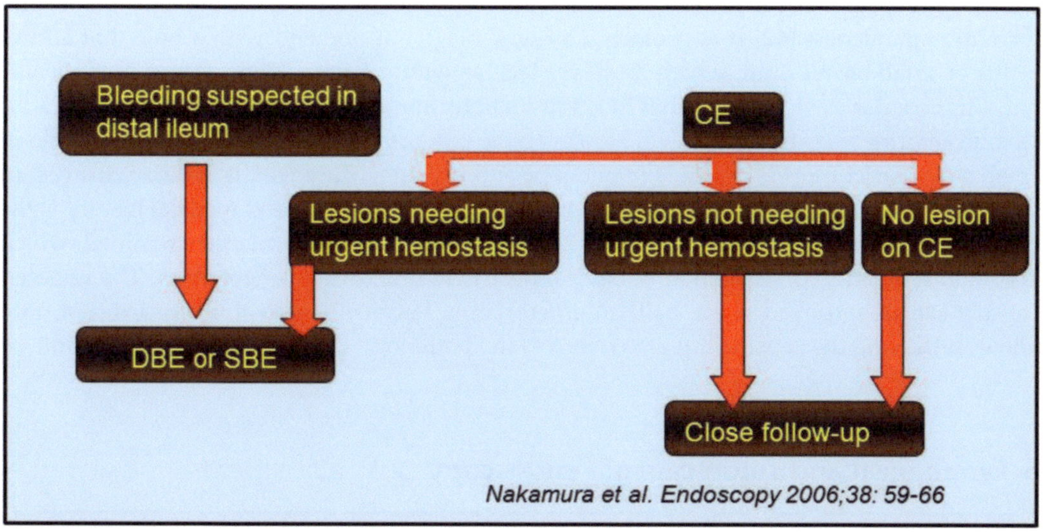

Figure 4. An outline of diagnostic algorithm of patients with obscure gastrointestinal bleeding.

4. Contraindications of capsule endoscopy

Contraindications of capsule endoscopy include suspected intestinal stricture (in which patency capsule may be used to evaluate tightness of the stricture),[39] cardiac pacemaker (recently capsule has been found safe and Capsovision type of capsule is quite safe),[40], [41] gastroparesis and esophageal motility disorders (capsule can be endoscopically delivered in the small bowel).[27] Even if capsule gets retained in stricture, it can be retrieved by single balloon and double balloon enteroscopy. Moreover, precipitation of small bowel obstruction by retained capsule is rare.[27] Pregnancy is also a contraindication to capsule endoscopy.

5. Complications of capsule endoscopy

Capsule retention is considered as a complication of capsule endoscopy. Capsule retention is defined as having a capsule remain in the digestive tract for a minimum of two weeks. Frequency of capsule retention in various studies varies from 0-13%.[42], [43] In a large series of 900 patients undergoing capsule endoscopy for obscure gastrointestinal bleeding, seven (0.77%) had capsule retention.[43] Interestingly, six of these seven patients had retention in spite a normal barium series. Several subsequent studies showed that normal barium does not prevent possible capsule retention.[27] Hence, a barium small bowel series is not indicated before capsule endoscopy. Moreover, yield of small bowel barium series is low to pick up causes of obscure gastrointestinal bleeding.[23] In an attempt to prevent capsule retention, patency capsule has been developed. This self-dissolving capsule (Fig. 1) of size same as endoscopy capsule, consists of a cellophane-walled cylinder filled with lactose and 10% barium for radio-opaqueness.[42] It is protected by wax plague at one end with a hole that allows influx of small bowel fluid, which dissolves lactose within 5 days. The patency capsule also has a transpoder device inside that helps in its detection using a hand-held scanner placed close to anterior abdominal wall.[42] However, the patency capsule can itself gets impacted in small bowel stricture.[44] Hence, it may not be entirely safe. Moreover, it increases the cost of capsule endoscopy. Hence, it has been suggested that obtaining a good medical history is the best method to avoid capsule retention.[44] Moreover, even if capsule gets retained, which occurs infrequently, precipitation of clinical obstruction is further uncommon. The retained capsule can be retrieved using balloon enteroscopy. Surgical removal, if needed, not only allows retrieving the capsule but also removes the pathology that led to capsule retention.

6. Esophageal and colon capsule endoscopy

Table 2 summarizes technical differences between esophageal and small bowel capsule endoscopy. Initial studies on esophageal capsule endoscopy did not find it very rewarding for detection of esophageal varices and Barrett esophagus in comparison to conventional esophagogastroduodenoscopy.[45], [46] Subsequently, string-controlled esophageal capsule endoscopy was tried to overcome some of the limitations.[47] However, it has to be noted that esophageal capsule endoscopy is expensive as compared to conventional esophagogastroduodenoscopy, will not have therapeutic potential and is not maneuverable. Hence, esophagogastroduodenoscopy remains the modality of choice for screening for Barrett's esophagus.[48]

Table 2 summarizes technical specifications of colon capsule endoscopy. Colon capsule endoscopy may score over conventional colonoscopy as it will reduce patients discomfort and need for sedation. However, its efficacy for colon cancer screening, which is likely to be its major indication,[49] remains to be proved in large studies though a few meta-analysis have been reported.[50], [51] If it is effective, it may be useful to improve compliance with colorectal cancer screening. However, this technology is currently only a diagnostic method, any positive finding requires conventional colonoscopy for tissue sampling or polypectomy. There is currently no video capsule device cleared by the US Food and Drug Administration for dedicated colon imaging. This technology requires more research before it can become clinically applicable as standard of care.

Future of capsule endoscopy: Limitations of the current system of capsule endoscopy include inability to steer the capsule, inability to biopsy lesions, and lack of therapeutic potential. Localization and estimation of size of the lesions using capsule endoscopy is often inaccurate. False negative and false positive diagnoses are other limitations. Moreover, in almost 20% of procedures the capsule does not reach the cecum while it is active. However, advances have been made to overcome these limitations. For example, now some of the capsules can be magnetically steered to pass through gastrointestinal tract.[52] Some capsules also provide ability to real time imaging so that the operator can see while the capsule is passing down the

http://dx.doi.org/10.5772/52732

GI tract.[6] Works are also ongoing to provide therapeutic potential to the imaging capsules.[53] Several methods are being developed to improve image quality by improvement in the software or by chromoendoscopy (FICE).[54]

Author details

Uday C Ghoshal*

Address all correspondence to: udayghoshal@gmail.com

Dept. of Gastroenterology, Sanjay Gandhi Postgraduate Institute of Medical Sciences, Lucknow, India

References

[1] Iddan, G, Meron, G, Glukhovsky, A, & Swain, P. Wireless capsule endoscopy. Nature (2000).

[2] Vazquez-iglesias, J. L. Capsule endoscopy: a new era in the history of endoscopy. Rev Esp Enferm Dig (2004). , 96, 3-9.

[3] Iddan, G. J, & Swain, C. P. History and development of capsule endoscopy. Gastrointest Endosc Clin N Am (2004). , 14, 1-9.

[4] Carey, E. J, & Fleischer, D. E. Investigation of the small bowel in gastrointestinal bleeding--enteroscopy and capsule endoscopy. Gastroenterol Clin North Am (2005). , 34, 719-34.

[5] Moglia, A, Menciassi, A, Dario, P, & Cuschieri, A. Capsule endoscopy: progress update and challenges ahead. Nat Rev Gastroenterol Hepatol (2009). , 6, 353-62.

[6] Lai, L. H, Wong, G. L, Lau, J. Y, Sung, J. J, & Leung, W. K. Initial experience of real-time capsule endoscopy in monitoring progress of the videocapsule through the upper GI tract. Gastrointest Endosc (2007). , 66, 1211-4.

[7] Rondonotti, E, Herrerias, J. M, Pennazio, M, Caunedo, A, Mascarenhas-saraiva, M, & De Franchis, R. Complications, limitations, and failures of capsule endoscopy: a review of 733 cases. Gastrointest Endosc (2005). quiz 752, 754., 62, 712-6.

[8] Villa, F, Signorelli, C, Rondonotti, E, & De Franchis, R. Preparations and prokinetics. Gastrointest Endosc Clin N Am (2006). , 16, 211-20.

[9] Dai, N, Gubler, C, Hengstler, P, Meyenberger, C, & Bauerfeind, P. Improved capsule endoscopy after bowel preparation. Gastrointest Endosc (2005). , 61, 28-31.

[10] Ben-soussan, E, Savoye, G, Antonietti, M, Ramirez, S, Ducrotte, P, Lerebours, E, & Is, a. liter PEG preparation useful before capsule endoscopy? J Clin Gastroenterol (2005). , 39, 381-4.

[11] Caddy, G. R, Moran, L, Chong, A. K, Miller, A. M, Taylor, A. C, & Desmond, P. V. The effect of erythromycin on video capsule endoscopy intestinal-transit time. Gastrointest Endosc (2006). , 63, 262-6.

[12] Endo, H, Kondo, Y, Inamori, M, Ohya, T. R, Yanagawa, T, Asayama, M, Hisatomi, K, Teratani, T, Yoneda, M, Nakajima, A, & Matsuhashi, N. Ingesting 500 ml of polyethylene glycol solution during capsule endoscopy improves the image quality and completion rate to the cecum. Dig Dis Sci (2008). , 53, 3201-5.

[13] Lapalus, M. G. Ben Soussan E, Saurin JC, Favre O, D'Halluin PN, Coumaros D, Gaudric M, Fumex F, Antonietti M, Gaudin JL, Jacob P, Heresbach D, Pilichos C, Fan R, Mozer M, Heyries L, Dumortier J, Ponchon T. Capsule endoscopy and bowel preparation with oral sodium phosphate: a prospective randomized controlled trial. Gastrointest Endosc (2008). , 67, 1091-6.

[14] Niv, E, Bonger, I, Barkay, O, Halpern, Z, Mahajna, E, Depsames, R, Kopelman, Y, & Fireman, Z. Effect of erythromycin on image quality and transit time of capsule endoscopy: a two-center study. World J Gastroenterol (2008). , 14, 2561-5.

[15] Fireman, Z, Kopelman, Y, Fish, L, Sternberg, A, Scapa, E, & Mahaina, E. Effect of oral purgatives on gastric and small bowel transit time in capsule endoscopy. Isr Med Assoc J (2004). , 6, 521-3.

[16] Kalantzis, C, Triantafyllou, K, Papadopoulos, A. A, Alexandrakis, G, Rokkas, T, Kalantzis, N, & Ladas, S. D. Effect of three bowel preparations on video-capsule endoscopy gastric and small-bowel transit time and completeness of the examination. Scand J Gastroenterol (2007). , 42, 1120-6.

[17] Niv, Y. Efficiency of bowel preparation for capsule endoscopy examination: a meta-analysis. World J Gastroenterol (2008). , 14, 1313-7.

[18] Albert, J, Gobel, C. M, Lesske, J, Lotterer, E, Nietsch, H, & Fleig, W. E. Simethicone for small bowel preparation for capsule endoscopy: a systematic, single-blinded, controlled study. Gastrointest Endosc (2004). , 59, 487-91.

[19] Fang, Y. H, Chen, C. X, & Zhang, B. L. Effect of small bowel preparation with simethicone on capsule endoscopy. J Zhejiang Univ Sci B (2009). , 10, 46-51.

[20] Postgate, A, Tekkis, P, Patterson, N, Fitzpatrick, A, Bassett, P, & Fraser, C. Are bowel purgatives and prokinetics useful for small-bowel capsule endoscopy? A prospective randomized controlled study. Gastrointest Endosc (2009). , 69, 1120-8.

[21] Buscaglia, J. M, Kapoor, S, Clarke, J. O, Bucobo, J. C, Giday, S. A, Magno, P, Yong, E, & Mullin, G. E. Enhanced diagnostic yield with prolonged small bowel transit time during capsule endoscopy. Int J Med Sci (2008). , 5, 303-8.

[22] Aparicio, J. R, Martinez, J, & Casellas, J. A. Right lateral position does not affect gastric transit times of video capsule endoscopy: a prospective study. Gastrointest Endosc (2009). , 69, 34-7.

[23] Triester, S. L, Leighton, J. A, Leontiadis, G. I, Fleischer, D. E, Hara, A. K, Heigh, R. I, Shiff, A. D, & Sharma, V. K. A meta-analysis of the yield of capsule endoscopy compared to other diagnostic modalities in patients with obscure gastrointestinal bleeding. Am J Gastroenterol (2005). , 100, 2407-18.

[24] Leighton, J. A, Triester, S. L, & Sharma, V. K. Capsule endoscopy: a meta-analysis for use with obscure gastrointestinal bleeding and Crohn's disease. Gastrointest Endosc Clin N Am (2006). , 16, 229-50.

[25] Gupta, R, Lakhtakia, S, Tandan, M, Banerjee, R, Ramchandani, M, Anuradha, S, Ramji, C, Rao, G. V, Pradeep, R, & Reddy, D. N. Capsule endoscopy in obscure gastrointestinal bleeding--an Indian experience. Indian J Gastroenterol (2006). , 25, 188-90.

[26] Carey, E. J, Leighton, J. A, Heigh, R. I, Shiff, A. D, Sharma, V. K, Post, J. K, & Fleischer, D. E. A single-center experience of 260 consecutive patients undergoing capsule endoscopy for obscure gastrointestinal bleeding. Am J Gastroenterol (2007). , 102, 89-95.

[27] Ghoshal, U. C, Lakshmi, C. P, Kumar, S, Das, K, Misra, A, Rai, P, Mohindra, S, Saraswat, V. A, Kumar, A, & Choudhuri, G. Capsule endoscopy for obscure gastrointestinal bleeding in the tropics: report from India. Dig Endosc (2011). , 23, 17-23.

[28] Bar-meir, S, Eliakim, R, Nadler, M, Barkay, O, Fireman, Z, Scapa, E, Chowers, Y, & Bardan, E. Second capsule endoscopy for patients with severe iron deficiency anemia. Gastrointest Endosc (2004). , 60, 711-3.

[29] Viazis, N, Papaxoinis, K, Vlachogiannakos, J, Efthymiou, A, Theodoropoulos, I, & Karamanolis, D. G. Is there a role for second-look capsule endoscopy in patients with obscure GI bleeding after a nondiagnostic first test? Gastrointest Endosc (2009). , 69, 850-6.

[30] Green, P. H, & Rubin, M. Capsule endoscopy in celiac disease: diagnosis and management. Gastrointest Endosc Clin N Am (2006). , 16, 307-16.

[31] Ciorba, M. A, & Prakash, C. Wireless capsule endoscopy in the diagnosis of small bowel Crohn's disease. Inflamm Bowel Dis (2003).

[32] Bailey, A. A, Debinski, H. S, Appleyard, M. N, Remedios, M. L, Hooper, J. E, Walsh, A. J, & Selby, W. S. Diagnosis and outcome of small bowel tumors found by capsule endoscopy: a three-center Australian experience. Am J Gastroenterol (2006). , 101, 2237-43.

[33] Cobrin, G. M, Pittman, R. H, & Lewis, B. S. Increased diagnostic yield of small bowel tumors with capsule endoscopy. Cancer (2006). , 107, 22-7.

[34] Burke, C. A, Santisi, J, Church, J, & Levinthal, G. The utility of capsule endoscopy small bowel surveillance in patients with polyposis. Am J Gastroenterol (2005). , 100, 1498-502.

[35] De Palma, G. D, Rega, M, Masone, S, Persico, F, Siciliano, S, Patrone, F, Matantuono, L, & Persico, G. Mucosal abnormalities of the small bowel in patients with cirrhosis and portal hypertension: a capsule endoscopy study. Gastrointest Endosc (2005). , 62, 529-34.

[36] Goulas, S, Triantafyllidou, K, Karagiannis, S, Nicolaou, P, Galanis, P, Vafiadis, I, Tzivras, M, & Mavrogiannis, C. Capsule endoscopy in the investigation of patients with portal hypertension and anemia. Can J Gastroenterol (2008). , 22, 469-74.

[37] Christodoulou, D. K, Sigounas, D. E, Katsanos, K. H, Dimos, G, & Tsianos, E. V. Small bowel parasitosis as cause of obscure gastrointestinal bleeding diagnosed by capsule endoscopy. World J Gastrointest Endosc (2010). , 2, 369-71.

[38] Das, K, Sarkar, R, Dasgupta, J, Ray, S, Ghatak, S, Mridha, A. R, Dhali, G. K, & Chowdhury, A. Obscure GI bleeding in the tropics: impact of introduction of double-balloon and capsule endoscopies on outcome. Gastrointest Endosc (2010). , 72, 292-300.

[39] Spada, C, Shah, S. K, Riccioni, M. E, Spera, G, Marchese, M, Iacopini, F, Familiari, P, & Costamagna, G. Video capsule endoscopy in patients with known or suspected small bowel stricture previously tested with the dissolving patency capsule. J Clin Gastroenterol (2007). , 41, 576-82.

[40] Leighton, J. A, Sharma, V. K, Srivathsan, K, Heigh, R. I, Mcwane, T. L, Post, J. K, Robinson, S. R, Bazzell, J. L, & Fleischer, D. E. Safety of capsule endoscopy in patients with pacemakers. Gastrointest Endosc (2004). , 59, 567-9.

[41] Payeras, G, Piqueras, J, Moreno, V. J, Cabrera, A, Menendez, D, & Jimenez, R. Effects of capsule endoscopy on cardiac pacemakers. Endoscopy (2005). , 37, 1181-5.

[42] Lewis, B. Capsule endoscopy--transit abnormalities. Gastrointest Endosc Clin N Am (2006). vii., 16, 221-8.

[43] Barkin, J. S, & Loughlin, O. C. Capsule endoscopy contraindications: complications and how to avoid their occurrence. Gastrointest Endosc Clin N Am (2004). , 14, 61-5.

[44] Delvaux, M. Ben Soussan E, Laurent V, Lerebours E, Gay G. Clinical evaluation of the use of the M2A patency capsule system before a capsule endoscopy procedure, in patients with known or suspected intestinal stenosis. Endoscopy (2005). , 37, 801-7.

[45] Lin, O. S, Schembre, D. B, Mergener, K, Spaulding, W, Lomah, N, Ayub, K, Brandabur, J. J, Bredfeldt, J, Drennan, F, Gluck, M, Jiranek, G. C, Mccormick, S. E, Patterson, D, & Kozarek, R. A. Blinded comparison of esophageal capsule endoscopy versus conventional endoscopy for a diagnosis of Barrett's esophagus in patients with chronic gastroesophageal reflux. Gastrointest Endosc (2007). , 65, 577-83.

[46] Chavalitdhamrong, D, Jensen, D. M, Singh, B, Kovacs, T. O, Han, S. H, Durazo, F, Saab, S, & Gornbein, J. A. Capsule endoscopy is not as accurate as esophagogastroduodeno-

scopy in screening cirrhotic patients for varices. Clin Gastroenterol Hepatol (2012). e1., 10, 254-8.

[47] Ramirez, F. C, Akins, R, & Shaukat, M. Screening of Barrett's esophagus with string-capsule endoscopy: a prospective blinded study of 100 consecutive patients using histology as the criterion standard. Gastrointest Endosc (2008). , 68, 25-31.

[48] Bhardwaj, A, Hollenbeak, C. S, Pooran, N, & Mathew, A. A meta-analysis of the diagnostic accuracy of esophageal capsule endoscopy for Barrett's esophagus in patients with gastroesophageal reflux disease. Am J Gastroenterol (2009). , 104, 1533-9.

[49] Iobagiu, S, Ciobanu, L, & Pascu, O. Colon capsule endoscopy: a new method of investigating the large bowel. J Gastrointestin Liver Dis (2008). , 17, 347-52.

[50] Rokkas, T, Papaxoinis, K, Triantafyllou, K, & Ladas, S. D. A meta-analysis evaluating the accuracy of colon capsule endoscopy in detecting colon polyps. Gastrointest Endosc (2010). , 71, 792-8.

[51] Spada, C, Hassan, C, Marmo, R, Petruzziello, L, Riccioni, M. E, Zullo, A, Cesaro, P, Pilz, J, & Costamagna, G. Meta-analysis shows colon capsule endoscopy is effective in detecting colorectal polyps. Clin Gastroenterol Hepatol (2010). , 8, 516-22.

[52] Carpi, F. Magnetic capsule endoscopy: the future is around the corner. Expert Rev Med Devices (2010). , 7, 161-4.

[53] Van Gossum, A, & Ibrahim, M. Video capsule endoscopy: what is the future? Gastroenterol Clin North Am (2010). , 39, 807-26.

[54] Crespo-perez, L, & Vazquez-sequeiros, E. Virtual chromoendoscopy as an adjuvant to capsule endoscopy: a step ahead? Rev Esp Enferm Dig (2012). , 104, 227-30.

[55] Albert, J. G, Schulbe, R, Hahn, L, Heinig, D, Schoppmeyer, K, Porst, H, Lorenz, R, Plauth, M, Dollinger, M. M, Mossner, J, Caca, K, & Fleig, W. E. Impact of capsule endoscopy on outcome in mid-intestinal bleeding: a multicentre cohort study in 285 patients. Eur J Gastroenterol Hepatol (2008). , 20, 971-7.

[56] Almeida, N, Figueiredo, P, Lopes, S, Freire, P, Lerias, C, Gouveia, H, & Leitao, M. C. Urgent capsule endoscopy is useful in severe obscure-overt gastrointestinal bleeding. Dig Endosc (2009). , 21, 87-92.

[57] Apostolopoulos, P, Liatsos, C, Gralnek, I. M, Giannakoulopoulou, E, Alexandrakis, G, Kalantzis, C, Gabriel, P, & Kalantzis, N. The role of wireless capsule endoscopy in investigating unexplained iron deficiency anemia after negative endoscopic evaluation of the upper and lower gastrointestinal tract. Endoscopy (2006). , 38, 1127-32.

[58] Apostolopoulos, P, Liatsos, C, Gralnek, I. M, Kalantzis, C, Giannakoulopoulou, E, Alexandrakis, G, Tsibouris, P, Kalafatis, E, & Kalantzis, N. Evaluation of capsule endoscopy in active, mild-to-moderate, overt, obscure GI bleeding. Gastrointest Endosc (2007). , 66, 1174-81.

[59] Ben Soussan EAntonietti M, Herve S, Savoye G, Ramirez S, Lecleire S, Ducrotte P, Lerebours E. Diagnostic yield and therapeutic implications of capsule endoscopy in obscure gastrointestinal bleeding. Gastroenterol Clin Biol (2004). , 28, 1068-73.

[60] Bresci, G, Parisi, G, Bertoni, M, Tumino, E, & Capria, A. The role of video capsule endoscopy for evaluating obscure gastrointestinal bleeding: usefulness of early use. J Gastroenterol (2005). , 40, 256-9.

[61] Calabrese, C, Liguori, G, Gionchetti, P, Rizzello, F, Laureti, S, Simone, M. P, Poggioli, G, & Campieri, M. Obscure gastrointestinal bleeding: single centre experience of capsule endoscopy. Intern Emerg Med (2011).

[62] Carlo, J. T, Demarco, D, Smith, B. A, Livingston, S, Wiser, K, Kuhn, J. A, & Lamont, J. P. The utility of capsule endoscopy and its role for diagnosing pathology in the gastrointestinal tract. Am J Surg (2005). , 190, 886-90.

[63] Chao, C. C. Ng Jao YT, Mo LR. Capsule endoscopy for gastrointestinal bleeding with an obscure etiology. J Formos Med Assoc (2005). , 104, 659-65.

[64] Chong, A. K, Taylor, A. C, Miller, A. M, & Desmond, P. V. Initial experience with capsule endoscopy at a major referral hospital. Med J Aust (2003). , 178, 537-40.

[65] De Leusse, A, Landi, B, Edery, J, Burtin, P, Lecomte, T, Seksik, P, Bloch, F, Jian, R, & Cellier, C. Video capsule endoscopy for investigation of obscure gastrointestinal bleeding: feasibility, results, and interobserver agreement. Endoscopy (2005). , 37, 617-21.

[66] Enns, R, Go, K, Chang, H, & Pluta, K. Capsule endoscopy: a single-centre experience with the first 226 capsules. Can J Gastroenterol (2004). , 18, 555-8.

[67] Estevez, E, Gonzalez-conde, B, & Vazquez-iglesias, J. L. de Los Angeles Vazquez-Millan M, Pertega S, Alonso PA, Clofent J, Santos E, Ulla JL, Sanchez E. Diagnostic yield and clinical outcomes after capsule endoscopy in 100 consecutive patients with obscure gastrointestinal bleeding. Eur J Gastroenterol Hepatol (2006). , 18, 881-8.

[68] Fireman, Z, Eliakim, R, Adler, S, & Scapa, E. Capsule endoscopy in real life: a four-centre experience of 160 consecutive patients in Israel. Eur J Gastroenterol Hepatol (2004). , 16, 927-31.

[69] Fireman, Z, & Friedman, S. Diagnostic yield of capsule endoscopy in obscure gastro-intestinal bleeding. Digestion (2004). , 70, 201-6.

Section 2

Upper Gastrointestinal Tract

Chapter 6

Diagnostic Value of Upper Gastrointestinal Endoscopy Prior to Cholecystectomy

Waleed Al-Khyatt, Farhan Rashid and S.Y. Iftikhar

Additional information is available at the end of the chapter

http://dx.doi.org/10.5772/52520

1. Introduction

Gallstone disease remains one of the most common medical problems leading to surgical intervention. It occurs in up to 20% of men and 35% of women in Western societies [1, 2]. Every year, more than 500,000 cholecystectomies are performed in the US [3]. The resultant direct and indirect cost of gallbladder disease represents a consumption of ~$6.2 billion annually in the U.S., constituting a major health burden that has increased more than 20% over the last 3 decades [4]. Hence, the treatment of gallstones and its complications (cholecystitis, pancreatitis and bile duct obstruction) contributes substantially to healthcare costs [2]. The term "symptomatic gallstones" is widely used to describe symptoms arising secondary to presence of gallstones. There are wide range of gastrointestinal symptoms have been linked to gallstones but causal relationship has not been established yet [3, 5]. Although, gallstone disease is asymptomatic in the vast majority of individuals, it is commonly accepted that removal of the gallbladder is the best treatment for symptomatic gallstone disease [6]. However, less focus has been on patient selection and typical or common symptoms of this disease in order to understand prevailing symptoms after surgery. Cholecystectomy is a commonly performed abdominal surgical procedure performed for treatment of symptomatic gallstones and prevention of complications. Nevertheless, given the high proportion of non-specific abdominal symptoms in the people with known gallstones may lead to unjustifiable cholecystectomies [3, 7].

2. Is it a biliary pain or not?

Gallstones found incidentally in the investigation of gastrointestinal symptoms may become falsely incriminated to explain pathology that arises outside the biliary tree [8]. The majority of patients presenting to general practitioners with chronic or colicky upper abdominal pain undergo ultrasound examination. Ultrasound is non-invasive, readily available and inexpensive. After ultrasound detection of gallstones the main focus of the attending clinician stays around treating the gallstones and further investigations to rule out other pathologies that may produce similar symptoms are seldom considered. Almost all of the patients with proven gallstones are referred to surgeons with a view to performing laparoscopic cholecystectomy [6]. With the advancement in laparoscopic skills, laparoscopic cholecystectomy has become a very common and safe operation [9]. As cholecystectomy become a safer and a more routine laparoscopic procedure [9], patients may consent to surgery without as much consideration as they had done in the past, when it was performed with a much more invasive open technique [10].

The finding of gallstones on imaging studies but without symptoms is the most common presentation [3, 6]. On the other hand patients with gallstones can be presented with one of the known complications like acute cholecystitis, acute pancreatitis or obstructive jaundice. Typically patients with symptomatic cholilithiasis complain of recurrent epigastric pain which happens one or two hours after meals and could last for few hours[3, 6]. These recurrent attacks are normally aggravated by fatty meal and may associate with nausea and vomiting. Although biliary colic was specific for gallstones, 80% of the referred patients with gallstones presented with other abdominal symptoms [11]. Sometimes, patients have mixture of atypical upper GI symptoms and discovered to have gallstones on imaging studies [5]. The latter group where inappropriate cholecystectomies thus performed are likely to be associated with poor symptomatic outcome [6].

Persistent pain or the so-called 'postcholecystectomy syndrome' is a common occurrence and varies in frequency between 6% and 47% [12-15]. Therefore, the identification of patients most likely to benefit from cholecystectomy is critically important [8, 10]. Other causes of persistent postoperative pain may be peptic ulcer disease, hiatus hernia or other gastrointestinal diseases. These patients should first have been investigated to rule out gastroduodenal pathology before undergoing operation to remove gallstones [5]. This approach will not only decrease persistence of symptoms but can also be helpful in detecting gastroduodenal pathologies at an early stage [5, 6].

4. OGD prior surgical treatment of gallstones: Is it of a value?

Many studies have emphasized on the potential therapeutic role of upper gastrointestinal tract endoscopy in the presence of overlapping upper GI symptoms (table 1)[16]. For instance, Rassek et al. suggests that endoscopic examination of the upper gastrointestinal tract is highly recommended prior to an elective cholecystectomy. In his study, 589 of 960 patients underwent gastroscopy ahead of elective cholecystectomy. Although, 56% had normal gastroscopy, 11.3% (113 patients) underwent a change in plan of management because of the OGD findings and 11 patients were discharged after conservative medical therapy (1.1%) [17].

In another prospective study, the routine OGD of the upper gastrointestinal tract was carried out in 100 patients before they underwent elective cholecystectomy for gallstones, Diettrich et al. found that 31/100 patients had abnormal OGD which changed their subsequent plan of treatment. In 18% of patients, the cholecystectomy was differed for 4 to 8 weeks, after additional medical treatment and 7 patients were discharged on only conservative medical treatment. Therefore, he recommended that preoperative endoscopy of the upper gastrointestinal tract should be used in patients undergoing cholecystectomy to rule out other gastrointestinal disorders [18]. Likewise, another study by Schwenk et al, 1143 patients underwent preoperative OGD or upper gastrointestinal series prior cholecystectomy. The incidence of pathological findings was 30.2% (345 patients), with 68.3% of findings was of inflammatory in nature. In 28 patients (2.5%) cholecystectomy or bile duct exploration was combined with an additional gastrointestinal surgical procedure. In 227 cases (19.8%) biliary surgery was followed by medical treatment of co-existing gastrointestinal diseases. Because of the high incidence of simultaneous Upper GI diseases, they recommended that routine preoperative gastroscopy is indicated before elective surgical treatment of gallstones disease [19].

Thybusch et al. also evaluated the role and therapeutic implications of routine OGD before cholecystectomy. In his study, endoscopy of the upper digestive tract was performed in 338 consecutive patients undergoing cholecystectomy. Nearly 50% of patients had pathological findings on OGD examination. These findings varied from peptic ulcers (6.8%), gastric erosions (1.8%), gastritis (25.7%), polyps (3.2%), hiatal hernias (4.7%), oesophagitis(3%) and gastric cancer (0.6%). The management plan had to be changed in 8.3% of patients based on those OGD findings. Although these findings did not correlate with patients' symptoms, 26 patients received medical treatment prior to undergoing cholecystectomy. Two patients with gastric cancer underwent gastrectomy. These results underline the importance of a routine gastroscopy before elective cholecystectomy [20].

In their retrospective review of 143 patients who presented with atypical abdominal pain, gallstones, and underwent EGD before their cholecystectomy, Yavorski et al, recommend that patients who present with cholelithiasis and atypical abdominal pain undergo preoperative OGD, as they found that at least 9 per cent of the patients in their study had significant findings that altered their management [21]. On the hand, Sosada et al. recommended the performance of routine OGD for each patient who is elected to undergo laparoscopic cholecystectomy [22]. He suggested that in patients with asymptomatic gallstones, abdominal pain is most likely secondary to underlying peptic ulcer disease. In this study, OGD which was performed 1–4 days prior to surgery in 2800 patients. Pathological findings were identified in 1187(42%) patients; gastric ulcer in 179 (6.4%), duodenal ulcer in 127 (4.5%), gastritis in 375 [(26.3%), polyps in 143 [(5.1%) and cancer in 3 [(0.1%) patients. The surgery was delayed for patients with ulcers and they were treated appropriately. 16 patients had complete resolution of symptoms after medical treatment, therefore cholecystectomy was not performed [22]. Similarly, selective endoscopy has also been recommended by Beyermann et al. [23]. However, only 11% of their total study cohort had endoscopy out of 610 patients. But even with those figures they have suggested that routine OGD should be performed in patients with history of upper abdominal pain and discomfort [23].

In the same way, Rashid et al evaluated the routine use of OGD prior laparoscopic cholecystectomy [24]. In his retrospective analysis, the routine use of OGD resulted in detection of other coexisting pathologies in about one third (33%) of patients. All of these OGD findings lead to a change in the management plan for these patients. Also they noticed that, the recurrence or persistence of symptoms was significantly higher in patients who were not scoped prior surgery (33 %) in comparison to patients who were scoped where only (3.3%) had recurrent or persistent symptoms. Therefore they suggested that, OGD should be considered as a routine investigation before laparoscopic cholecystectomy especially in those selected group of patients, who do present with overlapping upper GI symptoms. The data suggest that routine use of OGD before laparoscopic cholecystectomy will help to reduce postoperative persistence of symptoms and may reduce overall cholecystectomy rates with beneficial clinical and economical outcomes [24].

Although there is growing evidence that preoperative OGD is useful in identifying medically treatable diseases in patients undergoing surgical removal of gallstones, few studies however suggested that OGD prior surgical removal of gallstones has little or no influence on the postoperative outcome [25, 26]. For instance, Ure el al, suggested that routine endoscopy before laparoscopic cholecystectomy is neither clinically useful nor cost effective in patients with symptomatic gallstone disease [25]. Nevertheless this suggestion was related exclusively to patients with typical gallstone symptoms. Besides, even in patients typical biliary, OGD abnormalities were found in 60 patients (16.0 %); these included peptic ulcer (n = 14), gastric erosions (n = 15) and oesophagitis (n = 11). Thirty patients were treated medically and two by endoscopic polypectomy. In four patients endoscopy led to cancellation of cholecystectomy [25]. Similarly, the significance of preoperative OGD in patients scheduled for laparoscopic cholecystectomy was also evaluated by Al-Azawi et al [26]. They compared a group of patients who underwent OGD before laparoscopic cholecystectomy and a group of patients who underwent laparoscopic cholecystectomy with no preoperative OGD. In this study, 218[(54.5%) of 400 patients underwent OGD prior cholecystectomy. In the OGD group, there were normal findings in 98 (45%) patients. Disorders such as hiatus hernia (21%), acute duodenal ulcers (3.6%), esophagitis (3.6%), gastric ulcer (0.4%), and Barrett's oesophagus(0.4%) were among the findings. Laparoscopic cholecystectomy was avoided in six patients with chronic cholecystitis. However, in this study, the use of preoperative OGD had no apparent benefit in reducing the incidence of postoperative residual abdominal pain. Therefore they suggest that OGD prior to laparoscopic cholecystectomy does not have an impact on postoperative residual abdominal pain. Despite that, they have also concluded that OGD can disclose other gastrooesophageal disorders with similar symptoms to gallstones and may change the course of the planned surgery in chronic cholecystitis[26].

Study	Study population	Results/ recommendation
Rassek et al, 1988 [17]	589 patients	11.3% (113 patients) underwent a change in plan of management because of the OGD findings and 11 patients were discharged after conservative medical therapy (1.1%)
Diettrich et al, 1990 [18]	100 patients	31/100 patients had abnormal OGD, 18% of patients had their cholecystectomy differed for 4 to 8 weeks, after additional medical treatment, 7 patients were discharged on only conservative medical treatment
Beyermann et al, 1992 [23]	660 patients	Routine OGD should be performed in patients with history of upper abdominal pain and discomfort
Schwenk et al, 1992 [19]	1143 patients	30.2% (345 patients) had abnormal findings, 28 patients (2.5%) cholecystectomy or bile duct exploration was combined with an additional gastrointestinal surgical procedure. In 227 cases (19.8%) biliary surgery was followed by medical treatment of co-existing gastrointestinal diseases.
Ure et al, 1992 [25]	376 patients	OGD abnormalities were found in 60 patients (16.0 %), Thirty patients were treated medically and two by endoscopic polypectomy. In four patients endoscopy led to cancellation of cholecystectomy
Thybusch et al, 1996 [20]	338 patients	Nearly 50% of patients had pathological findings on OGD examination. The management plan had to be changed in 8.3% of patients based on those OGD findings. 26 patients received medical treatment prior to undergoing cholecystectomy. Two patients with gastric cancer underwent gastrectomy.
Yavorski et al, 1995 [21]	143 patients	9 per cent of the patient population will have significant findings that may alter their management. Patients who present with cholelithiasis and atypical abdominal pain is recommended to undergo preoperative OGD.
Sosada et al, 2005 [22]	2800 patients	Pathological findings were identified in 1187(42%) patients, surgery was delayed for patients with ulcers until they finished their medical treatment. 16 patients had complete resolution of symptoms after medical treatment, therefore cholecystectomy was not performed
Al-Azawi et al, 2006 [26]	400 patients	Preoperative OGD did not reduce the incidence of postoperative residual abdominal pain.
Rashid et al, 2010 [24]	121 patients	The recurrence or persistence of symptoms was significantly higher in patients who were not scoped prior surgery (33 %) in comparison to patients who were scoped where only (3.3%) had recurrent or persistent symptoms.

Table 1. Studies evaluated the role of oesophagogastrocopy prior cholecystectomy.

5. Conclusion

Cholelithiasis can present with a complex combination of clinical symptoms which may resemble the presentation of other gastrointestinal diseases. Hence, the use of routine preoperative investigations like OGD prior planning surgical treatment of cholelithiasis may help to identify other potentially treatable medical conditions and hence may reduce overall cholecystectomy rates. Besides its cost effectiveness, it may potentially help in reducing the incidence of postoperative persistence of symptoms.

Author details

Waleed Al-Khyatt[1], Farhan Rashid[2] and S.Y. Iftikhar[1]

1 Division of Surgery, Royal Derby Hospital, Uttoxeter Road, Derby, UK

2 Specialist Surgical Registrar, Cambridge/East of England Higher Surgical Training Rotation, UK

References

[1] Borch K, Jonsson KA, Zdolsek JM, Halldestam I, Kullman E. Prevalence of gallstone disease in a Swedish population sample. Relations to occupation, childbirth, health status, life style, medications, and blood lipids. Scand J Gastroenterol. 1998 Nov; 33[(11)]:1219-25.

[2] Romero Y, Thistle JL, Longstreth GF, Harmsen WS, Schleck CD, Zinsmeister AR, et al. A questionnaire for the assessment of biliary symptoms. Am J Gastroenterol. 2003 May;98[(5)]:1042-51.

[3] Schirmer BD, Winters KL, Edlich RF. Cholelithiasis and cholecystitis. J Long Term Eff Med Implants. 2005;15[(3)]:329-38.

[4] Stinton LM, Shaffer EA. Epidemiology of gallbladder disease: cholelithiasis and cancer. Gut Liver. Apr;6[(2)]:172-87.

[5] Kraag N, Thijs C, Knipschild P. Dyspepsia--how noisy are gallstones? A meta-analysis of epidemiologic studies of biliary pain, dyspeptic symptoms, and food intolerance. Scand J Gastroenterol. 1995 May;30[(5)]:411-21.

[6] Berger MY, Olde Hartman TC, Bohnen AM. Abdominal symptoms: do they disappear after cholecystectomy? SurgEndosc. 2003 Nov;17[(11)]:1723-8.

[7] Glambek I, Arnesjo B, Soreide O. Correlation between gallstones and abdominal symptoms in a random population. Results from a screening study. Scand J Gastroenterol. 1989 Apr;24[(3)]:277-81.

[8] Halldestam I, Kullman E, Borch K. Defined indications for elective cholecystectomy for gallstone disease. Br J Surg. 2008 May;95[(5)]:620-6.

[9] Fenster LF, Lonborg R, Thirlby RC, Traverso LW. What symptoms does cholecystectomy cure? Insights from an outcomes measurement project and review of the literature. Am J Surg. 1995 May;169[(5)]:533-8.

[10] Lublin M, Crawford DL, Hiatt JR, Phillips EH. Symptoms before and after laparoscopic cholecystectomy for gallstones. Am Surg. 2004 Oct;70[(10)]:863-6.

[11] Berger MY, van der Velden JJ, Lijmer JG, de Kort H, Prins A, Bohnen AM. Abdominal symptoms: do they predict gallstones? A systematic review. Scand J Gastroenterol. 2000 Jan;35[(1)]:70-6.

[12] Bates T, Ebbs SR, Harrison M, A'Hern RP. Influence of cholecystectomy on symptoms. Br J Surg. 1991 Aug;78[(8)]:964-7.

[13] Peterli R, Schuppisser JP, Herzog U, Ackermann C, Tondelli PE. Prevalence of postcholecystectomy symptoms: long-term outcome after open versus laparoscopic cholecystectomy. World J Surg. 2000 Oct;24[(10)]:1232-5.

[14] Jorgensen T, Teglbjerg JS, Wille-Jorgensen P, Bille T, Thorvaldsen P. Persisting pain after cholecystectomy. A prospective investigation. Scand J Gastroenterol. 1991 Jan; 26[(1)]:124-8.

[15] Luman W, Adams WH, Nixon SN, McIntyre IM, Hamer-Hodges D, Wilson G, et al. Incidence of persistent symptoms after laparoscopic cholecystectomy: a prospective study. Gut. 1996 Dec;39[(6)]:863-6.

[16] Coleman MJ, Hugh TB, James J, Kelly TA, Leslie GJ. Routine upper gastrointestinal endoscopy in elective cholecstectomy. Med J Aust. 1981 Nov 28;2[(11)]:600-1.

[17] Rassek D, Osswald J, Stock W. [Routine gastroscopy before cholecystectomy]. Chirurg. 1988 May;59[(5)]:335-7.

[18] Diettrich H, Wundrich B, Kobe E, Noack S, Weber K. [Gastroscopy before cholecystectomy]. Gastroenterol J. 1990;50[(4)]:173-4.

[19] Schwenk W, Bohm B, Badke A, Zarras K, Stock W. [Preoperative esophagogastroduodenoscopy before elective surgical therapy of symptomatic cholelithiasis]. LeberMagenDarm. 1992 Nov;22[(6)]:225-9.

[20] Thybusch A, Schaube H, Schweizer E, Gollnick D, Grimm H. [Significant value and therapeutic implications of routine gastroscopy before cholecystectomy]. J Chir (Paris). 1996 Jun;133[(4)]:171-4.

[21] Yavorski CC, Acosta JA, Ragland JJ. Precholecystectomy esophagogastroduodenoscopy: is it of value? Am Surg. 1995 Dec;61[(12)]:1032-4.

[22] Sosada K, Zurawinski W, Piecuch J, Stepien T, Makarska J. Gastroduodenoscopy: a routine examination of 2,800 patients before laparoscopic cholecystectomy. SurgEndosc. 2005 Aug;19[(8)]:1103-8.

[23] Beyermann K, Stinner B, Hasselmann U, Rothmund M. [Consequences of routine gastroscopy before cholecystectomy]. Langenbecks Arch Chir. 1992;377[(5)]:314-6.

[24] Rashid F, Rashid N, Waraich N, Ahmed J, Iftikhar SY. Role of routine oesophagogastroduodenoscopy before cholecystectomy. Int J Surg. 2010;8[(3)]:236-8.

[25] Ure BM, Troidl H, Spangenberger W, Lefering R, Dietrich A, Sommer H. Evaluation of routine upper digestive tract endoscopy before laparoscopic cholecystectomy. Br J Surg. 1992 Nov;79[(11)]:1174-7.

[26] Al-Azawi D, Rayis A, Hehir DJ. Esophagogastroduodenoscopy prior to laparoscopic cholecystectomy. J LaparoendoscAdvSurg Tech A. 2006 Dec;16[(6)]:593-7.

Chapter 7

Endoscopic Management of Oesophageal and Gastric Varices

Neil Rajoriya and David A. Gorard

Additional information is available at the end of the chapter

http://dx.doi.org/10.5772/52524

1. Introduction

Chronic liver disease of any aetiology can result in portal hypertension. Portal hypertension leads to the formation of porto-systemic collaterals including gastro-oesophageal varices. The development of portal hypertension can also herald the development of other complications of liver cirrhosis such as ascites formation, hepatic encephalopathy and when varices occur, their bleeding. However it should be noted that portal hypertension also occurs in non-cirrhotic conditions, such as: Budd-Chiari, myeloproliferative diseases and extra-hepatic portal vein obstruction.

Variceal haemorrhage is a serious life-threatening complication of portal hypertension, with overall mortality rates historically reported as 30-50% [1]. Although mortality can be up to 40% at 6 weeks, it can be up to 70% at 1 year [2]. With the generally improved management of the critically ill cirrhotic patient, together with vasoactive therapy and new endoscopic techniques for managing variceal haemorrhage, overall mortality has reduced, with one centre in Europe showing a reduction from 42% in 1980 to 14% in 2000 [3]. The treatment of gastric varices has also evolved over recent years with the introduction of adhesive compounds such as N-butyl-2-cyanoacrylate and thrombin, and the increased use of Transjugular Intrahepatic Portosystemic Shunts (TIPS) in variceal bleeding and early in rebleeding. New self-expanding oesophageal stents have been developed for oesophageal haemorrhage in the ever expanding endoscopic armamentarium against variceal bleeding. Earlier emergency access to endoscopy performed by skilled endoscopists has coincided with the decline in use of tamponade equipment such as Sengstaken-Blakemore tubes, and the virtual extinction of emergency surgical procedures of oesophageal transection or porto-caval shunt formation.

This chapter addresses the aetiology and pathogenesis of oesophageal and gastric varices, the strategy of primary prophylaxis against variceal bleeding, and reviews the medical and endoscopic treatment of variceal haemorrhage and rebleeding thereafter.

2. Portal hypertension and the development of varices

Portal hypertension is a key factor in the development of oesophageal or gastric varices. The endoscopic appearances of oesophageal and gastric varices can be seen in Figures 1 and 2 respectively.

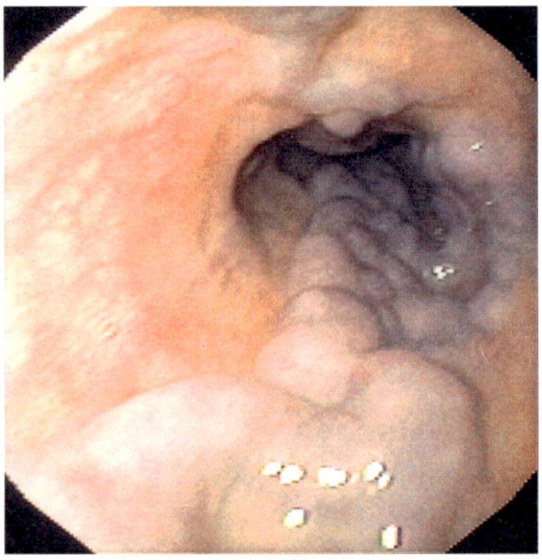

Figure 1. Quiescent column of oesophageal varices

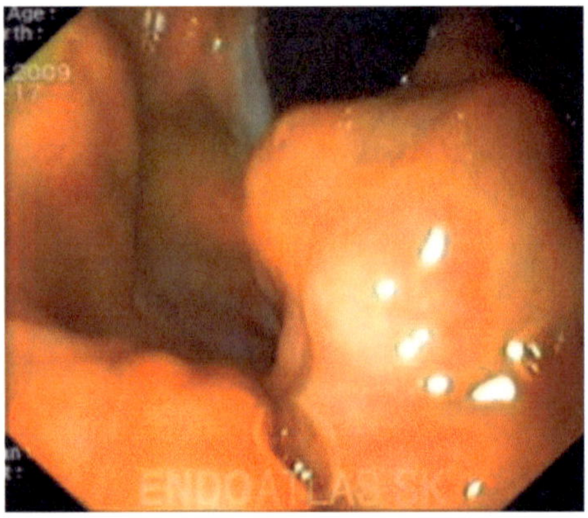

Figure 2. Gastric varix seen on retroflexion of the endoscope in fundus of the stomach with the classical "hanging grapes" appearance (courtesy of Dr Branislav Kunčak, University of Trnava and Nové Zámky Hospital, Nové Zámky, Slovakia at www.Endoatlas.sk)

http://dx.doi.org/10.5772/52524

The portal pressure is the pressure in the portal vein and portal vein tributaries. Normal portal pressure is 1-5 mmHg. When the portal pressure gradient (difference in pressure between the pressure in the portal vein and hepatic vein) exceeds 10-12mmHg, varices will form. The causes of portal hypertension categorised by anatomical site are summarised in Table 1.

SITE	CAUSES
PRE-HEPATIC	Portal vein/ splenic vein thrombosis Extrinsic compression of portal vein Portal vein congenital abnormalities (stenosis)
INTRA-HEPATIC	Any cause of cirrhosis (alcoholic, metabolic, viral, biliary, autoimmune) Acute alcoholic hepatitis Veno-occlusive disease Hepatocellular carcinoma Chronic active hepatitis Acute fatty liver of pregnancy Amyloidosis Chronic Hypervitaminosis A Polycystic disease Nodular regenerative hyperplasia Granulomatous liver diseases (TB, sarcoidosis, schistosomiasis)
POST-HEPATIC	Tricuspid valve disease / severe right heart failure Constrictive pericarditis Inferior vena cava thrombosis/ congenital malformations Hepatic vein thrombosis (Budd Chiari)

Table 1. Causes of portal hypertension related to site of increased resistance to portal blood flow

Irrespective of the site of resistance to portal blood flow, there are different mediators involved in the development of portal hypertension as outlined in Figure 3.

Portal hypertension can develop from structural changes within the liver, altering the architecture and thus leading to distortion of the blood flow through the liver. This results in increased vascular resistance. Such structural changes are the main cause for increased intrahepatic vascular resistance. Nodule generation, sinusoidal capillarization (development of a basal membrane around the sinusoid in the Space of Disse and fibrous tissue accumulation), sinusoidal collapse and hepatocyte enlargement all lead to shrinking and narrowing of the sinusoid unit leading to increased intrahepatic vascular resistance. Once these pathological changes occur, they can be an irreversible / fixed component of the development of portal hypertension. Depending on the aetiology and thus treatment of disease, degrees of fibrosis can in some cases be partially reversed.

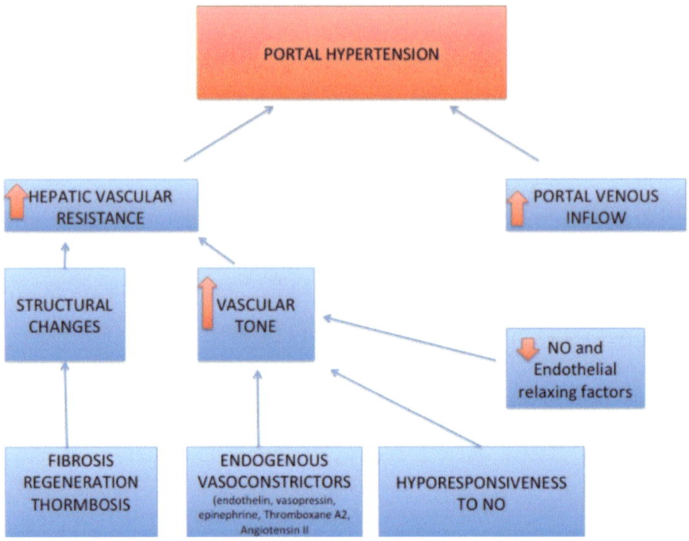

Figure 3. Overview of the mechanisms in the development of portal hypertension. (NO = nitric oxide)

Activated hepatic stellate cells (HSCs) are key mediators in the production of peri-sinusoidal hepatic fibrous tissue and the laying down of extracellular matrix [4]. Such deposition of fibrous tissue around the sinusoids can be the initial event in sinusoidal capillarization [5]– whereby extracellular matrix is deposited in the Space of Disse, and furthermore this can result in sinusoidal endothelial cells producing less nitric oxide (NO), which activates HSCs further. Any underlying liver disease promoting a fibrosis architecture of the liver can lead to portal hypertension [6]. As the fibrosis persists and progresses, liver cirrhosis can ensue.

The development of portal hypertension leading to collateral formation and varices relies not only on structural changes within the liver, but also on increased vascular tone within the liver. The alterations in vascular tone are dynamic changes. The HSCs are activated and can constrict as fibrosis and cirrhosis develop leading to a further vasoconstriction at the sinusoidal level. The mechanisms by which this occurs are multifactorial but include a change of HSC from a quiescent phenotype to a myofibroblast-like phenotype [6], which has greater contractile properties, and an up-regulation of calcium-channel receptors that mediate constriction [6, 7]. In addition to the activation of HSCs, there is an increase in mediators of vasoconstriction including Thromboxane A2, Angiotensin II, RhoA, endothelin, and eicanosoid, which have been shown at experimental level to increase intravascular intrahepatic tone [8-11]. The increase in vasoconstrictors is coupled with a reduction of vasodilators such as homocysteine and NO, with the latter being a key mediator in portal circulation vasodilatation [12] and in the formation of collateral vessels [13,14]. The production of NO is promoted by vascular endothelial growth factor, which also promotes porto-collateral vessel formation [15].

Vasodilatation of the arterial splanchnic vessels is an important factor in the development of portal hypertension. Chronic vasodilatation leads to increased blood flow to the porto-venous system and development of porto-systemic collateral formation and varices [16]. Increased portal pressure is the most important risk factor for the development of varices [2]. Varices develop once a hepatic venous pressure gradient (HVPG), a surrogate marker for sinusoidal portal hypertension, exceeds 10-12mm Hg [17]. Lowering the portal pressure is a key target in the prevention of variceal formation, in the prevention of variceal bleeding, and in the management of acutely bleeding varices [18]. One other major feature in portal hypertension is the development of the hyperdynamic circulatory syndrome, which is associated with the development of varices [16]. This is characterised by a decreased mean arterial pressure, increased cardiac output and decreased systemic vascular resistance. The hyperdynamic circulation again is a target for drug therapies including beta-blockers to reduce portal hypertension, with the main driver for the vasodilatation and subsequent hyperdynamic circulation being NO [16].

3. Growth, classification and location of varices

Once portal hypertension ensues, there is development of porto-systemic collateral formation in an attempt to decompress the rising portal pressure. Two basic mechanisms lead to: (1) neo-angiogenesis and (2) dilatation of pre-existing embryonic channels between the portal and systemic circulations [19, 20]. Gastro-oesophageal varices develop as part of cephalad collaterals formed after dilatation of the left gastric (coronary) vein and the short gastric veins. Once established, varices can remain indolent or grow in size, and also cause life-threatening haemorrhage. When the portal pressure is above 10 mmHg, the median time for the development of varices is 4 years [21] while some studies show a *de novo* formation rate of 4-6% per year [22, 23].

Variceal size is a predictor of haemorrhage, as predicted by La Place's law, whereby wall tension increases with variceal radius and transmural variceal pressure. The mean risk of haemorrhage from larger varices (>5mm) is 30% at 2 years, compared to 10% from small varices at 2 years [24,25]. Risk factors for the dilatation of varices include: an increase in portal pressure [26], alcohol consumption [27], circadian rhythm [28], prandial blood flow bursts [29] and also Child-Pugh class at baseline and its deterioration during follow-up [30, 31]. The rate of yearly increase in size of varices varies from a range of 8% to 31% [32, 33].The two main locations of varices that may rupture are the lower oesophagus and the stomach.

3.1. Oesophageal varices

Oesophageal varices are long columns of dilated veins (Figure 1), usually occurring within the lower third of the oesophagus, immediately above the gastro-oesophageal junction (GOJ). Oesophageal varices can be graded endoscopically according to size [34] (Table 2/ Figure 4), while the American Association for the Study of Liver Diseases (AASLD) recommends the classification into small and large oesophageal varices based on a cut-off of 5mm [35].

GRADE OF OESOPHAGEAL VARIX	DESCRIPTION
1 (small)	Small straight varices
2 (medium)	Enlarged tortuous varices occupying less than one third of the lumen
3 (large)	Large coil-shaped varices occupying more than one third of the lumen

Table 2. Grading of oesophageal varices according to Italian liver cirrhosis project. (Reference 34)

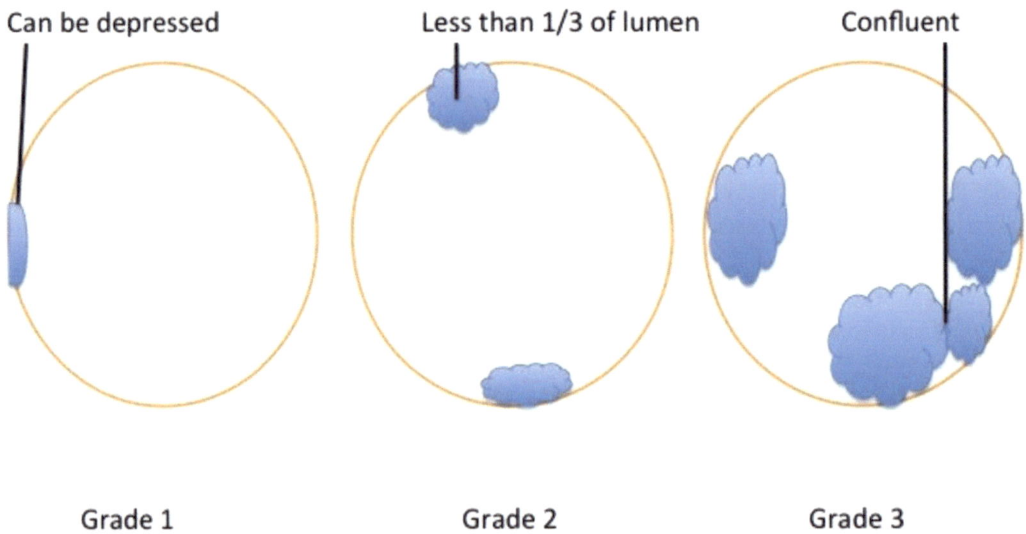

Figure 4. Grading of oesophageal varices endoscopically (adapted from reference 24)

The major blood supply to oesophageal varices is from the left gastric vein. There are 4 layers of veins in the oesophagus (Figure 5). The intra-epithelial veins are the most superficial veins and correlate with the red spots seen at time of endoscopy. These red spots have been shown to be predicative of variceal rupture (along with variceal size and Child-Pugh class [25]). Deeper to these veins is the superficial venous plexus, which then drains into deeper intrinsic veins. These in turn are then connected via perforating veins to the deepest adventitia plexus. It is the main trunks of the deep adventitia plexus that large oesophageal varices arise from.

An area of common oesophageal variceal rupture is at the GOJ - the palisade zone – an area of venous tributaries between the gastric zones and perforating zone (in the oesophagus). This area is a watershed between the azygous and portal blood flow systems, where venous flow is bidirectional with turbulent flow – which may explain frequent rupture [36] – and thus why when banding, oesophageal bands should be applied as close to the GOJ as possible.

http://dx.doi.org/10.5772/52524

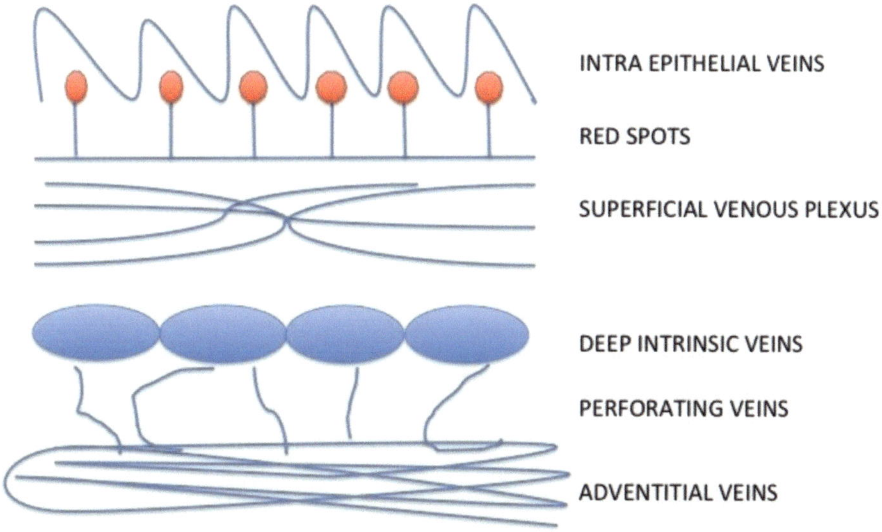

Figure 5. The anatomy of veins within the oesophagus from which oesophageal varices arise.

3.2. Gastric varices

Gastric varices are supplied by the short gastric veins, draining into the deep intrinsic veins of the lower oesophagus, and can be classified according to site by the Sarin classification of gastric varices [37] (Figure 6 / Table 3).

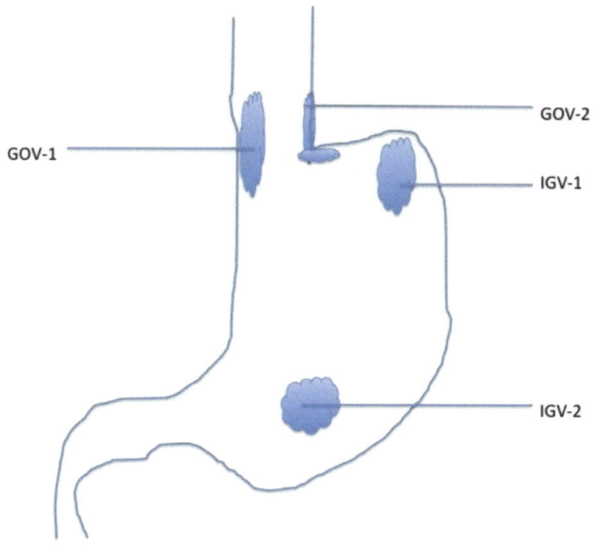

Figure 6. Sarin classification of gastric varices (adapted from reference 37)

Gastric varices account for 10-30% of variceal haemorrhage and can occur in up to 20% of patients with portal hypertension [17, 38]. Management of bleeding gastric varices differs from that of the more common situation of bleeding oesophageal varices (see later in chapter).

SARIN TYPE OF GASTRIC VARIX	DESCRIPTION/LOCATION
Gastro-Oesophageal Varices -1 (GOV-1)	Continuation from oesophageal varices and extend on lesser curve
Gastro-Oesophageal Varices -2 (GOV-2)	Extend along lesser curve and more tortuous than GOV-1
Isolated Gastric Varices-1 (IGV-1)	Occur in absence of oesophageal varices, and occur in the fundus, and are tortuous and complex
Isolated Gastric Varices-2 (IGV-2)	Occur in absence of oesophageal varices, in the body, antrum or pylorus

Table 3. Sarin classification of gastric varices (adapted from reference 37).

4. Prevention of 1st variceal haemorrhage – Primary prophylaxis

Since patients with cirrhosis may have portal hypertension and varices, there is a rationale for screening of such patients to identify those with varices who might benefit from primary prophylaxis against variceal haemorrhage. Thus those patients who have a diagnosis of cirrhosis either clinically, biochemically or on liver biopsy, should be offered Oesopho-Gastro-Duodenoscopy (OGD) looking for gastro-oesophageal varices [39]. When cirrhosis is diagnosed, any factors causing the continuing insult to the liver must be addressed – such as treatment of the underlying condition (e.g. viral /autoimmune or ongoing alcohol intake in alcoholic liver disease). In those cirrhotic patients who do not have varices diagnosed on initial endoscopy, a follow up endoscopy has been recommended after 2-3 years [40] particularly if hepatic synthetic function worsens (i.e. worsening in Child-Pugh status). Primary prophylaxis aims to prevent variceal haemorrhage in patients who have varices but who have not had a previous bleeding episode. Strategies used in primary prophylaxis can be broadly divided into pharmacological and endoscopic therapies.

4.1. Pharmacological therapies as primary prophylaxis

Drug therapies are used to prevent variceal bleeding, and if well tolerated by patients can be effective. Isosorbide mononitrate (ISMN) is a potent vasodilator used in ischaemic heart disease and reduces vascular tone. There are theoretical reasons why ISMN should help to prevent variceal bleeding. In randomised control trials ISMN has been shown to reduce HVPG by 7.5% [41,42], and to augment the splanchnic vasoconstrictive effects of the non-selective beta-blocker propranolol [42]. It has been used when there are contra-indications to, or intolerance of beta-blocker drugs in patients with varices. However a double-blind randomised controlled trial in patients intolerant of beta-blockers, compared ISMN with placebo and found that ISMN was ineffective at preventing a first variceal bleed [43].

Non-selective beta-blockers are the mainstay of treatment in the prevention of variceal bleeding once varices have been identified. Non-selective beta-blockers not only block beta-1 receptors, reducing cardiac output and thus portal blood flow, but also block the adrenergic dilatory tone in the mesenteric arterioles, resulting in unopposed alpha-adrenergic vasoconstriction and a decrease in portal blood flow [44]. Nadolol or propanolol can reduce HVPG measurements by up 10% [45,46] and are effective in reducing variceal bleeding rates and mortality when compared to placebo [47,48]. Their roles have been firmly established in guidelines [2,35] with the choice between them dependent on institutional practice. Carvedilol is a potent non-selective beta-blocker, with weak vasodilating effects due to alpha-1-blockade [49]. This leads to a reduction in hepatic vascular tone and hepatic resistance [50]. Carvedilol has been shown in multiple studies to reduce portal pressure and HVPG significantly more than propranolol [51-54], but its role in primary prophylaxis is not yet been established [2]. Once beta-blocker therapy has been instituted, patients with varices who are compliant with their medication do not require further endoscopy unless bleeding occurs. However some US centres prefer to repeat endoscopy annually in varices patients on beta-blockers and consider changing to a programme of endoscopic variceal band ligation (EVBL) if the varices increase in size. This latter strategy, however, is non-evidence based.

Side-effects of beta-blockers include bronchoconstriction, heart failure and impotence, and these can often limit a patient's tolerability of the drug. The safety of beta-blockers in cirrhotic patients with refractory ascites has also been questioned in a prospective study of 151 patients in such a cohort [55]. The 1-year probability of survival was significantly lower in patients who received propranolol [19% (95% CI = 9%-29%)] versus those who did not [64% (95% CI = 52%-76%), $p < 0.0001$]. Further studies in this area are required as this initial study was not a randomised controlled trial. It has been postulated that beta-blockers are only beneficial during a set time window in the progression of cirrhosis with portal hypertension [56]. There may be no benefit in early cirrhosis when there is less risk of bacterial translocation, no increase in sympathetic nervous system activity and when the cardiac compensatory reserve remains intact. However as cirrhosis progresses with increasing bacterial translocation and increased sympathetic nervous system activity, there is an increased risk of variceal haemorrhage, and beta-blockers become beneficial in not only reducing variceal bleeding but also reducing bacterial translocation. The window then closes in advanced cirrhosis as beta-blockers exert a negative impact on cardiac compensatory reserve.

4.2. Endoscopic therapies as primary prophylaxis

Endoscopic treatments can be used to obliterate/thrombose oesophageal varices. Injection sclerotherapy involves the injection of a sclerosant (usually ethanolamine) via a needle-catheter directly into a varix to thrombose it. Although intuitively the obliteration of varices before they have a chance to bleed would seem to be a logical strategy, injection sclerotherapy is not without complication. In fact when sclerotherapy for primary prophylaxis against variceal bleeding was formally studied in a randomised trial, patients with varices randomised to sclerotherapy had a higher mortality than patients with varices in the control arm [57]. Consequently injection sclerotherapy should not be used as primary prophylaxis against variceal bleeding. Injection sclerotherapy for oesophageal varies has largely been superseded by EVBL in the past 2 decades. EVBL is an alternative to non-selective beta-blockers, in those intolerant to the medication or for those often with medium or large varices (Figure 7). EVBL should be performed by an endoscopist who has expertise in variceal band ligation to minimise complications in day-case endoscopy patients.

EVBL can be used to treat acutely or recently bleeding oesophageal varices, or can be performed electively to obliterate varices and thus prevent bleeding or rebleeding. Once a diagnostic OGD has been performed and has identified oesophageal varices, the most distal level of variceal location is noted, and the endoscope removed. A single-use, multiband ligator incorporating up to 10 bands, is then loaded onto the endoscope. A cap fitting over the endoscope's tip holds the mounted bands, and is connected through the accessory port of a standard endoscope, with the firing handle mounted close to the endoscope's operating wheels. Once the ligator has been loaded onto the endoscope, the oesophagus is re-intubated. The ligator's cap may make intubation and subsequent endoscopic views a little more difficult.

The first varix to be banded should be the largest one with stigmata of recent/active haemorrhage, or if quiescent then the most distal varix just above the GOJ, since varices at/just above the GOJ are those most likely to bleed. Furthermore, if a proximal varix is banded first, it may be difficult to then pass the endoscope beyond it without dislodging the band. Suction is applied, aspirating the varix into the cap, until the varix is completely sucked up (as seen by a red-out on the screen). Operating the firing handle releases a band onto the varix neck, and release of suction allows the banded varix to be viewed (Figure 7). Thereafter, additional variceal banding can be continued in a cranial direction. Complications of EVBL include band-induced ulceration (which may present as a re-bleed requiring urgent endoscopy), transient dysphagia or chest pain, and rarely oesophageal stricturing.

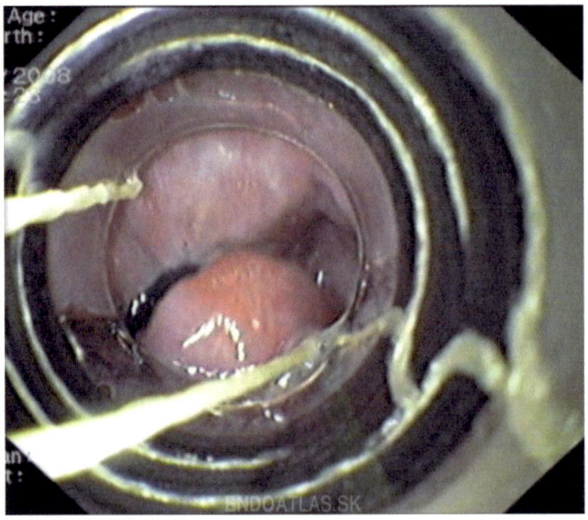

Figure 7. Endoscopic variceal band ligation of oesophageal varices (courtesy of Dr Branislav Kunčak, 2nd Dept. of Internal Medicine, Faculty of Health and Social Work, University of Trnava and Nové Zámky Hospital, Nové Zámky, Slovakia. at www.Endoatlas.sk)

The role of EVBL in patients with medium or large varices has been studied in several trials, and has also been compared to beta-blockers. Meta-analyses show that for primary prophylaxis, both beta-blockade and EVBL have similar efficacy and mortality [53, 58-63]. Guidelines currently do not recommend combination therapies with both EVBL and non-selective beta-blockers [2,35,40]. Local factors including availability of endoscopic procedures, and technicians able to perform EVBL may influence choices between beta-blockade and EVBL as primary prophylaxis. The cost of endoscopy with EVBL is higher than the cost of beta-blocker medication, particularly since banding programmes require follow-up endoscopies to ensure variceal eradication (with up to 22% recurrence post-EVBL reported in one study [59]). Guidelines recommend EVBL every 1-2 weeks after initial OGD until the varices are obliterated, and then 6-12 monthly check endoscopies [35].

Current Baveno V guidelines on portal hypertension [2] recommend primary prophylaxis with non-selective beta-blockers for patients with small oesophageal varices and red wale marks or Child C cirrhotic patients. These guidelines also suggest that patients with small oesophageal varices but without signs of increased risk of haemorrhage or Child C cirrhosis could be considered for treatment with non-selective beta-blockers, although further studies are necessary. Patients with medium or large oesophageal varices can be treated with either beta-blockers or EVBL. Current American Association for the Study of Liver Diseases (AASLD) guidelines [35] similarly recommend prophylaxis with non-selective beta-blockers for patients with compensated cirrhosis and small oesophageal varices with or without features of likely increased haemorrhage risk. The AASLD guidelines also recommend non-selective beta-blockers or EVBL for those with medium or large varices.

For gastric varices, injection of N-Butyl-2-Cyanoacrylate glue has been studied in the primary prophylaxis setting. This long-chain cyanoacrylate glue polymerises and solidifies within seconds following contact with aqueous media such as blood within a varix. This leads to obliteration of the varix from which the cast extrudes after 2-4 weeks. Mixing the cyanoacrylate with the oily agent Lipiodol delays polymerisation. The glue treatment was compared with beta-blockers or no therapy in a randomised controlled trial [64], with significantly reduced probabilities of bleeding in patients treated with glue compared to beta-blockers or no therapy (13% v 28% and 45% respectively). However the use of the glue for gastric varices has complications (see later in chapter in "Endoscopic treatment of acute gastric variceal haemorrhage" section) and its role in primary prophylaxis against gastric variceal bleeding has not yet been established [2]. Although there is a paucity of data from prophylactic studies on gastric variceal bleeding, there is current consensus that using beta-blockers to reduce portal pressure is appropriate in this setting [2].

5. General management strategies in acute variceal haemorrhage

Variceal haemorrhage is a life-threatening emergency with a mortality of 20-40% at 6-weeks (65). Factors predictive of death within 6 weeks of index bleeding in patients with cirrhosis include: site of bleed is varices (instead of other pathology), level of bilirubin, underlying alcoholic liver disease, presence of encephalopathy or coagulopathy and the need for balloon tamponade [2,40,65]. If haematemesis or melena occurs in patients known to have cirrhosis or stigmata of chronic liver disease, variceal bleeding should be considered. AASLD guidelines recommend such patients should be managed in an intensive care setting [35]. Tracheal intubation should be considered if the patient has a reduced Glasgow Coma Scores (GCS) or signs of hepatic encephalopathy, since these increase the risk of aspiration. Furthermore, subsequent endoscopy to diagnose and treat the bleeding point is safer in an intubated patient. General measures include wide-bore venous access or central venous access, and fluid resuscitation with either colloid or blood products. Blood resuscitation to maintain a haemoglobin level of approximately 8g/dl has been recommended [40], as experimental studies have shown the total restoration of all lost blood may raise portal pressure higher than that of baseline [66], with subsequent higher rates of re-bleeding and mortality [67]. There must however be adequate arterial pressure to maintain renal perfusion (and prevent acute kidney injury and the development of hepato-renal syndrome). Clotting and platelet deficiencies should be corrected.

Bacterial infections are common in cirrhotic patients, and antibiotics have been shown to reduce bacterial infections, recurrent bleeding and mortality in patients bleeding from oesophageal varices [68,69]. Broad-spectrum antibiotic prophylaxis is recommended [35]. Local antibiotic policy and a patient's nil-by-mouth status are important influences, but the antibiotic used should be either an oral quinolone, or else a 3rd generation intravenous cephalosporin in patients who have advanced cirrhosis, or previously received quinolone prophylaxis, or live in areas of high quinolone resistance [2].

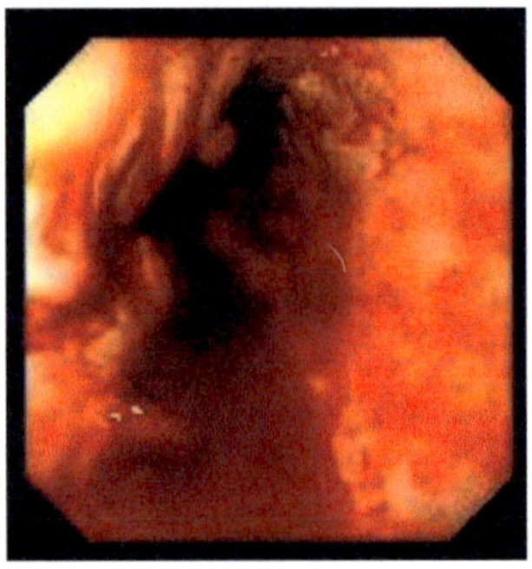

Figure 8. Bleeding oesophageal varices (courtesy of ELLA-CS, Hradec Kralove, Czech Republic)

The use of vasoactive drugs to lower portal pressure is paramount in the initial management of variceal bleeding. Such drugs should be given prior to endoscopy if the source of upper gastrointestinal bleeding is suspected to be varices [2, 70]. Vasopressin and terlipressin cause constriction of the splanchnic arterioles, thus leading to increased resistance to inflow of blood to the gut. This leads to a lowering of portal venous pressure. Side effects however include myocardial ischaemia and these vasoconstrictors are contraindicated in peripheral vascular disease. Vasopressin has been shown to achieve haemostasis in 60-80% of patients, but has limited effects on reducing early rebleeding and does not improve survival from active variceal haemorrhage [71]. Vasopressin has largely been superseded by terlipressin in countries where it is available (not the USA). Terlipressin (triglycyl-lysine vasopressin) is a synthetic analogue of vasopressin administered at an initial dose of 2mg, then 1mg intravenously every four hours. Meta-analysis shows that terlipressin reduces all-cause mortality when compared to placebo [71, 72] and it should be instituted early and continued for up to 5 days, as this is the period during which rebleeding is common. When compared to somatostatin analogues such as octreotide, the haemodynamic effects of terlipressin on portal pressure are more sustained [73], suggesting terlipressin may have a more prolonged benefit in bleeding varices.

Somatostatin and somatostatin analogues (e.g. the long-acting analogue octreotide) act by increasing splanchnic arterial resistance, and inhibit vasoactive peptides such as glucagon. Octreotide is used as first-line vasoactive therapy in the USA (where terlipressin is unavailable). It is given intravenously as a 50 microgram bolus followed by a continuous infusion of 50 micrograms per hour. Octreotide causes a transient reduction in portal pressure and azygous blood flow lasting up to only 5 minutes despite continuous infusion [74]. However additional effects are via inhibition of glucagon and other peptides that increase post-prandial mesenteric blood flow [75]. The mesenteric blood flow increases in variceal bleeding due to the high protein gut loading from the intraluminal blood [76], and octreotide can reduce the hormone-induced changes for up to 38 hours [77]. Somatostatin has fewer side effects than terlipressin (0% vs. 10%) and a higher relative risk (1.62) for achieving initial control of bleeding, but no survival benefit [78]. Thus vasoactive drugs are part of the initial therapy in variceal haemorrhage and one of these drugs should be continued for 2- 5 days [2].

Prior to endoscopy a tamponading balloon such as the Sengstaken-Blakemore tube or Minnesota tube can be considered, but the advent of 24-hour endoscopy services, vasoactive drugs and TIPS has largely obviated the need for this intervention. Balloon tamponade should be only be used in massive haemorrhage as a bridge to endoscopy [2]. Complications of tube insertion include upper airway obstruction, inadvertent tracheal intubation, lower oesophagus ulceration and even oesophageal rupture if the gastric balloon is wrongly inflated in the oesophagus.

6. Endoscopic treament of acute oesophageal variceal haemorrhage

OGD is the investigation of choice in the diagnosis of variceal bleeding, and it offers endoscopic therapeutic capability at the time. After general measures covered earlier in the chapter have been instituted in a patient with variceal bleeding, an urgent OGD should be carried out within 12 hours of presentation [2]. Some experts recommend tracheal intubation prior to OGD in all patients suspected of having variceal bleeding, to prevent aspiration of blood into the airway. Endoscopic therapy for bleeding varices largely depends on the type of varix that is bleeding – oesophageal or gastric. The mainstays of endoscopic therapy for bleeding oesophageal varices include injection sclerotherapy and EVBL.

Endoscopic sclerotherapy for oesophageal varices has mainly been performed using the sclerosant ethanolamine. Cyanoacrylate glue and thrombin have also been used. Sclerotherapy is done using a catheter with a retractable needle introduced through the endoscope's operating channel. Under endoscopic vision, the sclerosant is directly injected into the bleeding oesophageal varix. Local complications can include bleeding, stricture formation, ulceration, oesophagitis, mediastinitis and oesophageal perforation.

Sclerotherapy controls active bleeding from oesophageal varices in 62-100% of patients and is more effective than treatment with placebo, vasoactive therapy or balloon tamponade [40]. A meta-analysis of 5 studies (Laine L, personal communication in Baveno IV consensus statements [40]) of 251 patients comparing sclerotherapy with sham sclerotherapy, balloon tamponade and/or vasopressive therapies showed significant benefits of sclerotherapy in terms of initial haemostasis, in patient re-bleeding (OR=0.36, 0.21-0.62) and mortality (OR=0.57, 0.33-0.98) [79-83]. A meta-analysis suggested that sclerotherapy was the "gold standard" in acute variceal bleeding [84]. Despite the efficacy of endoscopic sclerotherapy for actively bleeding oesophageal varices, endoscopic therapy has switched to EVBL. In part this switch may have been extrapolated from the negative outcomes when sclerotherapy was used as primary prophylaxis against variceal bleeding[57], but subsequent comparative trials detailed below have pointed to a superiority of EVBL.

EVBL has evolved as the recommended standard of treatment for bleeding oesophageal varices (Baveno IV guidelines) [40], and sclerotherapy is only recommended if ligation is technically difficult. In a meta-analysis of 10 randomized controlled trials comparing EVBL with sclerotherapy, there was an almost significant benefit of EVBL in achieving initial haemostasis compared to sclerotherapy (pooled relative risk of 0.53 with CI 0.28-1.01) [85]. In one of the studies in the meta-analysis, HVPG increased significantly immediately after both EVBL and sclerotherapy, but the HVPG remained elevated for the duration of the study (5 days) in the sclerotherapy group while returning to baseline levels by 48 hours after EVBL group [86]. Another meta-analysis however found no difference in initial haemostasis rates between sclerotherapy and EVBL (RR 1.1, 95% CI: 0.4-2.9) [87], but the actively bleeding patients represented a small subset from larger trials, and were thus not truly from pure randomized controlled trials in this population [40]. EVBL is associated with fewer adverse effects than sclerotherapy. By consensus, EVBL is the preferred form of endoscopic therapy for acute oesophageal variceal bleeding, although sclerotherapy is recommended in patients in whom EVBL is not technically feasible.

Combination therapies of vasoactive drugs and direct endoscopic therapies have been studied, with dual therapy conferring the potential benefits of pharmacological reduction in portal pressure together with the direct local haemostasing effects of either sclerotherapy or EVBL. Combination is now recommended as a standard of care in oesophageal variceal bleeding [2,40]. The combined effect of initial haemostasis was initially difficult to assess due to heterogeneity of trials and definitions of immediate haemostasis. A meta-analysis of 4 trials including 559 patients, concluded that combined therapy was associated with a higher rate of initial haemostasis than endoscopic therapy alone (88% v 76%, RR: 1.12, 95% CI: 1.02-1.23) [88]. Five-day haemostasis rates were studied in the Baveno IV consensus statements [40]. Pooling of results of 939 patients demonstrated that combination therapy achieved greater haemostasis rates than endoscopic therapy alone (77% v 58%, RR: 1.28, 95% CI: 1.18-1.39) with a number needed to treat of 5 (95% CI 4-8) [89-96]. However no significant differences were found in 5-day or 42-day mortality when combined vasoactive drug and endoscopic therapy was compared to endoscopic therapy alone in 2 meta-analyses [88, 89].

http://dx.doi.org/10.5772/52524

Two pooled randomized controlled trial results of combination therapy versus pharmacological therapy alone showed combination therapy improved control of bleeding (RR: 3.1, 95% CI: 1.2-8.3) but with no influence on mortality [88, 89].

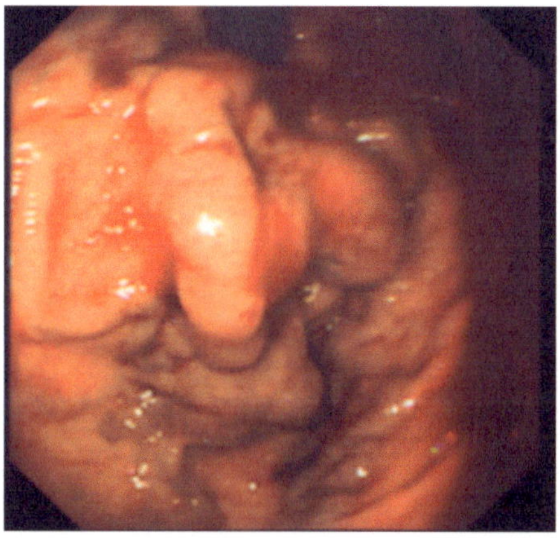

Figure 9. A bleeding gastric varix seen on retroflexion of the gastroscope (courtesy of Dr Adrian Stanley, Glasgow Royal Infirmary, 2006)

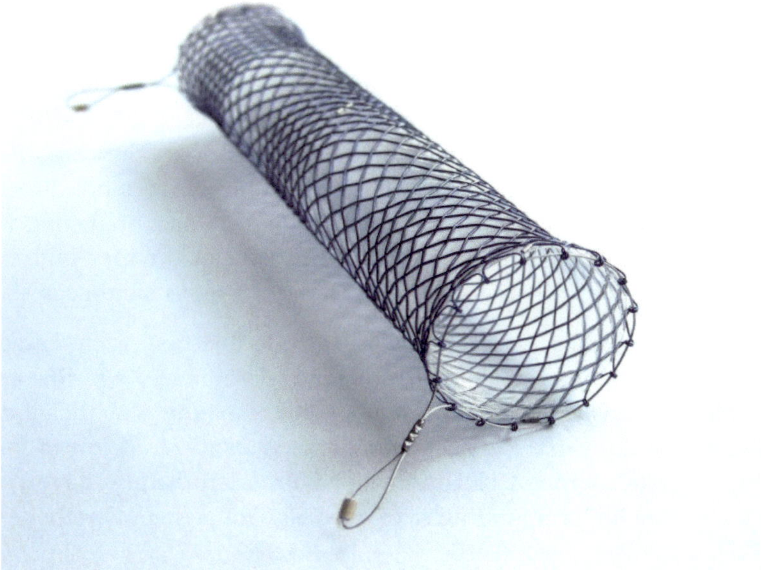

Figure 10. Self-expanding oesophageal metallic stent (courtesy of ELLA-CS, Hradec Kralove, Czech Republic)

More recently self-expanding oesophageal metallic stents have been developed and used in oesophageal variceal bleeds. They have been developed from their role in oesophageal malignancy, and act by applying direct tamponading pressure to the distal oesophageal mucosa and any associated varices. Stents were used in a pilot study in 20 patients who failed to achieve haemostasis with pharmacological or endoscopic techniques [92]. Immediate haemostasis was achieved in 100% of these patients. Such stents seem a promising option in the situation of refractory oesophageal haemorrhage, but further evaluation is needed.

Radiological therapies have been used in acute oesophageal variceal bleeding, with TIPS the most commonly studied and available radiological modality. TIPS involves the placement of a needle catheter via the transjugular route into the hepatic vein, and wedging it there under fluoroscopic guidance. The needle is then advanced through the liver parenchyma to the intrahepatic portion of the portal vein, creating a "side-to-side" anastomotic shunt. A stent is then positioned across the liver, connecting the portal vein and hepatic veins, and allowing blood to flow normally from the portal vein through the liver with a drop in the portal pressure. TIPS was initially used as therapy for uncontrolled bleeding and achieved control of bleeding in 90-95% of patients and a 4-week survival of 50-60% [93]. Early TIPS placement has been shown to have beneficial effect in patients with a HVPG > 20mmHg presenting with a variceal bleed [94]. TIPS reduced treatment failures, hospital stay and 1-year mortality. Other studies have confirmed the role of TIPS in variceal bleeding which cannot be controlled by endoscopy or vasoactive drugs [95-97]. Complications of TIPS include haemorrhage, infection, intravascular haemolysis and worsening of hepatic encephalopathy [95-97].

7. Endoscopic treatment of acute gastric variceal haemorrhage

Although less common than oesophageal variceal bleeding, gastric variceal haemorrhage is often torrential with an associated high mortality (Figure 9). Re-bleeding is also common with reported figures of up to 43-89% after a gastric variceal bleed [37, 98-101]. Gastric varices can occur alone or in combination with oesophageal varices. They are often large and located deep in the submucosa, making EVBL or injection therapy more difficult than that for oesophageal varices. Gastric varices can remain quiescent and predicting which gastric varix is likely to bleed can be difficult. Factors that are associated with a high risk of gastric variceal bleeding include: red colour sign, large varices, or a rapid increase in size [102-104].

Therapeutic options for bleeding gastric varices include injection sclerotherapy, banding, TIPS and other radiological interventions. Endoscopic sclerotherapy was first applied in the treatment of a bleeding gastric varix in 1984 [105] and results in endothelial damage with subsequent sclerosis of the varix. Variceal obliteration rates of 71.6% (mean follow up 24.2 +/-22.9 months) in gastric variceal bleeds treated with sclerotherapy have been reported [101], but there are often high re-bleeding rates of 60-90% following sclerotherapy for gastric varices [106, 107].

There are limited data on EVBL in the management of gastric variceal bleeding. EVBL can be useful for varices extending from the oesophagus along the proximal lesser curve (Sarin

GOV-1), but it is problematic for other types of gastric varices. High rates of gastric variceal recurrence following EVBL may be due to a more superficial effect compared with obturation therapy [108]. This, together with the technical difficulty of banding in a retroflexed endoscope position has meant EVBL for gastric varices has largely been superseded by obturation therapies using cyanoacrylate and thrombin injection.

Cyanoacrylate injection is effective for bleeding gastric varices, yet remains unapproved in the USA. Injection of cyanoacrylate is not without complications including endoscope damage due to blockage of the injection channel, detachment of the injection needle into a varix, cerebral embolism, pulmonary embolism, splenic infarcts, mediastinitis and local abscesses. Although most reports of this therapy for gastric varices have limited follow-up, immediate haemostasis rates of 92-100% have been reported with variable re-bleeding rates [108-113]. Cyanoacrylate glue has been compared with ethanol injection in a randomised study with the former showing faster rates of variceal obliteration with a smaller injection volume, improved efficacy in control of acute gastric oesophageal variceal bleeding and reduced need for rescue surgery [114]. Another randomised study concluded that the obliteration of gastric varices using EVBL was more difficult and less effective than cyanoacrylate glue injection [115]. Early haemostasis rates were 87% with cyanoacrylate and 45% with EVBL, and re-bleeding rates were 31% and 54% respectively. Cyanoacrylate injection is also superior to beta-blockers in preventing gastric variceal re-bleeding [116]. When 77 patients who had bled from gastric varices were assigned to either beta-blockers or cyanoacrylate, those whose varices were injected with cyanoacrylate had lower rebleeding rates (15% v 55%), and lower mortality (3% v 25%) [116]. The addition of beta-blockers to cyanoacrylate therapy for secondary prevention after a cyanoacrylate-treated index bleed, does not confer any additional benefit [117].

Thrombin is another obturation therapy advocated for acutely bleeding gastric varices in some United Kingdom centres. It converts fibrinogen to a fibrin clot and causes platelet aggregation [118]. There have been small case-series of its use with haemostasis rates between 70-100% using bovine thrombin [119-122]. However there was concern that this material of bovine origin might present a potential risk of prion transmission. Short-term small studies of human-derived thrombin have demonstrated initial haemostasis rates of 100% but a high mortality from re-bleeding [123-125].

Interventional radiological procedures for the treatment of gastric varices include TIPS [126-128] and Balloon-occluded Retrograde Transvenous Obliteration (BRTO) [127-129] as salvage or rescue therapy when obturation therapy fails. BRTO is an interventional radiological technique used mostly in Far East Asia for gastric variceal bleeding. The gastro-renal shunts often seen in such patients can be occluded with sclerosant via a balloon catheter approach via the left renal vein [129]. BRTO may become an alternative to TIPS in patients with active gastric variceal bleeding in whom a gastrorenal shunt is present [130].

Current Baveno V guidelines [2] suggest early TIPS within 72 hours (ideally < 24 hours) in patients at high risk of treatment failure (Child-Pugh class C < 14 points or Child-Pugh class B with active bleeding) after initial pharmacology and endoscopic therapy in patients with variceal bleeding. This recommendation is derived from the pivotal study from Barcelona in which 63 cirrhotic patients with variceal bleeding were treated with vasoactive drugs and endoscopic therapy and then randomised to treatment with a TIPS within 72 hours ("early-TIPS") or else continuation of vasoactive drugs for 3 to 5 days followed by non-selective beta-blockers and long-term EVBL with insertion of a TIPS only if required as a rescue therapy [132]. Rebleeding or failure to control bleeding occurred in only 1 of the "early-TIPS" patients and in 14 of the vasoactive drug/EVBL group (p<0.001). Overall mortality was lower in the "early-TIPS" group (12 patients versus 4, p = 0.01) with 1-year survival 61% in the vasoactive drug/EVBL group versus 86% in the "early-TIPS" group (p <0.001).

8. Prevention of rebleeding (secondary prophylaxis)

The improvement in survival from index variceal bleeds using the therapies discussed has focussed attention on prevention of rebleeding. 60-80% of patients who bleed from varices will rebleed if not treated [18, 40,133, 134], and the risk of rebleeding is greatest in the first 10 days (131,132), during which 50% of those who are going to rebleed, do so. The risk of rebleeding gradually falls over the first month when an additional 10% rebleed [133, 134]; the risk after the first six weeks then plateaus out. Despite the advent of endoscopic therapies and early pharmacological therapies, rebleeding rates are still higher early on, with factors predictive of early rebleeding /treatment failure at 5 days including: active bleeding at index endoscopy, severity of liver disease (Child-Pugh class), severity of bleed, and severity of portal hypertension [132, 135]. HVPG is one of the best predictors of identifying those who will re-bleed. After an index variceal bleed, a reduction of HVPG to less than 12mm Hg or by at least 20%, reduces the risk of rebleeding from 46-65% to 0.13% [136]. HVPG measurement is usually limited to specialist centres.

Strategies to prevent rebleeding historically included surgical portocaval shunts, but currently involve pharmacological and endoscopic therapies. Pharmacological therapies include non-selective beta-blockers, and endoscopic therapies include sclerotherapy or EVBL. Beta-blockers significantly reduce rebleeding rates and improve survival at 2 years when compared to placebo [24,137]. Factors associated with a risk of rebleeding in patients treated with beta-blockers included a lack of compliance or a lack of reduction of heart rate [138]. Injection sclerotherapy reduces the risk of rebleeding from 65% to 35% but does not appear to reduce overall mortality and is associated with complications such as oesophageal ulceration [40]. When sclerotherapy was compared with beta-blockers there was less rebleeding in the sclerotherapy group, but significantly more side effects and no impact on mortality [136, 139]. EVBL has been shown to be superior to sclerotherapy in reducing the risk of rebleeding to a greater level with fewer side effects [87]. The combination of EVBL and sclerotherapy was no more effective than EVBL alone [140]. A combination of beta-blocker therapy with either EVBL or sclerotherapy has been found to reduce all bleeding, rebleeding from varices and variceal recurrence but not mortality, when compared to any single modality of therapy [141]. TIPS has been studied in early rebleeding with excellent results as mentioned previously in the chapter [132].

In summary, current Baveno V guidelines [2] suggest secondary prophylaxis should start on day 6 of the index bleed. A combination of beta-blocker therapy and EVBL is recommended

http://dx.doi.org/10.5772/52524

over either treatment alone as there are lower re-bleed rates with combination therapy. In patients who are unwilling to have EVBL, beta-blockers with ISMN is recommended [2]. In patients intolerant of beta-blockers, EVBL alone is recommended. In patients who re-bleed despite endoscopic and pharmacological therapies, TIPS is recommended. Transplantation should be considered in those who are appropriate candidates.

9. Conclusions

Variceal haemorrhage remains a life-threatening emergency, and a cause of decompensation of patients with portal hypertension or cirrhosis. Prevention of the development of portal hypertension where possible remains key in halting the development of oesophageal or gastric varices. However when portal hypertension has developed, it is important to identify those at risk of varices and enter them into a screening programme. Those found to have varices should be offered primary prophylaxis if required. Once a varix bleeds, urgent specialist care is required to potentially save life. In addition to fluid and blood resuscitation to stabilise conditions before endoscopy, vasoactive medications to reduced portal pressure and antibiotics should be administered. At urgent endoscopy performed by an experienced endoscopist, EVBL is the preferred endoscopic technique to achieve haemostasis in oesophageal variceal haemorrhage, and injection of cyanoacrylate glue is the preferred endoscopic technique to achieve haemostasis in gastric variceal haemorrhage. If endoscopic therapy is difficult, or does not halt the bleeding then TIPS can be performed, although self-expanding tamponading stents may be useful in refractory oesophageal variceal bleeding and BRTO may be useful in refractory gastric variceal bleeding. Survivors of variceal bleeding should receive secondary prophylaxis with beta-blocker medication, together with EVBL in the case of oesophageal varices.

Acknowledgements

The authors would like to acknowledge those permitting the reprint of images in the chapter: Dr Adrian Stanley, Consultant Gastroenterologist, Glasgow Royal Infirmary, Scotland; the company ELLA-CS, Hradec Kralove, Czech Republic; and Dr Branislav Kunčak, 2nd Dept. of Internal Medicine, Faculty of Health and Social Work, University of Trnava and Nové Zámky Hospital, Nové Zámky, Slovakia.

Author details

Neil Rajoriya and David A. Gorard

Department of Gastroenterology, Wycombe Hospital, High Wycombe, Buckinghamshire, UK

References

[1] D'Amico G, Pagliaro L, Bosch J. The treatment of portal hypertension: a meta-analytic review. Hepatology 1995;22(1):332-54

[2] De Franchis R. Baveno V consensus faculty. Revising consensus in portal hypertension: report of the Baveno V consensus workshop on methodology of diagnosis and therapy in portal hypertension. J Hepatol 2010;53(4): 762-768

[3] Carbonell N, Pauwels A, Serfaty L, et al. Improved survival after variceal bleeding in patients with cirrhosis over the past 2 decades. Hepatology 2004;40(3):652-659

[4] Pinzani M, Failli P, Ruocco C, Casini A, Milani S, Baldi E, Giotti A, et al. Fat storing cells as liver-specific pericytes. Spatial dynamics of agonist-stimulated intracellular calcium transients. J Clin Invest 1992;90(2):642-646

[5] Deleve LD, Wang X, Guo Y. Sinusoidal endothelial cells prevent rat stellate cell activation and promote reversion to quiescence. Hepatology 2008;48(3):920-30

[6] Freidman SL. Mechanisms of hepatic fibrogenesis. Gastroenterology 2008;134:1655-1669

[7] Bataller R, Gasull X, Gines P, et al. In vitro and in vivo activation of rat hepatic stellate cells results in de novo expression of L-type voltage operated calcium channels. Hepatology 2001;33(4):956-962

[8] Bataller R, Sancho-Bru P, Gines P, et al. Activated human hepatic stellate cells experss the renin-angiotensin system and synthesize angiotensin II. Gastroenterology 2003;125(1):117-125

[9] Rockey D. The cellular pathogenesis of portal hypertension: stellate cell contractility, endothelin and nitric oxide. Hepatology 1997;25:2-5

[10] Zhou Q, Hennenberg M, Trebicka J, Jochem K, Leifield L, Biecker E, Saurbruch T, et al. Intrahepatic upregulation of RhoA and Rho-kinase signalling contributes to increased hepatic vascular resistance in rats with secondary biliary cirrhosis. Gut 2006;55(9):1296-1305

[11] Gracia-Sancho, Lavina B, Rodriquez-Vilarrupla A, et al. Enhanced vasoconstrictor prostanoid production by sinusoidal endothelial cells increases portal perfusion pressure in cirrhotic rat livers. J Hepatol 2007;47(2):220-227

[12] Lee CH, Loureiro-Silva MR, Abraldes JG, et al.. Decreased intrahepatic response to alpha(1)-adrenergic agonists in lipopolysaccharide-treated rats is located in the sinusoidal area and depends on Kupffer cell function. J Gastroenterol Hepatol 2007;22(6):893-900

[13] Carmeliet P. Mechanisms of angiogenesis and arteriogenesis. Nat Med 2000;6(4): 389-395

[14] Fukumura D, Yuan F, Endo M, Jain RK. Role of nitric oxide in tumour microcirculation. Blood flow, vascular permeability, and leucocyte-endothelial interactions. Am J Pathol 1997;150(2):713-725

[15] Fernandez M, Vizzutti F, Garcia-Pagan JC, Rodes J, Bosch J. Anti-VEGF receptor-2 monoclonal antibody prevents porto-systemic collateral vessel formation in portal hypertensive mice. Gastroenterology 2004;126(3):886-894

[16] Wiest R, Groszmann RJ. Nitric oxide and portal hypertension: its role in the regulation of intrahepatic and splanchnic vascular resistance. Sem Liver Dis 1999;19(4): 411-426

[17] Garcia-Tsao G, Groszmann RJ, Fisher RL, et al. Portal pressure, presence of gastro-oesophageal varices and variceal bleeding. Hepatology 1985;5(3):419-24

[18] D'Amico G. The role of vasoactive drugs in the treatment of oesophageal varices. Expert opinion pharmcother 2004;5(2):349-360

[19] Noda T. Angioarchitectural study of oesophageal varices (with special reference to variceal rupture). Virchows Archiv A 1984;404:381-392

[20] Vianna A. Anatomy of the portal venous system in portal hypertension. In: McIntyre N, Benhamou JP, Birhcer J, Rizzetto M, Rodes J (eds). Oxford textbook of clinical hepatology, Oxford University press, Oxford 1991; 393-399

[21] Grozsmann RJ, Garcia-Tsao G, Bosch J, et al. Multicentre randomised placebo controlled trial of non-selective beta-blockers in the prevention of the complications of portal hypertension: final results and identification of predictive factor. AASLD, Boston, Hepatology 2003;38(4) (suppl 1):206A

[22] Primignani M, Albe R, Preatoni P, et al. "De-novo" development of esophageal varices in patients with a recent histological diagnosis of liver cirrhosis. Gastroenterology 1998;114:A1234

[23] Polio J, Grozsmann RJ. Hemodynamic factors involved in the development and rupture of esophageal varices: a pathophysiological approach to treatment. Semin Liv Dis 1986;6:318-331

[24] D'Amico G, Pagliaro L, Bosch J. Pharmacological treatment of portal hypertension: An evidence-based approach. Semin Liv Diseas 1999;19(4):475-505

[25] The North Italian Endoscopic Club for the Study and Treatment of Esopheageal Varices. Predictors of the first variceal haemorrhage in patients with cirrhosis of the liver and esophageal varices. N Engl Med J 1988;13:983-989

[26] Dell'Era A, Bosch J. review article: the relevance of portal pressure and other risk factors in acute gastro-oesophageal variceal bleeding. Aliment Pharmaco Ther 2000; 20 (suppl 3): 8-15, discussion 16

[27] Luca A, Garcia-Pagan JC, Bosch J, et al. Effects of ethanol consumption on hepatic haemodynamics in patients with alcoholic cirrhosis. Gastroenterology 1997;112(4): 1284-1289

[28] Garcia-Pagan JC, Feu F, Castells A, et al. Circadian variations of portal pressure and variceal haemorrhage in patients with cirrhosis. Hepatology 1994;16(3):595-601

[29] Lee SS, Hadengue A, Moreau R, et al. Postprandial hemodynamic responses in patients with cirrhosis. Hepatology 1988;8(3):647-651

[30] Cales P, Desmorat H, Vinel JP, et al. Incidence of large oesophageal varices in patients with cirrhosis: application to prophylaxis of first bleeding. Gut 1990;31:1298-1302

[31] Merli M, Nicolini G, Angeloni S, et al. Incidence and natural history of small esophageal varices in cirrhotic patients. J Hepatol2003;38:266-278

[32] Merkel C, Marin R, Angeli P, et al. A placebo-controlled trial of nadolol in the prophylaxis of growth of small esophageal varices in cirrhosis. Gastroenterology 2004;127(2):476-84

[33] Zoli M, Merkel C, Magalotti C, et al. Natural history of cirrhotic patients with small esophageal varices: a prospective study. Am J Gastroenteterol 2000;95(2):503-508

[34] Italian liver cirrhosis project. Reliability of endoscopy in the assessment of variceal features. J Hepatol 1987;4:93-98

[35] Garcia-Tsao G, Sanyal AJ, Grace ND, Carey W Prevention and management of gastroesophageal varices and variceal hemorrhage in cirrhosis. Hepatology. 2007;46(3): 922-38.

[36] McCormack TT, Rose JD, Smith PM, Johnson AG. Perforating veins and blood flow in oesophageal varices. Lancet 1983; 2: 1442-1444

[37] Sarin SK, Lahoti D, Saxena SP, Murthy NS, Makwana UK. Prevalence, classification and natural history of gastric varices: a long-term follow-up study in 568 portal hypertension patients. Hepatology 1992;16 (6):1343–1349.

[38] Feu F, Garcia-Pagan JC, Bosch J, et al. Relation between portal pressure response to pharmacotherapy and risk of recurrent variceal haemorrhage in patients with cirrhosis. Lancet 1995;346:1056–9

[39] Bosch J, Berzigotti A, Garcia-Pagan JC, Abraldes JG. The management of portal hypertension: Rational basis, available treatments and future options. J Hepatol 2008;S68-92

[40] de Franchis R. Evolving consensus in portal hypertension report of the Baveno IV consensus workshop on methodology and therapy in portal hypertension. J Hepatol 2005;43:167-176

[41] Navasa M, Chesta J, Bosch J, Rodes J. Reduction of portal pressure by isosrbide-5-mononitrate in patients with cirrhosis. Effects on splanchnic and systemic hemodynamics and liver function. Gastroenterology 1989;96(4):1110-1118

[42] Garcia-Pagan JC, Navasa M, Bosch J, et al. Enhancement of portal pressure reduction by the association of isosorbide-5-mononitrate to propranolol administration in patients with cirrhosis. Hepatology 1990;11(2):230-238

[43] Garcia-Pagan JC, Villanueva C, Vila MC et al. Isosorbide mononitrate in the prevention of fist bleed in patients who cannot receive beta-blockers. Gastroenterology 2001;121(4):908-914

[44] Sanyal AJ, Shiffman ML. The pharmacological treatment of portal hypertension. Annu Rev Gastrointest Pharmacol 1996;242

[45] Bosch J, Masti R, Kravetz D, et al. Effects of propranolol on azygous venous blood flow and hepatic and systemic hemodynamics in cirrhosis. Hepatology 1984;4(6): 1200-1205

[46] Garcia-Tsao G, Grace ND. Groszmann RJ, et al. Short-term effects of propranolol on portal venous pressure. Hepatology 1986;6(1):101-106

[47] Cheng JW, Zhu L, Gu MJ, Song ZM. Meta-analysis of propranolol effects on gastrointestinal haemorrhage in cirrhotic patients. World J Gastroenterol 2003;9(8):1836-1839

[48] Hayes PC, Davis JM, Lewis JA, Bouchier IA. Meta-analysis of value of propranolol in prevention of variceal haemorrhage. Lancet 1990;336:153-156

[49] Bartsch W, Sponer G, Strein K, Muller-Beckman B, von Mollendorf E, Abshagen U. Pharmacologie und klinische pharmakologie des neunen vasodila tierenden beta-rezeptoren blockers. BM 14190. Therapiewoche 1982;32:5714

[50] Bosch J. Carvedilol for portal hypertension in patients with cirrhosis. Hepatology 2010;51(6):2214

[51] Forrest EH, Bouchieria, Hayes PC. Acute haemodynamic changes after oral carvedilol, a vasodilating beta-blocker, in patients with cirrhosis. J Hepatol 1996;25(6): 909-915

[52] Stanley AJ, Therapondos G, Helmey A, Hayes PC. Haemodynamic effects of acute and chronic administration of low dose carvedilol in patients with cirrhosis. J Hepatol1999;30(3):479-484

[53] Tripathi D, Ferguson JW, Kochar N, et al. Randomised controlled trial of carvedilol versus variceal band ligation for the prevention of fist variceal bleed. Hepatology 2009;50(3):825-833

[54] Tripathi D, Therapondos G, Lui HF, Stanley AJ, Hayes PC et al. Haemodynamic effects of acute and chronic administration of low-dose carvedilol, a vasodilating beta-blocker, in patients with cirrhosis and portal hypertension. Aliment Pharmacol Ther 2002;16(3):373-80

[55] Serste T, Melot C, Francoz C, et al. Deleterious effects of beta-blockers on survival in patients with cirrhosis and refractory ascites. Hepatology 2010;52(3):1017-22

[56] Krag A, Wiest R, Albillos A, Gluud LL. The window hypothesis: haemodynamic and non-haemodynamic effects of β-blockers improve survival of patients with cirrhosis during a window in the disease. Gut. 2012;61(7):967-9.

[57] The Veterans Affairs Cooperative Variceal Sclerotherapy Group. Prophylactic Sclerotherapy for Esophageal Varices in Men with Alcoholic Liver Disease — A Randomized, Single-Blind, Multicenter Clinical Trial..N Engl J Med 1991; 324:1779-1784

[58] Lay CS, Tsai YT, Teg CY, et al. Endoscopic variceal ligation in prophylaxis of first variceal bleeding in cirrhotic patients with high-risk esophageal varcies. Hepatology 1997;25(6):1346-1350

[59] Sarin SK, Lamba GS, Kumar M, et al. Comparison of endoscopic ligation and propranolol for the primary prevention of variceal bleeding. N Engl Med 1999;340(13): 988-993

[60] Lui HF, Stanley AJ, Forrest EH, et al. Primary prophylaxis of variceal haemorrhage: a randomised controlled trial comparing band ligation, propranolol, and isosorbide mononitrate. Gastroenterology 2002;123(3):735-744

[61] Imperiale TF, Chalasni N. A meta-analysis of endoscopic variceal ligation for primary prophylaxis of esophageal variceal bleeding. Hepatology 2001;33(4):802-807

[62] Khuroo MS, Khuroo NS, Farahat KL, et al. Meta-analysis: endoscopic variceal ligation for primary prophylaxis of oesophageal variceal bleeding. Aliment Pharmaco Ther 2005;21(4):347-361

[63] Gluud LL, Klingenberg S, Nikolova D, Gluud C. Banding ligation versus Beta-blockers as primary prophylaxis in esophageal varices: a systematic review of randomised trials. Am J Gastroentertol 2007;102(12):2842-2848

[64] Mishra SR, Sharma BC, Kumar A, Sarin SK. Primary prophylaxis of gastric variceal bleeding comparing cyanoacrylate injections and beta-blockers: a randomised controlled trial. J Hepatol 2011;54(6):1161-1167

[65] Chalasani N, Kahi C, Francois F, et al. Improved patient survival after acute variceal bleeding: a multicentre cohort study. Am J Gastroenterol 2003;98(3):653-9

[66] Kravetz D, Sikuler E, Groszmann RJ. Splanchnic and systemic hemodynamics in portal hypertensive rats during hemorrhage and blood volume restitution. Gastroenterology 1986;90(5 Part 1):1232-1240

[67] Castaneda B, Morales J, Lionetti R, et al. Effects of blood volume restitution following a portal hypertensive-related bleeding in anesthetized cirrhotic rats. Hepatology 2001;33(4):821-825.

[68] Hou MC, Lin HC, Liu TT, et al. Antibiotic prophylaxis after endoscopic therapy prevents rebleeding in acute variceal haemorrhage: a randomised controlled trial. Hepatology 2004;39(3):746-53

[69] Soares-Weiser K, Brezis M, Tur-Kaspa R, et al. Antibiotic prophylaxis of bacterial infections in cirrhotic inpatients: a meta-analysis of randomised controlled trials. Scand J Gastroenterol 2003;38(2):193-200

[70] Burroughs AK, Planas S, Svoboda P. Optimising care of upper gastrointestinal bleeding in cirrhotic patients. Scand J Gastroenterol 1998;226:14-24

[71] Ianno G, Doust J, Rockey DC. Terlipressin for acute esophageal variceal haemorrhage. Cochrane Database Syst Rev. 2003;(1):CD002147

[72] Gotzsche PC, Hrobjartsson A. Somatostatin analogues for acute bleeding oesophageal varices. Cochrane Database Syst Rev 2008;3:CD000193

[73] Baik SK, Jeong PH, Ji SW, et al. Acute hemodynamic effects of octreotide and terlipressin in patients with cirrhosis: a randomized comparison. Am J Gastroenterol 2005;100(3):631-5

[74] Escorsell A, Bandi JC, Andreu V, et al. Desensitisation to the effects of octreotide in cirrhotic patients with portal hypertension. Gastroenterology 2001;120(1):161-169

[75] Spahr L, Giostra E, Frossard JL, et al. A 3-month course of long-acting repeatable octreotide (sandostatin LR) improves portal hypertension in patients with cirrhosis: a randomized controlled study. Am J Gastroenterol 2007;102(7):1397-1405

[76] Chen J, Grozsmann RJ. Blood in the gastric lumen increases splanchnic portal flow and portal pressure in portal-hypertensive rats. Gastroenterology 1986;111:1103-

[77] Ludwig D, Schadel S, Bruning A, Schiefer B, Stange EF.et al. 48-hour hemodynamic effects of octreotide on postprandial splanchnic hyperemia in patients with liver cirrhosis and portal hypertension: double-blind, placebo-controlled study. Dig Dis Sci 2000;45(5):1019-1027

[78] Imperiale TF, Teran JC, McCullough AJ. A meta-analysis of somatostatin versus vasopressin in the management of acute esophageal variceal haemorrhage. Gastroenterology 1995;109(4):1289-1294

[79] Hartigan PM, Gebhard RL, Gregory PB. Sclerotherapy for actively bleeding esophageal varices in male alcoholics with cirrhosis. Veterans Affairs Cooperative Variceal Sclerotherapy Group. Gastrointest Endoscop 1997;46(1):1-7

[80] Piquet KJ, Flessner H, Endoscopic sclerosis and esophageal balloon tamponade in acute haemorrhage from esophagogastric varices: a prospective controlled randomized trial. Hepatology 1985; 5(4): 580-583

[81] Westaby D, Hayes PC, Gibson AE, Polson RJ, Williams R. Controlled clinical trial of injection sclerotherapy for active variceal bleeding. Hepatology 1989;9(2):272-277

[82] Larson AW, Cohen H, Zweiban B, et al. Acute esophageal variceal sclerotherapy. Results of a prospective randomized controlled trial. JAMA 1986;255(4):497-500

[83] Moreto M, Zaballa M, Bernal A, et al. A randomized trial of tamponade or sclerotherapy as immediate treatment for bleeding esophageal varices. Surg Gynecol Obstet 1988;167(4):331-334

[84] Traintos CK, Goulis J, Patch D, et al. An evaluation of emergency sclerotherapy of varices in randomized trials: looking the needle in the eye. Endoscopy 2006;38(8): 797-807

[85] Garcia-Pagan JC, Bosch J. Endoscopic band ligation in the treatment ofportal hypertension. Nat.Clin Pract.Gastroenterol Hepatol 2005;2(11):526-535.

[86] Avgerinos A, Armonis A, Stefanidis G, et al. Sustained rise of portal pressure after sclerotherapy, but not band ligation, in acute variceal bleeding in cirrhosis. Hepatology 2004;39(6):1623-1630.

[87] Laine L, Cook D. Endoscopic ligation compared to sclerotherapy for treatment of esophageal variceal bleeding. A meta-analysis. Ann Inter Med 1995;123(4):280-287

[88] Banares R, Albillos A, Rincon D, et al. Endoscopic treatment versus endoscopic plus pharmacologic treatment for acute variceal bleeding: a meta-analysis. Hepatology 2002;35(3):609-615

[89] D'Amico G, Criscuoli V, Fili D, Mocciaro D, F, Pagliaro L. Meta-analysis of trials for variceal bleeding. Hepatology 2002;36(4 Pt 1):1023-1024

[90] Novella MT, Villanueva C, Ortiz J, et al. Octreotide vs sclerotherapy and octreotide for acute variceal bleeding. A pilot study. Hepatology 1996;24(suppl): 207A

[91] Villanueva C, Ortiz J, Sabat M, et al. Octreotide in acute bleeding esophageal varices: a prospective randomized trial. Hepatology 1999;30(2):384-389

[92] Hubmann R, Bodlaj G, Czompo M, Benko L, Pichler P, et al. The use of self-expanding metal stents to treat acute esophegeal variceal bleeding. Endoscopy 2006; 38: 896-901

[93] Teres J, Planas R, Panes J, et al. Vasopressin/nitroglycerine infusion vs esophageal tamponade in the treatment of acute variceal bleeding: a randomized controlled trial. Hepatology 1990;11(6):964-968

[94] Monescillo A, Martinez-Lagares F, Ruiz-Del-Arbol L, et al. Influence of portal hypertension and its early decompression by TIPS placement on the outcome of variceal bleeding. Hepatology 2004;40:793-801

[95] Burroughs AK, Triantos CK. Predicting failure to control bleeding, and mortality in acute variceal bleeding. J Hepatology 2008;48(2):185-188

[96] Sanyal A, Freedman Am, Luketic VA, et al. Transjugular intrahepatic portosystemic shunts for patients with active variceal hemorrhage unresponsive to sclerotherapy. Gastroenterology 1996;111(1): 138-146

[97] Chau TN, Patch D, Chan YW, et al. "Salvage" transjugular intrahepatic portosystemic shunts: gastric fundal compared with esophageal variceal bleeding. Gastroenterology 1998;114(5):981-987

[98] Trudeau W, Prindville T. Endoscopic injection sclerosis in bleeding gastric varices. Gastrointest Endosc 1986;32(4):264-268

[99] Thakeb F, Salem SA, Abdallah M, el Batanouny M. Endoscopic diagnosis of gastric varices. Endoscopy 1994;26(3):287-291.

[100] Bretagne JF, Dudicourt JC, Morisot D, et al. Is endoscopic variceal sclerotherapy effective for the treatment of gastric varices.(abstr) Dig Dis Sci 1986;31:505S

[101] Sarin SK. Long term follow up gastric variceal sclerotherapy: an eleven-year experience. Gastrointest Endosc 997;46(1):8-14

[102] Ogawa K, Ishikawa S, Naritaka Y, et al. Clinical evaluation of endoscopic injection sclerotherapy using N-Butyl-2-Cyanoacrylate for gastric variceal bleeding. J Gastroenterol Hepatol 1999; 14(3):245-50

[103] Hirota S, Matsumoto S, Tomita, Sako M, Kono M.. Retrograde transvenous obliteration of gastric varices. Radiology 1999 ;211(2) :349-356

[104] Kim T, Shijo H, Kokawa H, et al. Risk factors for hemorrhage from gastric fundal varices. Hepatology 1997 ;25(2) :307-312

[105] Gotlib JP, Zimmerman P. Une nouvelle technique de traitement encoscopique des varices oesophagiennes: l'obriteration. Endosc Dig 1984;7:10-12

[106] Sarin SK, Sachdev G, Nanda R, Misra SP Broor Sl. Endoscopic Sclerotherapy in the treatment of gastric varices. Br J Surg 1988;75(8):747-750

[107] Jalan R, Hayes PC. UK Guidelines on the management of variceal haemorrhage in cirrhotic patients. British Society of Gastroenterology. Gut 2000;46 (Suppl. 3-4):III1-III5

[108] Lee MS, Shim CS. Is endoscopic ligation therapy with large detachable snare and elastic bands really safe and effective? Response. Gastrointest Endosc 2003;57:439-440

[109] Billi P, Milandri GL, Borioni D, Fabbri C, Baroncini D, Cennamo V, et al. Endoscopic treatment of gastric varices with N-butyl-2-cyanoacrylate: a long term follow up (abstract). Gastrointest Endosc 1998; 47:AB26

[110] Huang YH, Yeh HZ, Chen GH, et al. Endoscopic treatment of bleeding gastric varices by N-butyl-2-cyanoacrylate (Histoacryl) injection: long term efficacy and safety. Gastrointest Endosc 2000;52:160-7

[111] Seewald S, Naga M, Onar S, et al. Standardised injection technique and regimen minimises complication and ensures safety of N-Butyl-2-Cyanoacrylate injection for the treatment of Gastric Fundal Varices. GastroIntest Endosc 2005; 61 (5): AB91-372

[112] Iwase H, Maeda O, Shinida M, et al. Endoscopic ablation with cyanoacrylate glue for isolated gastric variceal bleeding. Gastrointest Endosc 2001; 53(6):585-596

[113] Rajoriya N, Forrest EH, Gray J, et al. Long-term follow-up of endoscopic Histoacryl glue injection for the management of gastric varicieal bleeding. QJM. 2011 Jan;104(1): 41-47.

[114] Sarin SK, Jain AK, Jain M, Gupta R. A randomised controlled trial of cyanoacrylate versus alcohol injection in patients with isolated fundic varices. Am J Gastroenterol 2002;97(4):1010-1015

[115] Lo GH, Lai KH, Cheng JS, Chen MH, Chiang HT. A prospective, randomised trial of butyl cyanoacrylate injection versus band ligation in the management of bleeding gastric varices. Hepatology 2001;33(5):1060-1064

[116] Mishra SR, Chander Sharma B, Kumar A, Sarin SK. Endoscopic cyanoacrylate injection versus beta-blocker for secondary prophylaxis of gastric variceal bleed: a randomised controlled trial. Gut 2010;59(6):729-735

[117] Hung HH, Chang CJ, Hou MC, et al. Efficacy on non-selective B-Blockers as adjunct to endoscopic prophylactic treatment for gastric variceal bleeding: A randomized controlled trial. J Hepatol 2012;56(5):1025-1032

[118] Tripathi D, Ferguson JW, Therapondos G, Pleveris JN, Hayes PC. Review article: recent advances in the management of bleeding gastric varices. Aliment Pharmaco Therp 2006;24(1):1-17

[119] Kitano S, Hashizume M, Yamaga H, et al. Human thrombin plus 5 per cent ethanolamine oleate injected to sclerose oesophageal varices: a prospective randomized trial. Br J Surg 1989; 76(7): 715–718.

[120] Przemioslo RT, McNair A, Williams R. Thrombin is effective in arresting bleeding from gastric variceal hemorrhage. Dig Dis Sci 1999; 44(4): 778–781.

[121] Snobl J, Van Buuren HR, Van Blankenstein M. Endoscopic injection using thrombin: an effective and safe method for controlling oesophagogastric variceal bleeding. Gastroenterology 1992;102: A891 (abstract).

[122] Williams SG, Peters RA, Westaby D. Thrombin – an effective treatment for gastric variceal haemorrhage. Gut 1994; 35(9): 1287–1289.

[123] Heneghan MA, Byrne A, Harrison PM. An open pilot study of the effects of a human fibrin glue for endoscopic treatment of patients with acute bleeding from gastric varices. Gastrointest Endosc 2002; 56(3): 422–426.

[124] Datta D, Vlavianos P, Alisa A, Westaby D. Use of fibrin glue (beriplast) in the management of bleeding gastric varices. Endoscopy 2003; 35(8): 675–678.

[125] Yang WL, Tripathi D, Therapondos G, Todd A, Hayes PC. Endoscopic use of human thrombin in bleeding gastric varices. Am J Gastroenterol 2002; 97(6): 1381–1385.

[126] Albillos A, Ruiz Del Arbol L, "Salvage" transjugular intrahepatic portosystemic shunt: gastric fundal compared with esophageal variceal bleeding. Gastrointest Endosc 1999;50(2):294–295.

[127] Stanley AJ, Jalan R, Ireland HM, et al. A comparison between gastric and oesophageal variceal haemorrhage treated with transjugular intrahepatic portosystemic stent shunt (TIPSS). Aliment Pharmacol Ther 1997;11(1):171–176.

[128] Barange K, Peron JM, Imani K, et al. Transjugular intrahepatic portosystemic shunt in the treatment of refractory bleeding from ruptured gastric varices. Hepatology 1999;30(5):1139–1143.

[129] Kiyosue H. Mori H. Matsumoto S. Yamada Y. Hori Y. Okino Y. Transcatheter obliteration of gastric varices. Part 1. Anatomic classification. Radiographics. 2003;23(4): 911-920

[130] Choi YH. Yoon CJ. Park JH. Chung JW. Kwon JW. Choi GM. Balloon-occluded retrograde transvenous obliteration for gastric variceal bleeding: its feasibility compared with transjugular intrahepatic portosystemic shunt. Korean Journal of Radiology. 2003;4(2):109-116,

[131] Matsumoto A, Haramoto N, Nomura T, Hongou Y, Arisaka Y, Morikawa H, Hirata I, Katsu K. Balloon-occluded retrograde transvenous obliteration of high risk gastric varices. Am Journal of Gastroenterol; 94(3):643-649

[132] Garcia-Pagan JC, Caca K, Bureau C, et al. Early use of TIPS in patients with cirrhosis and variceal bleeding. N Engl J Med 2010;362(25):2370-2379.

[133] Graham DY, Smith JL. The course of patients with variceal hemorrhage. Gastroenterology 1981;80(4):800-809

[134] D'Amico G, de Franchis R.. Upper digestive bleeding in cirrhosis. Post-therapeutic outcome and prognostic indicators. Hepatology 2003;38(3):599-612

[135] Bambha K, Kim WR, Pedersen R, et al. Predictors of early rebleeding and mortality after acute variceal hemorrhage in patients with cirrhosis. Gut 2008;57(6):814-820

[136] Bosch J, Garcia-Pagan JC. Prevention of variceal rebleeding. Lancet 2003; 361:952-954

[137] Bernard B, Lebrec D, Mathurin P,Opolon P, Poynard T. Beta-adrenergic antagonists in the prevention of gastrointestinal rebleeding in patients with cirrhosis: a meta-analysis. Hepatology 1997;25(1):63-70

[138] Poynard T, Lebrec D, Hillon P, et al. Propanolol for the prevention of recurrent gastrointestinal bleeding in patients with cirrhosis: a prospective study of factors associated with rebleeding. Hepatology 1987;7(3):447-451

[139] Bernard B, Lebrec D, Mathurin P, Opolon P, Poynard T. Propanolol and sclerotherapy in the prevention if gastrointestinal rebleeding in patients with cirrhosis. J Hepatol 1997;26(2):312-324

[140] Karsan H, Morton SC, Shekelle PG, et al. Combination of endoscopic band ligation and sclerotherapy compared with endoscopic band ligation alone for the secondary prophylaxis of esophageal variceal haemorrhage: A meta-analysis. Dig Dis Sci 2005;50(2):399-406

[141] Gonzalez R, Zamora J, Gomez-Camerero J, et al. Meta-analysis: Combination endoscopic and drug therapy to prevent variceal rebleeding in cirrhosis. Ann Intern Med 2008;149(2):109-22

Chapter 8

Diagnosis and Management of Barrett's Esophagus with and Without Dysplasia

Borislav Vladimirov, Radina Ivanova and
Ivan Terziev

Additional information is available at the end of the chapter

http://dx.doi.org/10.5772/52735

1. Introduction

Barrett's esophagus (BE) is the partial replacement, from the gastro-esophageal junction (GEJ) proximally, of esophageal squamous epithelium with metaplastic columnar epithelium. It develops in patients with gastroesophageal reflux disease (GERD) because of chronic injury and inflammation of the esophageal epithelium. Many other factors have also significance. BE is the only known precursor to esophageal adenocarcinoma (EAC), the incidence of which has been increased faster in Western world in the past four decades [1, 2]. In the United States, the incidence of EAC increased from 3.6 cases per 1,000,000 in 1973 to 25.6 per 1,000,000 in 2006 [1]. Since EAC is frequently detected at an advanced stage, the prognosis remains poor. The 5-year survival rate of patients with locally advanced EAC undergoing curative resection is around 15–20% [3]. So detection at an early stage of neoplastic progression may be important in improving survival. The risk of developing EAC is 30–40-fold higher in patients with BE compared with the general population [4, 5]. The development of EAC in BE has been shown to occur through a multistep process of increasing grades of epithelial dysplasia, from no dysplasia to low-grade dysplasia (LGD), high-grade dysplasia (HGD) and finally EAC [6]. In two studies of 136 and 170 patients with nondysplastic Barrett's esophagus (NDBE), followed for approximately 4 years, the rate of progression to EAC was 0.5% per patient-year [7, 8]. The risk additionally increases if Barrett's dysplasia is present. The annual incidence of EAC in patients with LGD and HGD is about 1.7% and 6.6% respectively [9]. In another study of 75 BE patients with HGD, 16% developed EAC over a mean follow-up period of 7.3 years [10]. In last years, there are many new data for the pathogenesis and the natural history of BE, which raise many points regarding surveillance of BE and risk stratification for EAC, and current role of anti-reflux therapy. Many enhanced imaging technologies and new endoscopic modalities for detection or management of any grade dysplasia and early cancer have been developed.

2. Definitions and diagnosis of BE

2.1. Definitions of BE

There is universal agreement that the underlying component of the definitions of Barrett's esophagus is the partial replacement, from the GEJ proximally, of esophageal squamous epithelium with metaplastic columnar epithelium. A mosaic of several histologic types of columnar metaplasia can be seen on biopsies from BE, including cardia type metaplasia, gastric fundus type metaplasia and specialized intestinal metaplasia (IM) type, containing goblet cells. The term BE is currently confusing because of varying definitions used for the diagnosis of BE [11, 12]. There is a lack of consensus among various professional organizations whether goblet metaplasia should be a requirement for the diagnosis of BE. According to the British Society of Gastroenterology (BSG), BE represents an endoscopically apparent area of columnar mucosa proximal to the GEJ, proven on histologic examination [13]. The American College of Gastro-enterology(ACG) and the American Gastroenterological Association (AGA) recommend documentation of IM for the diagnosis of BE [14, 15]. Several arguments can be made in favor of requiring IM for the diagnosis of BE. This definition is related with the concept of more malignant potential of IM compared to the risk of neoplastic progression in patients with metaplastic nongoblet columnar epithelium [14]. Some studies have also suggest that a diagnosis of BE may have a negative impact on overall quality of life of the patients. Patients with BE tend to overestimate their risk of EAC, and this leads to higher utilization of healthcare resources. A diagnosis of BE can result in higher health insurance premium and difficulty in obtaining health insurance [16, 17]. The varying definitions of BE lead to difficulties in the interpretation of know ledges for BE, because of the selection and follow-up of different cohorts of cases [12]. The "only IM type" definition of BE dominates the literature, but in many publications the diagnosis is made on the basis of varying endoscopic criteria unsupported by histopathology or on the presence of any type of columnar metaplasia. In 2006 the definition of BE was considered by the Global Evidence-Based Consensus Workshop on the Definition and Classification of Reflux Disease (the Montréal workshop) [18]. The experts reached consensus that the label BE should be used when any type of columnar metaplasia (CM) is confirmed by histology, with description of presence or absence of IM. There are different evidence –based considerations which support this non-restrictive definition of BE. The density of goblet cells in any segment of CM is dependent on a variety of factors, such as patient age, length of the columnar-lined segment, and number or location in which biopsies are obtained [19-22]. The most endoscopists in routine practice do not take enough biopsies to screen adequately for IM so many patients are being incorrectly assigned to diagnosis "not BE" on the basis of a technically inadequate diagnostic process. The analysis of 1646 biopsies from 125 consecutive patients with suspected endoscopic CM showed that goblet cells were identified in 68% of patients when a mean of 8 biopsies were obtained but only in 34.7%, when a mean of 4 biopsies were evaluated [22]. The goblet cell density is greater near the proximal neo-squamocolumnar compared to the distal area of CM [21]. The findings that the nongoblet columnar epithelium possess "intestinal" features and exhibit molecular and genetic abnormalities similar to those seen in BE with IM are other data supporting the use of non-restrictive definition of BE [23, 24]. The immunohistochemical study of the expression of different markers of intestinal differentiation as DAS-1, villin, and CDX-2 showed reactivity in both types of metaplastic (goblet and nongoblet) epithelium [23]. Abnormal DNA has been found recently to be present to similar degrees in esophageal CM of all types, making the malignant potential of "negative for IM-type" BE also probable [24]. In confirmation of Montreal definition of BE are the data that dysplasia and cancer may arise in nongoblet CM [25, 26]. It was found that there is no statistical difference in the risk of dysplasia or EAC in patients either without (n= 322) or with (n= 612) IM in index biopsies from metaplastic CM [25]. In another study endoscopic surveillance (median follow-up of 12 years) of patients with BE according "any metaplasia" was evaluated. It was reported that EAC developed in the 399 patients in whom IM was not found, at a rate that did not differ significantly from the 379 patients in whom IM had been demonstrated [26].

All these data confirm that the more correct definition of BE is that of Montreal definition.

2.2. Diagnosis of BE

BE is diagnosed by both endoscopy and histology. On endoscopy, it is suspected by the presence of "tongues" as extensions of salmon-colored mucosa above the GEJ. According to Montreal classification endoscopically suspected esophageal metaplasia (ESEM) describes the endoscopic findings consistent with BE that await histological evaluation [18]. The term BE should not be used before histological confirmation. Multiple, closely spaced biopsies are necessary to characterize ESEM. Standard protocol includes four quadrant biopsies performed at every 1 or 2 cm intervals from the proximal GEJ extending to the squamocolumnar junction. It was decided that all types of histologically proven oesophageal CM, including gastric or specialized IM should be included in the diagnosis of BE. The presence or absence of dysplasia should be evaluated. Morphologically, dysplasia is defined as "unequivocal neoplastic epithelium confined to the basement membrane, classified as LGD and HGD. Because of significant interobserver variations, the diagnosis of dysplasia should be confirmed by at least one additional pathologist, preferably one who is an expert in gastrointestinal (GI) pathology.

2.2.1. Endoscopy in BE

Endoscopy is the only practical option for the routine diagnosis and surveillance of esophageal CM. The first steps of endoscopic assessment are the recognition of BE and the grading of it's extent. BE has been divided into long-segment (>3 cm), short-segment (1-3 cm), and ultra-short-segment (< 1cm) categories [27]. The first systematic and standardized method for description of the extent of BE, which was carried out by the International Working Group for the Classification of Oesophagitis (IWGCO), resulted in the Prague C & M Criteria [28]. They were developed on the base of interpretations of purpose-recorded and standardized endoscopic video recordings. The C-value describes the length of circumferential metaplasia, whilst the M (for maximum) value describes the most upper point of any tongue of metaplasia. These values are referenced to the position of the GEJ and are given in centimeters. The validation of the Prague C&M Criteria showed good inter-observer agreement on the position of the GEJ and also on C&M-values greater than 1 cm. The agreement on presence of metaplastic segments less than 1 cm in length was unacceptably poor. A second, independent validation study of the Prague Criteria was done in several Asian countries [29]. It confirmed the data of the IWGCO and showed that the endoscopist can use the criteria successfully also in regions with a low prevalence of BE.

The most misdiagnoses of BE are related with the endoscopic features in patients with a hiatus hernia. This is due to failure to spend enough time in observing the region of the diaphragmatic hiatus and the upper end of the gastric mucosal folds at a relatively low level of distension [12]. Accurate location of the GEJ is of diagnostic importance, since mucosa of columnar appearance above this level has to be concluded to be metaplastic. The histological examination cannot reliably differentiate between metaplastic esophageal mucosa and the mucosa of the extreme upper stomach. Correct interpretation of biopsies around the GEJ depends on the accuracy of their location by endoscopy. Current guidelines recommend use of the Seattle protocol as the primary approach to assessment of the mucosa in BE with and without dysplasia [14, 15]. It was found that the protocol, with biopsies from all visible abnormalities and random four-quadrant biopsies every 1cm starting from the top of the gastric folds up to the GEJ, is superior to random biopsies or 2-cm biopsies in detecting early cancers arising in BE with HGD. In a study of 45 patients with BE with HGD, the 2-cm protocol (four-quadrant biopsies every 2 cm) missed 50% of cancers that were detected by a 1-cm protocol in Barrett's segments of 2 cm or more length without visible lesions [30]. In last years, with the improvement of image resolution of endoscopes, there is convincing evidence that guided biopsy is more sensitive for detection of dysplasia and EAC than blind biopsies [31-33].

The significant increase in image resolution by high-resolution endoscopy and high definition monitors (HDTV) is the most important recent improvement in endoscopic imaging in general, and particularly with regard to detection of early neoplastic lesions [34].

These require updating to place greater emphasis on visually guided biopsy with a high-resolution endoscopic system [12]. Given that general endoscopists are currently inadequately skilled and equipped for recognition of mucosal areas of concern, it is probably best that blind biopsies are also taken at least for the present [12]. Many imaging modalities as chromoendoscopy/magnifying chromoendoscopy, narrow band imaging (NBI) with/without magnification, autofluorescence imaging (AFI), and confocal microendoscopy can improve identification of abnormal areas and their targeting biopsy, and finally increase identifying HGD and early neoplasia [32, 34, 35].

Chromoendoscopy involves the topical application of stains or pigments to improve tissue localization, characterization, or diagnosis during endoscopy [36]. Methylene blue chromoendoscopy (MBC) has been reported to improve the detection of dysplasia in BE [37]. However, other authors found that MBC may be less effective in detecting dysplasia and also labor-intensive, and operator-dependent [38-41]. A meta-analysis of nine studies showed that staining with methylene blue did not significantly increase the detection of specialized IM and dysplasia compared with random biopsies [41]. In addition, methylene blue has been shown to induce cellular DNA damage when is photoexcited by endoscopic light and therefore it may be potentially carcinogenic [42]. It has been demonstrated that combination of chromoendoscopy with magnifying endoscopy improves the inspection of the mucosal surface pattern and may differentiate HGD from NDBE [43]. Our experience shows that magnifying chromoendoscopy with methylene blue and indigo carmine is helpful for more correct distinguishing between the focal metaplastic as well as dysplastic epithelial lesions in patients with BE [44]. It also increased the diagnostic rate of islands with Barrett's IM or dysplasia after endoscopic therapy (figure 1, 2, 3). *NBI* is a high-resolution endoscopic technique that enhances the fine structure of the mucosal surface. The improved imaging of mucosal patterns is resulted from the relatively high-intensity of blue light in NBI which reveals superficial structures because of its shallow penetration depth. In addition, absorption of blue light by hemoglobin enables detailed inspection of the microvasculture [45]. Using high-resolution endoscopy and NBI, the same authors have proposed a classification of mucosal surface characteristics of BE, which may be useful in the characterization of dysplastic and nondysplastic tissues. In their study of 200 mucosal areas in 63 patients with Barrett's, a regular mucosal and vascular patterns, and flat mucosa (i.e. without any villi or pits) were significantly associated with IM, while all areas with HGD exhibited irregular mucosal and irregular vascular patterns, or abnormal blood vessels. *AFI* is based on the tissue autofluorescence in exposition to light of a short wavelength and certain endogenous biological substances (fluorophores). In BE, normal and early neoplastic tissues have different autofluorescence properties [34]. According to our experience, delta-aminolevulinic acid/Protoporphyrin IX (5-ALA/PpIX) is a very good fluorescent marker for dysplasia and tumor detection in esophagus [46, 47]. AFI technology has been incorporated into high-resolution endoscopy systems. Using such a system, one study reported that the total number of detected lesions was doubled and one-third of the patients with HGD or early cancer were diagnosed with AFI when compared with high-resolution endoscopy alone [48]. The limitation of AFI was a relatively high rate of false positive findings. In later study the same authors used a combination of high-resolution white light imaging, AFI and NBI and they called endoscopic tri-modal imaging (ETMI) [49]. They found that AFI increased the sensitivity and NBI reduced the false positive rate, thus improving specificity. These findings were confirmed in two multicenter studies [50, 51]. The first study demonstrated that AFI increased the sensitivity for detecting early neoplasia in BE from 53% to 90%, and the inspection with NBI of suspicious areas reduced the false positive rate from 81% to 26% [50]. The other study, which was a multicenter randomized crossover study, compared ETMI to standard endoscopy in 87 patients referred for early neoplasia [51]. There was a significant increase of the targeted detection of early neoplastic lesions with AFI compared with standard video endoscopy. It was summarized that ETMI did not improve the overall detection of early neoplasia. *Confocal Endomicroscopy* derived from laser scanning confocal microscopy and allows subsurface analysis of the intestinal mucosa or *in-vivo* histology during the endoscopic procedure. The potential of this technique is to allow real-time histopathological diagnosis and eventually reducing the need of taking biopsy specimens. In a study of 63 patients using laser confocal microscopy, BE and associated neoplasia could be predicted with a sensitivity of 98.1% and 92.9% and a specificity of 94.1% and 98.4%, respectively [52]. But the limitation of this technique is the need of significant operator expertise in the use of the probe and in the interpretation of the real-time microscopic details. Further studies are needed to elucidate the clinical relevance and cost-effectiveness of in vivo pathology as a decision-making tool during endoscopy. The review on advanced endoscopic imaging in BE by M. Kara, W. Curvers and J. Bergman [34] may has practical importance. The authors summarized that the new endoscopic imaging techniques should be regarded as complementary to each other. High-resolution endoscopy should be the cornerstone and basic equipment for endoscopists who have a high volume of BE patients. On the basis of their own experience, the authors gave recommendations regarding advanced endoscopic imaging of BE. The first and the most important element is the use of a systematic and thorough approach for the initial endoscopic inspection. Targeted biopsy sampling is the main aim of this process. The use of a high-quality endoscope is of great importance in this aspect. Special attention should be given in the area between 12 and 6 o'clock in the endoscopic view, because in this region the neoplastic lesions are found very often. Most endoscopists are not familiar with the endoscopic appearance of early neoplastic lesions in BE and practical knowledge is required. Subtle lesions are generally shown but not necessarily recognized as such by the endoscopists ("the eyes see what the mind knows). Regarding new complementary imaging techniques, no technique improves sensitivity significantly above high-resolution endoscopy in BE surveillance. Autofluorescence imaging may improve targeted lesion detection but it may not improve overall sensitivity. Optical magnification with or without indigo carmine chromoendoscopy or NBI may be useful for precise delineation and characterization of lesions. Other techniques are of even more limited use.

Currently, *endoscopic ultrasonography (EUS)* is used to rule out lymph node metastasis. This method is accepted for the accurate locoregional staging. It's use is recommended in visible lesions and or in suspicion of early EAC. EUS is required in order to differentiate between patients with cancer in BE in whom endoscopic therapy is suitable and those in whom surgical treatment is required [53].

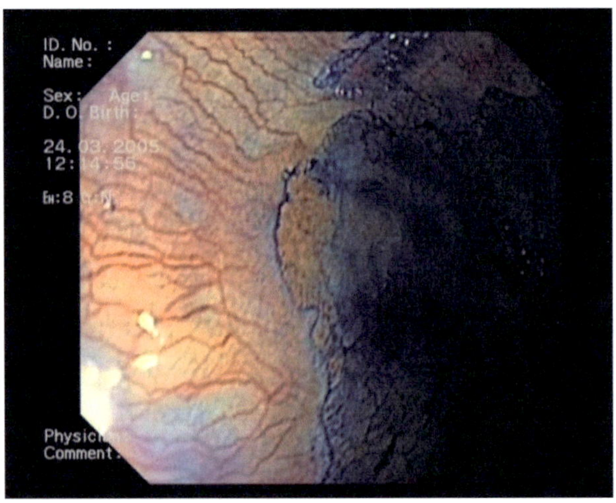

Figure 1. Magnifying chromoendoscopy with methylene blue in a BE patient.

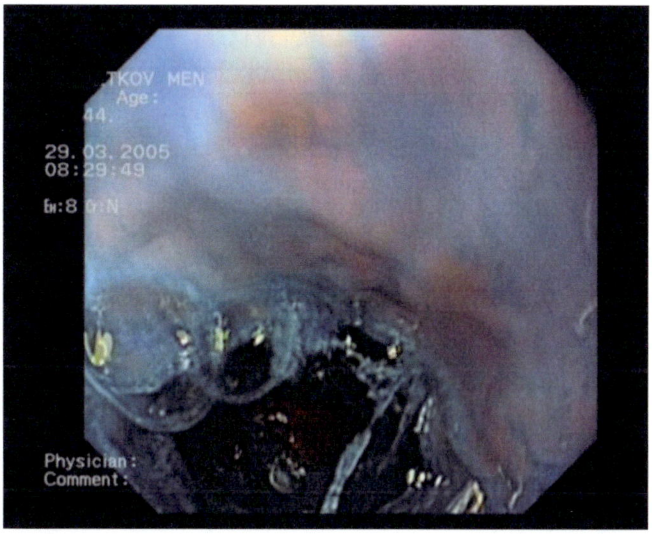

Figure 2. Magnifying chromoendoscopy with methylene blue after argon plasma coagulation of BE.

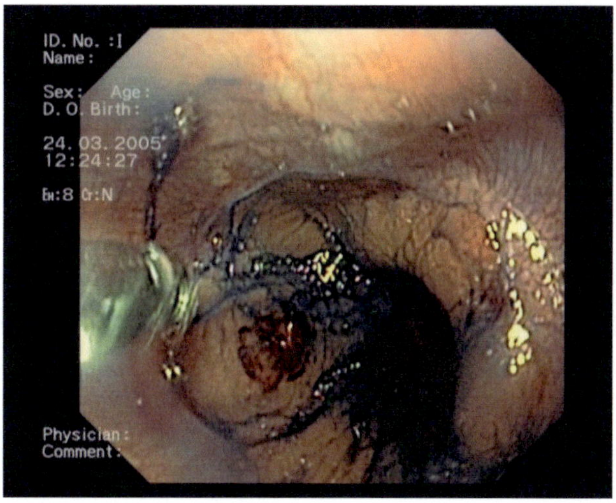

Figure 3. Magnifying chromoendoscopy with methylene blue after mucosal resection of BE.

2.2.2. Histology in BE

The normal squamous epithelium in BE is replaced by a mixture of cell types resembling gastric and or intestinal mucosa. The cardiac type BE contains mucus-secreting columnar cells; the fundic type BE is characterized with the parietal cells and chief cells; and the specialized intestinal epithelium is indicated by the presence of goblet cells. Morphologically, goblet cells can be identified by their large, cytoplasmic vacuole filled with abundant mucin on routine hematoxylin-eosin stain. The so called 'pseudogoblet cells" represent injured foveolar epithelial cells by concomitant GERD and resemble goblet cells with their abundant accumulation of cytoplasmic mucin [54]. But compared with true goblet cells, the mucin in pseudogoblet cells is neutral and stains slightly eosinophilic on hematoxylin-eosin stain. The biopsies specimens may also show a multilayered epithelium, which is characterized basally located squamous epithelium overlaid by superficial columnar epithelium. It is thought that this epithelium represents an early stage in the development of esophageal CM [55]. The cases with BE also exhibit stromal alterations as duplication and fragmentation of the muscularis mucosae (MM), increase in the number of blood vessels and lymphatics, and changes in the inflammatory cells [56, 57]. As already mentioned, the histological diagnosis of BE cannot be made when the exact site of biopsy is not known. Beside this, the IM of the distal esophagus and upper stomach are histologically indistinguishable. IM in a biopsy taken near the EGJ could be a part of a multifocal atrophic gastritis secondary to Helicobacter pylori. The etiology and significance of cardiac IM has become a topic of interest, because of rapidly rising incidence of gastric cardiac adenocarcinoma [58]. One study showed that the dysplasia risk of BE patients is significantly greater than in IM from the cardia, indicating two potentially different clinical processes [59]. Because of the difficulty in determining the precise site of a biopsy specimen in some cases and the inability to distinguish IM of the esophagus from gastric origin (cardiac IM) by routine methods, various immunohistochemical markers have been studied to be useful for this distinction. For example, cytokeratin (CK)7 and CK20 immunohistochemical staining has been used to differentiate IM of the esophagus versus gastric cardia [60]. It was found that Barrett's mucosa displays CK20 expression in the surface epithelium and superficial glands with no staining in the deep glands, but CK7 shows strong diffuse positivity in superficial and deep glands. On the other hand, gastric IM displays focal CK20 staining of both the superficial and deep glands, but only weak and variable CK7 labeling in the deep glands. Our results showed similar results [61]. Unfortunately, other studies have been unable to show the reliability of CK7 and CK20 immunoreactivity in distinguishing short-segment BE from IM in gastric cardia and corpus [62-64].

Histologic grading of dysplasia represents the "gold standard" method of estimating cancer risk and surveillance in patients with BE [14, 15]. The decision for subsequent patient management is also based on this evaluation. Clinically relevant diagnostic categories, include negative for dysplasia, indefinite for dysplasia, positive for dysplasia (either LGD or HGD), intramucosal adenocarcinoma (IMC), and invasive adenocarcinoma, which correspond to the Vienna classification of gastrointestinal epithelial neoplasia [65]. The term "dysplasia" is still used more widely than intraepithelial neoplasia [66]. In the 2000 WHO classification the term "dysplasia" was deserted for lesions which are characterized by morphological changes resulting from clonal alterations in genes and which carry a predisposition for progression [67]. But the new 2010 WHO classification brought back the term "dysplasia" officially and concluded that dysplasia is the more appropriate term for morphological changes indicative of precancerous lesions especially in the gastrointestinal tract [68]. Pathologic diagnoses of moderate dysplasia and in situ carcinoma (which is equivalent of HGD) are not recognized in current classification schemes.

Barrett's dysplasia is recognized histologically and graded into LGD or HGD by a combination of architectural and cytologic abnormalities. When no features of dysplasia are found, the diagnosis is negative for dysplasia. When the findings are uncertain, the category indefinite for dysplasia is applied. The grading in BE dysplasia is analogous to that of dysplasia complicating inflammatory bowel disease [69]. *NDBE* shows an absence of atypical cytologic or architectural features characteristic of dysplasia. Regenerating epithelium is characterized with "surface maturation", which included a progressive increase in mucin content and reduction in nuclear/cytoplasmic ratio from the bases of the glands to the mucosal surface. In some cases metaplastic epithelium may also demonstrate slight baseline architectural distortion, such as occasional branching and budding of crypts, atrophy, irregularity. *"Indefinite for dysplasia"* does not represent a discrete biologic entity. Biopsies that are classified in this category showed intact or mild distorted glandular architecture and the cytologic changes are also mild. The uncertainty whether or not dysplasia (generally low-grade) is present is usually due to the effects of active inflammation, erosion, or ulceration. This diagnosis may also be assigned to biopsies in which technical artifacts as thick or overstained sections or with lack of surface epithelium. These cases need rebiopsy after control of inflammation. *LGD* in BE is characterized mainly with cytologic changes. The nuclei are enlarged, elongated, hyperchromatic, and stratified, mostly confined to the basal half of the cell cytoplasm. In LGD, the nuclear polarity is preserved as the long axes of the nuclei remain perpendicular to the basement membrane. The cytoplasm is typically mucin-depleted and shows an increased nuclear/cytoplasmic ratio. These changes involve the crypts and there is lack of surface maturation. Glands may also demonstrate slight crowding or other mild architectural abnormalities. *HGD* in BE exhibits a greater degree of cytologic and/or architectural aberration. Characteristic architectural changes include increased budding, branching, and crowding, villiform surface configuration, and the presence of intraluminal bridges or papillae. Cytologic features include marked nuclear pleomorphism, loss of polarity, and full-thickness nuclear stratification. Mitotic figures, especially atypical ones, are often present and may involve the surface epithelium. *IMC* is diagnosed when single or small clusters of malignant cells infiltrate the lamina propria or MM but has not invaded the submucosa. This lesion is associated with a small risk of regional lymph node metastasis and, as such, is staged as T1a [70]. In contrast, AEC that invade into the submucosa are considered submucosal invasive carcinoma and the risk of lymph node metastases increases dramatically with depth of invasion. There is significant interobserver variation in the assessment of dysplasia in BE [39, 47, 56, 67-70]. This fact is related to various reasons. The reactive changes, particularly in the setting of active inflammation, overlap with those seen in dysplasia. Given the subtle gradation of changes from baseline atypia to LGD to HGD consecutively, it is not surprising that there is a variation in the diagnosis of degree of dysplasia. One study reported that the variation was most evident at the low end of the histologic spectrum or in distinguishing NDBE from changes that are indefinite for dysplasia or LGD [71]. In other study, 65% of 20 general pathologists misdiagnosed a case of LDG such as 25% classified it as normal, and the other as either moderate or HGD [72]. It was reported that general pathologists had only poor to fair interobserver agreement on the diagnosis of LGD [73]. In a study from the Netherlands, 85% of LHD cases diagnosed by general pathologists were downgraded to "not dysplasia" on review by expert pathologists [74]. These results lead to the recommendation that the diagnosis of LGD should be reviewed by an expert of GI pathology. At the other end of the spectrum, the differentiation between HGD and IMC is also difficult [75]. There are no objective criteria to distinguish HGD from IMC because endoscopic biopsies almost never sample the submucosa. The pathologic diagnosis of HGD or EAC shows excellent interobserver agreement among pathologists with extensive experience of BE but it is not so among general pathologists [72, 73]. In practice each biopsy report of HGD should also be review by an expert of GI pathology. Recent studies analyzed the histopathologic criteria in biopsies that appear to help the distinguishing between HGD and EAC, and those who have EAC elsewhere in the metaplastic mucosa [76, 77].

In last years, with the wide use of ablative and nonablative endoscopic therapy for BE with and without dysplasia, the role of histology increased. Because of ablation, patients develop islands of re-epithelialized squamous mucosa as it is called "neosquamous epithelium" (NSE). The last may also develop in patients treated with high-dose proton pump inhibitors (PPIs), but without ablation [78, 79]. The findings of various studies strongly suggest that NSE has no malignant potential and represents a successful outcome of ablation [19, 80]. A problem with NSE is that a residual Barrett's epithelium or dysplasia may persist underneath NSE, because they remain invisible on endoscopy. The prevalence rate of buried Barrett's or buried dysplasia is variable and dependent on the type of ablative therapy. The buried dysplasia is difficult to interpret because the maturation to the mucosal surface cannot be evaluated in the presence of NSE. The biologic potential of buried BE is the subject of many investigations [19, 81, 82]. The available data suggest that residual buried dysplasia, continues to be at risk for malignant progression. In contrast to non-tissue acquiring ablative therapies, endoscopic mucosal resection (EMR) is a modality designed to remove mucosa and superficial submucosal tissue [19]. In this way, it allows more accurate histologic evaluation and grading of dysplasia and determination of location and depth of invasion by adenocarcinoma when present. EMR is a valuable diagnostic tool which allows change of diagnosis of BE dysplasia when compared with mucosal biopsies. One study repoted that 37% of cases of BE with dysplasia showed a change of dysplasia grade in pre-EMR biopsies compared with EMR specimens. Of them, 21% of biopsies were with under-reported grade of neoplasia and 16% of biopsies were with over-reported grade [83]. In another study it was found that 24% of cases with HGD in biopsy specimens showed an increase in grade to IMC, and 40% of patients with IMC had their stage increased to submucosal invasive carcinoma by evaluation of EMR specimens [84]. There is also a greatly improved diagnostic agreement between pathologists when evaluating dysplasia in EMR specimens compared with biopsies [85]. This results is related to the larger tissue sampling compared with biopsy specimens and the ability to evaluate mucosal landmarks, such as double muscularis mucosae. Evaluation of depth of invasion in EMR specimens is important because the rate of lymph node metastasis has been shown to correlate with depth of invasion [19, 70]. The evaluations of the presence or absence of lymphovascular invasion and the status of the lateral and deep tissue margins are also of prognostic significance [85-88]. In this aspect, the method of processing EMR specimens and their orientation is very important. In summary, the problems in the diagnosis of dysplasia included difficulties relating to sampling errors, the distinction of reactive changes versus dysplastic ones, differences in observer interprepation of the diagnosis of dysplasia and in the differentiation of HGD from invasive carcinoma. Requiring confirmation of a diagnosis by a second pathologist is important in taking the decision for management.

The utility of many immunohistochemical and molecular markers has been studied as adjunctive tool for the diagnosis of dysplasia and also for identifying the cases of risk for malignant progression. Unfortunately, only a few markers show such a potential, including studies of DNA ploidy by computerized morphometric analysis, the expression of proliferation antigen Ki-67 (MIB-1) and of tumor suppressor proteins p53 and p16. By flow cytometry, it was found that patients with diploid baseline biopsies showed a significantly lower rate of cancer progression compared with patients with either aneuploidy or an increased 4N fraction (tetraploidy) [89]. Immunohistochemical staining for MIB-1 showed increased expression from normal squamous epithelium to CM to dysplasia and to invasive carcinoma [90, 91]. There are also alterations in the pattern of localization of staining. In NDBE the expression of MIB-1 is limited to the bases of the crypts, whereas in dysplasia it extends upward the mucosal surface. A recent study suggests that the combined use of MIB-1 and p53 staining reduces variations in the diagnosis of BE dysplasia [91]. Immunostaining for p53 has been widely studied, but the results have been controversial [19, 91, 92]. The frequency of positive immunostaining for p53 has been shown to correlate with higher grades of dysplasia, and, in some cases, is associated with an increased risk of cancer. Allelic loss of p16 (p16 LOH), which results in block of cell cycle in the G1-S phase and provides survival advantage of the cells, is common in EAC and appears to be an early event in the BE-dysplasia-adenocarcinoma sequences [94, 95]. It is well-known that the carcinogenesis is a multi-step process that occurs as a result of alterations in many different genes. Because of that, it is clear that there is no single molecular marker that will allow with high sensitivity to predict the neoplastic risk in BE.

3. Screening for BE

The most appropriate method for both diagnosis and surveillance of BE is upper GI endoscopy. There are no concrete guidelines for selecting patients who should undergo screening for BE, and this decision is currently made case by case.

The cost-effectiveness of upper GI endoscopy in patients with reflux symptoms, most of whom will never develop cancer is discussed. Approximately 40% of adults in the US experience symptoms of heart burn at least once a month and about 20% report these symptoms once a week [96]. So a large proportion of adult US population would be eligible for screening for BE based on this screening criteria. A study from Sweden estimated that BE was present in 1.6% of the general population [97]. BE patients are usually white, middle-aged males, often overweight [98]. The male-to-female ratio is 2:1 [99]. According to a retrospective study of 2100 patients undergoing upper GI endoscopy, the prevalence is higher among Whites (6.1%) as compared with Hispanics (1.7%) and African Americans (1.6%) [100]. The relationship between BE and gastroesophageal reflux symptoms is well known, but many patients with biopsy-proven BE do not report such symptoms. In one study, BE was identified in 50 of 300 consecutive patients (16.7%) undergoing screening or surveillance colonoscopies who also received upper GI endoscopy [101]. Among them, 19.8% reported GERD symptoms, whereas 14.9% were asymptomatic and the symptom questionnaires were unable to predict the presence of BE. It has been shown that 40% of patients with EAC also do not report heartburn or regurgitation [102]. By the other hand, even when BE is diagnosed, a vast majority of these patients will not develop EAC during their lifetime [10]. Studies have shown that the overall mortality rate in patients with BE is closely similar to that of the general population and EAC mortality is an uncommon cause of death in these patients [103, 104]. The most patients with BE die due to causes other than EAC. From this point of view, the current position of the AGA is that inadequate evidence exists to endorse endoscopic screening for BE based solely on the presence of GERD symptoms [14]. The decision regarding screening should be individualized after discussion about the benefits and limitations of screening with the patient. Other professional organizations also do not recommend routine screening for BE [13, 15, 105, 106]. The American Society of Gastrointestinal Endoscopy (ASGE) guidelines proposed that an initial screening endoscopy is appropriate in select patients with frequent, chronic, long-standing GERD (>5 years), who are white, males, aged >50 years, and those with nocturnal heart burn. No further screening is needed if the initial endoscopy is negative for BE [106]. Although the upper GI endoscopy with biopsy is the gold standard for the diagnosis of BE, other endoscopic and non- endoscopic alternative methods of the screening for BE are studied. One of them is capsule endoscopy, which is less invasive and offers increased acceptability of screening [107]. One study, using this technique for identifying BE, showed 67% sensitivity and 84% specificity [108]. A recent meta-analysis of nine studies including 618 patients, demonstrated pooled 77% sensitivity and 86% specificity for diagnosis of BE. When IM is used as the reference standard, the reported sensitivity and specificity are 78% and 73% respectively [109]. It was concluded that capsule endoscopy of esophagus has a moderate sensitivity and specificity for the diagnosis of BE in patients with GERD. The EGD remains the modality of choice for evaluation of suspected BE. Capsule sponge esophageal cytology appears to be one relatively low-cost, non-endoscopic screening method for BE which is not yet fully validated and not generally available [110-112]. A cytology sponge is compressed and encased in a gelatin capsule attached to a string. The capsule, but not the end of the string is swallowed. After a few minutes in the stomach, the liberated sponge is dragged back up the esophagus. The presence of BE is based on the expression of trefoil factor 3, which is a specific marker for esophageal CM. A pilot study in 96 controls and 36 BE patients found this test to have a sensitivity of 78% and a specificity of 94% for presence of BE [110].

According to the current data, there are no evidence that routine screening for BE will increase the rate of diagnosed cases of BE with or without dysplasia, or EAC.

4. Surveillance of patients with BE

Surveillance endoscopy is intended to detect neoplastic progression at an early stage and prevent cancer-related death. As pointed above, the histologic diagnosis and grading *of* dysplasia represents the "gold standard" method of assessing neoplastic risk in patients with BE. Despite limitations of the scientific evidence, several professional societies offer guidelines for endoscopic surveillance of patients with BE. Because the risk of EAC increases as NDBE progresses in a sequential manner to LGD and HGD, the frequency of surveillance is based on the grade of dysplasia. The recommendations of ACG, ASGE and AGA are very similar [13, 14, 106, 113]. Surveillance upper GI endoscopy should include 4 quadrant biopsies from every 1-2 cm of Barrett's mucosa and separate biopsies of areas of mucosal abnormalities if present. In cases with NDBE or LGD 2-cm protocol is recommended but for patients with HGD the 1-cm protocol is needed. MRE for all mucosal nodules or irregularities is recommended. When NDBE is found on biopsy, periodic endoscopic surveillance to rule out progression of disease is advocated. Current surveillance guidelines recommend 2 follow-up endoscopies with biopsy within 1 year of the diagnosis of BE and follow-up every 3 to 5 years thereafter. Surveillance endoscopy is also the mainstay of management for BE with LGD. The diagnosis of LGD has to be confirmed by en expert GI pathologist. If LGD is confirmed, an upper endoscopy should be repeated 6 months later to rule out a higher grade of dysplasia. If repeat biopsies show LGD as the worst histologic grade, annual follow-up endoscopies with biopsy are recommended thereafter as long as dysplasia persists. If regression is noted, surveillance every 3 to 5 years is recommended as with NDBE. For patients with HGD, the recommendations include expert confirmation of HGD and repeat endoscopy with biopsies within 3 months to exclude carcinoma. Patients should be counseled regarding their therapeutic options including continued 3 months surveillance, esophagectomy, or ablative therapies.

The effectiveness of surveillance of patients with BE is also discussed. By one hand, it has been demonstrated that patients with surveillance-detected EAC are diagnosed at an earlier stage and have a better prognosis than those who present with symptomatic tumours [114, 115]. These data support the effectiveness of endoscopic biopsy surveillance for early detection of EAC. However, there are no prospective data showing survival advantage with surveillance. As noted above, the majority of patients diagnosed with EAC have not a prior diagnosis of BE. A study reported that only 3.9% of the patients had a BE diagnosed before their EAC [116]. A review of reports on mortality in BE patients undergoing surveillance found that their risk of malignant progression is low and most of them die of other causes, especially cardiovascular, without development of HGD or EAC [117]. This undermines the cost-effectiveness of BE surveillance and supports the search for valid risk stratification tools to identify the minority of patients that are likely to benefit from surveillance. The majority of patients with LGD regressed and had a cancer incidence similar to all BE patients [9]. HGD is highly heterogeneous with regard to progression to EAC and rates of progression vary substantially in different studies. The reported 5-year cumulative incidences of EAC range from less than 10% to 59% [10, 89]. It may be concluded that even if current surveillance techniques are effective, they are unlikely to substantially impact the population's mortality from EAC and better methods are needed to identify at risk patients [116].

5. Therapy of BE

The management of patients with BE includes following major aims: treatment of the associated GERD, endoscopic surveillance to detect HGD or EAC, and treatment of dysplasia or IMC, as well as prevention of cancer.

5.1. Antireflux therapy

If one goal of this treatment is the control of GERD symptoms and heal esophagitis, anothers should be the regression of BE, and prevention of progression to EAC.

Lifestyle modifications can help control symptoms only in some patients with BE by increasing esophageal acid clearance and decreasing the incidence of reflux events [118]. *Acid suppressing medication* are the standard therapy for GERD in BE patients. Antisecretory treatment by PPIs or histamine-2 receptor antagonists (H2RAs) are usually used to decrease esophageal acid exposure, symptom relief, and to heal esophagitis. More complete esophagitis healing and heartburn relief is observed with PPIs versus H2RAs and occurs nearly twice as fast [119]. In addition, antisecretory effect of H2RAs failed to heal esophagitis in a high proportion of BE patients [12, 120]. Twice-daily standard dose of PPIs has been usually recommended for BE patients. A large meta-analysis of 136 randomized, controlled trials included 35978 patients with reflux esophagitis showed that taking twice-daily standard dose of PPIs showed modest benefit [121]. Once-daily standard dose PPIs fails to heal esophagitis or control reflux-induced symptoms in BE patients [12]. Esophageal pH monitoring studies have shown that many BE patients treated with once-daily PPIs in the morning still have high levels of esophageal acid exposure, especially at night [122]. A second dose, preferably before dinner, has been usually effective, given that BE patients have increased nocturnal esophageal acid exposure. Further increasing of PPIs dose is sometimes needed. The same authors showed that high-dose PPIs (esomeprazole 40 mg twice daily) for 6 months achieved higher levels of gastric acid suppression and control of oesophageal acid reflux and symptoms. When comparing GERD patients with and without BE, the BE group are characterized with abnormal oesophageal motility, reduced lower oesophageal sphincter pressures, more severe and prolonged pathological supine oesophageal reflux, as well as greater hiatal hernia size [123]. Patients with BE also have significant nocturnal gastric acid breakthrough. In patients with BE, oesophageal acid exposure is often difficult to control with commonly used dosages of PPIs [124, 125]. The underlying high levels of acid reflux may require greater levels of acid suppression. However, whether acid secretion is increased in BE is controversial [126, 127]. In 30–62% of BE patients on different PPIs have demonstrated abnormal oesophageal pH profiles, despite adequate control of reflux symptoms [123, 128, 129]. Esomeprazole up to three times daily decreases this value to 16% [130]. In one recent trial an adequate control of intra-oesophageal acidity in 97% (14/15) of patients with primarily short-segment BE treated by Omeprazole-sodium bicarbonate twice daily was demonstrated [131]. In addition a 100% control of nocturnal oesophageal reflux assessed as 48 h supine intra-oesophageal pH was found. These results demonstrated excellent suppression of daytime and nocturnal oesophageal pH.

Several observational and prospective studies have assessed *regression of BE* in response to antisecretopy therapy with conflicting results. At this time there is no evidence that H2RAs or PPIs can completely reverse this condition. Acid suppression with H2RAs has not been associated with significant regression of BE [132]. There are reports high-dose PPIs may decrease the length of BE, but not in all studies [133-135]. The incidence of complete regression in response to PPIs depends of length of Barrett's segment. It has been reported as approximately 2.4% in long-segment BE and 7.1% in short-segment BE [136, 137]. A small number of prospective studies showed that normalization of acid exposure leads to regression of BE, but other not confirmed these results [132]. It is discussed that control of pH alone may not be sufficient to cause significant regression. About half of patients on PPIs therapy demonstrated partial regression of BE. Development of new squamous islands or increasing number and size of islands within the metaplastic segment were observed [134, 135]. In one long-term endoscopic cohort study 188 BE patients treated with PPIs for 1 to 13 years were prospectively followed (mean follow-up 5 years). During the study period, no decrease in the length of BE was noted, but 48% of the patients developed squamous islands in the BE segments. The squamous islands development correlated with the duration of PPIs therapy but not with the PPIs dose [134]. The data suggest that very long PPI therapy is associated with a minor reduction of extent of metaplasia, but with appearance of more squamous islands. These changes are most unlikely to be associated with any useful reduction of cancer risk. Other authors discussed that chronic PPIs use can increase the risk of EAC or gastric cancer [138]. From other point of view, the increased incidence of these cancers might have been related to the original condition for which PPIs was prescribed rather than the PPI itself [135].

Some studies suggest that acid reflux plays a key role in the *progression* to dysplasia and EAC. There is indirect evidence that acid exposure increases proliferation and decrease apoptosis in BE [139]. Acid exposure may induce DNA double-strand break (DSB), increase reactive oxygen species (ROS), and activate mitogen-activated protein (MAP) kinase pathways in BE, suggesting its potential role in carcinogenesis [135]. Treatment with high-dose PPI was associated with a reduction in epithelial cell proliferation, as measured by proliferating cell nuclear antigen Ki67, in both the crypt and glands and the luminal surface cells [140]. The reduction of inflammation might have resulted from anti-inflammatory effects which may be exerted by PPIs independently of acid inhibition [141]. Another study showed that high-dose PPI (esomeprazole 40 mg twice daily) for 6 months significant decreased inflammation and epithelial proliferation, but without reversal of aberrant DNA methylation compared with the doses of PPIs before entering the study [142]. However, the clinical significance of the protective benefit of antisecretory therapy is not clear yet. Some data showed a persistence of mucosal markers for mucosal injury during partial control of esophageal acid exposure. The lack of detectable effect on risk for EAC from routine PPI therapy could be due to under-treatment. It has been proposed that twice-daily PPI, given at a dose to "normalize" levels of acid reflux, might reduce EAC risk [143]. This is an optimistic speculation, in light of the negative data for a cancer-protective effect of antireflux surgery [144, 145]. In addition, the study of [142] demonstrated that twice-daily PPIs therapy has no impact on mucosal markers of injury. Despite all, some observational studies showed that acid suppression with PPIs reduce the risk for development of dysplasia in patients with BE and therefore potentially reduce the risk of developing cancer [146-149]. These studies were uncontrolled and retrospective, and information on the effectiveness of the control of oesophageal acid exposure was not available because no pH monitoring was included. When compared with H2RAs, PPIs therapy has been shown to be more efficacious in preventing the progression of BE to both dysplasia and EAC [146, 149]. In one of these observational studies on 236 BE patients, the incidence of any grade dysplasia was significantly lower amongst patients receiving PPIs compared with those not treated by PPIs or treated by H2RAs [146]. A longer duration of PPIs use was associated with less frequent occurrence of dysplasia. Other authors demonstrated a lower incidence amongst patients being prescribed versus not being prescribed a PPI (7.4% versus 14.1%) [150].These data suggested that initiating PPI therapy soon after the diagnosis of BE may prevent this progression [148, 150]. In summary, acid suppressing therapy, especially by PPIs, is effective to treat GERD symptoms, heal reflux esophagitis and prevent related complications as it is for patients without BE. Evidence on the chemopreventive effect of PPIs for BE is indirect and not confirmed by a long-term prospective controlled data [14, 151]. The risks /benefit ratio of long-term PPIs therapy should be assessed and discussed carefully with BE patients in the context of their overall health status and medication use. In addition there is no evidence that higher than standard doses of PPIs are needed to reduce the cancer risk.

It has been discussed that *antireflux surgery* using fundoplication eliminates acid reflux and provides better control of GERD than PPIs in BE patients [132]. This effect is not different than those of PPIs. Optimal candidates for antireflux surgery include those who lack major comorbidities and demonstrate incomplete response to PPIs therapy [15]. Antireflux surgery should depend on patient preference and the severity of reflux symptoms despite PPIs therapy, but not for definitive management of Barrett's metaplasia. The concept that adequate reflux control following antireflux surgery is necessary to reduce the rate of progression of BE is supported by some studies [152, 153]. They suggest progression is significantly more likely to occur with a failed fundoplication and persistent reflux. The hypothesis that antireflux surgery could reduce the risk for development of EAC by transforming a highly aggressive esophageal luminal environment is not confirmed in the clinical practice. There are no data that antireflux surgery has detectable effect on adenocarcinoma risk. The incidence of EAC in the 14 102 patients having antireflux surgery in Sweden from 1965 to 2005 was evaluated and compared to controls [154]. Authors concluded that antireflux surgery cannot be able to prevent the development of esophageal or cardia adenocarcinoma. One randomized prospective trial compares antireflux surgery (n=58) and PPIs (n=43) in patients with BE [155]. No significant difference between the two groups was found with respect to preventing progression to dysplasia and adenocarcinoma. Given current knowledge, there are no confirming data that antireflux surgery is more effective than acid suppressing therapy for the prevention of HGD or cancer in BE Because of that antireflux surgery does not abolish the need for surveillance [132, 151].

5.2. Chemoprevention therapy

Except of antireflux medication and surgery, non-steroid anti-inflammatory drugs (NSAIDs) and acetyl-salicylic acid (ASA) as well as other drugs have been evaluated to be able to prevent cancer development in BE patients. It is well known that chronic inflammation has been associated with neoplasia formation in many organs, as well as esophagus. Chronic inflammation is characterised by production of cyclooxygenase (COX) and prostaglandins. COX-2 enzyme participates in several important tissue processes, for example cell proliferation, migration, apoptosis and angiogenesis. Overexpression of COX-2 has been found in patients with reflux esophagitis, BE, dysplasia, and EAC. NSAIDs and ASA as inhibitors of COX-1 and COX-2 enzymes attenuate cell growth and proliferation, inhibits angiogenesis, and restores apoptosis [156]. In addition to these findings, epidemiological studies suggest that ASA and other NSAID use may protect against cancers of several sites, especially colorectal cancer. Various studies suggest that NSAIDs and ASA use may reduce the risk of EAC but the other studies do not confirm these results [156-159]. Patients with exposure to NSAIDs or ASA had a 55% reduction of development of EAC [160-162]. A systematic review of 9 studies and meta-analysis assessed more than 1800 patients has been showed that NSAIDs or ASA had a 33% odds reduction of development of cancer [163]. Any use of ASA or NSAIDs was associated with a 43% reduced risk of cancer. Frequent use of ASA or NSAIDs decreased cancer risk with 46%, but intermittent use was associated with 18% risk reduction. Both ASA and NSAIDs use was associated separately with reduced risk of cancer. The associations were seen for both EAC and squamous cell carcinoma. In a recent study from Netherlands, 570 BE patients were prospectively followed for a median of 4.5 years. Use of NSAIDs (median duration 2 months) was associated with 53% lower risk of progression to HGD/EAC [164]. A cohort of 350 Barrett's patients from 20770 persons was followed up (median 65.5 months) [165]. The data showed that current NSAID and ASA users had 68% reduced risk of EAC, the past use decreased the risk with 30% compared with never-users of NSAIDs. The 5-year incidence of EAC was observed in 6.6% versus 14.3% in current versus never-users. It is discussed that NSAIDs and ASA may protect against EAC by reducing the risk of development of BE or by preventing progression from BE to EAC [132]. In a retrospective study, NSAIDs use was not found to be higher in BE patients when compare to EAC. However, ASA and NSAID use was lower in both of these groups compared with controls [161]. If there is a true protective effect of NSAIDs, this study suggests it may occur prior to the development of BE. A recent retrospective large population-based case-control study failed to find any benefit of aspirin use [157]. This study collected information of intake for ASA and NSAIDs during the past 5 years and other exposures from 285 patients with NDBE, 108 patients with dysplastic BE, and two separate control groups, including 313 endoscopy patients with acute inflammatory changes ('inflammation controls') and 644 population controls. Use of ASA was not associated with NDBE when compared with population or inflammation controls, but significant risk reductions for users of NSAIDs were found when compared with population controls. No dose-response effects were observed. These data showed little consistent evidence of an inverse association between use of ASA or NSAIDs and risk of BE. Authors concluded that the question of whether or not these medications prevent the onset of BE remains open. PPIs are usual concomitant medication in NSAID or ASA users with GERD. From this point of view, one study evaluated patients who take prescripted NSAIDs/ASA as well as PPIs. A decreased risk of EAC was demonstrated [161]. This protective effect may be due to the combination of each medication. On the other hand, the concomitant use of PPI in BE patients, should decrease the risk of serious GI complications associated with NSAIDs or ASA [151]. COX-2 inhibitors may be of benefit because of more specific inhibition of COX-2 receptors and fewer side effects on GI tract. In a multicenter, randomized trial of celecoxib versus placebo in 222 patients with BE and LGD or HGD, at 48 week follow up, no significant difference was observed in dysplasia or cancer between the groups [166]. Authors suggest that celecoxib does not prevents progression of BE, although further studies are needed. However the majority of these studies are associations and observations, because there are significant barriers in conducting a large clinical trial evaluating NSAIDs/ASA as potential chemoprotective agents [132]. Current evidence shows that NSAIDs may reduce the risk of EAC. Despite of this, most experts agree it is not clear that potential benefit overweighs the GI risks of this group of medication. On the other hand, there is also evidence that cardiovascular deaths became more common than deaths from EAC among BE patients. Because of that it is appropriate to screen these patients for cardiovascular risk. In addition, the proportion of cases that take low dose aspirin or statins for cardiovascular risk factors or events will be increase in the near future.

Possible chemopreventive properties of *statins* have been also suggested in some recent study [12, 135, 161]. Statins can increase apoptosis and inhibit proliferation in Barrett's epithelial cells because of reduction of serum-stimulated Ras activity, and inhibition of activation of extracellular signal-regulated kinase (ERK), and protein kinase B (Akt) [167, 168]. A case-control study of 12000 BE patients showed that statin use was associated with a reduction in EAC risk [161]. The risk reduction was higher in cases with longer duration of statin use. The Dutch data also confirmed that long-term use of statins (median duration of 5 years) leaded to 54% reduction in the risk of malignant progression of BE [164]. In addition a combination of NSAIDs and statins decreased this risk to 78%. Finally, the chemoprevention of BE is likely to remain an active area of research. There is a need of new evidence on the possible chemopreventive effects of novel options in prospective, randomized studies. Although, the positive results from chemopreventive studies will not change recommendations for endoscopic surveillance in the near future [12].

According to all current data, in the last version of AGA guidelines for the management of BE, AGA's experts strongly recommend: 1) Elimination of esophageal acid exposure by PPIs more than once daily. Esophageal pH monitoring is needed to define PPI dosing. Antireflux surgery is also recommended as a method to control esophageal acid exposure; 2) Screening of BE patients to assess cardiovascular risk and prescribe an ASA therapy is indicated. On the other hand using ASA solely to prevent EAC in the absence of other cardiovascular indications is not recommended [151].

5.3. Endoscopic treatment of BE

In recent years, endoscopic techniques used to eradicate BE with presence or absence of dysplasia or IMC include endoscopic resection and/ or ablations. The most commonly used technologies currently are EMR and RFA, applied alone or in combination. Evidence for their efficacy has emerged rapidly over the past decade [151, 169-171). The goal of endoscopic eradication therapy (EET) for BE patients, especially those with HGD or IMC is to complitelly eliminate all dysplastic and non-dysplastic Barrett's epithelium to get a complete reversion to normal squamous epithelium without islands of buried IM.

5.3.1. Non ablative modalities (endoscopic resection–EMR)

EMR has been provided both a diagnostic/ staging and therapeutic tool for Barrett's neoplasia. At now, EMR should be performed in BE patients who have dysplasia as macroscopically visible mucosal irregularities to determine the T stage of the neoplasia (151, 169-175). A large number of different techniques with or without suction or submucosal injection that raise the lesions can be used. EMR can be performed by the lift and snare technique, cap-assisted endoscopic resection, multiband mucosectomy, and Euroligator technique [169, 170, 172-175]. Endoscopic submucosal dissection (ESD) is also used. No data confirmed that one of these endoscopic techniques has proven to be superior to another. In a prospective randomized trial, both "cap-and-snare" and "band-and-snare" technique can provide adequate depth and histological staging and have similar safety profies [176, 177]. Studies have demonstrated that EMR is safe and effective for the treatment of superficial lesions for successful eradication of BE with varied degree of dysplasia and IMC [169, 178, 179]. Five-year follow-up data for 231 BE patients with IMC demonstrated a 95.7% complete response rate [180]. Focal EMR is associated with high recurrence rate up to 47%, and increased with longer observation times, may be due to multifocal synchronous lesions previously missed by biopsy, as well as the metachronous development of new lesions [169-172, 181-184]. Recent data suggests that the presence of submucosal invasion of occult adenocarcinoma in the setting of HGD was 6.7% - 12%, which was much lower than previously reported [171, 185]. One small, prospective study demonstrated an eradication rate of focal HGD or IMC more than 90% for small (< 2 cm) or low-risk lesions at a mean of 12 months follow-up [179]. On the opposite, a remission rate of only 59% and recurrence rates of 11% to 14% were observed for larger lesions (> 2 cm). Therefore, EMR has been accepted method for BE with small and/or raised lesions of HGD or IMC [172]. Independently of endoscopic techniques, the most common complications of EMR are bleeding and esophageal stricture formation, but most of them can be treated successfully by endoscopy [186-199]. Perforation has been reported in 1–2.6% of the patients, but seems to decrease with more experience. Despite known efficacy and a relatively good safety profile for small segments of neoplasia and raised lesions, the potential role of EMR in longer segments of BE remains limited because of several factors: piecemeal resections are needed a long time to complete; repeat sessions are often necessary; the risk of possible bleeding and perforation can be increased. EMR for long-segment BE appears to be associated with a relatively high stricture rates of 26% to 37% [196, 198]. *Complete Barrett's eradication EMR (CBE- EMR)* with aim to reduce the potential risk of synchronous or metachronous lesion has been performed in select centers. This more aggressive method is also known as circumferential EMR, stepwise radical endoscopic resection (SRER), and wide area EMR. All of these techniques have proven to eradicate all Barrett's epithelium curatively and give possibility for a more accurate pathology result when compared to pre-EMR biosy results [169, 170]. Complete eradication rate has observed from 76% to 100%, and recurrence of malignancy in up to 11%, without association with BE tissue recurrence [189, 196, 198, 200-202]. Only in one study recurrence rate of 36.5% was reported [196]. Short-term follow-up shows that CBE-EMR is effective in eradication of all BE and also eliminated the genetic alterations that are associated with early neoplasia [189, 202]. In a retrospective study recurrence of HGD or IMC was observed in 9% of patients and 15% had recurrent IM after a median follow-up of 23 months [197]. A multi-center European cohort study on 169 patients with BE and HGD or IMC treated by CBE- EMR showed a remission of neoplasia in 97.5%, and complete elimination of Barrett's metaplasia in 85% after 27 months of follow-up [200]. The recurrence rate for metachronous lesions was 1.8%. Complete eradication of HGD and/or IMC was observed in 100% at 11-month follow-up, while complete eradication of LGD and metaplasia was demonstrated in 89% [189]. In retrospective study of 41 patients with HGD or IMC on BE, a regression to normal squamous epithelium was found in 75% at a mean follow-up of 31 months [196]. The number increased to 90% in patients after repeat session of EMR after recurrence of metaplasia or carcinoma. A remission to normal squamous epithelium was recently observed in 96% with HGD and/or IMC at a median of 17 months after stepwise EMR [198]. These data demonstrated the efficacy of EMR for Barrett's dysplasia and IMC. On the other hand CBE-EMR seems to be associated with more complications [186-200]. Rates of bleeding and perforation in large EMRs increased up to 19% and 11% respectively, and appear to be higher than those for ablative modalities [195, 198]. A high stricture rate is the main limitation of CBE-EMR. In 34 patients, treated by SRER with median of two therapeutic sessions dysphagia occurred in 56%, necessitating dilations or stent placement [197]. Another prospective trial reported a stenosis rate of 26% after 88 SRER procedures [189]. A recent multicentre randomised study reported a stenosis rate of 88 % of cases [203]. Development of stenosis is highly dependent on the circumferential extent of the resection. Resections limited to 50% of the circumference rarely cause a significant stenosis. Risk of stricture formation is higher when more than three-quarters of the circumference of the mucosa is resected [204]. Because of that Japanese Society for Gastrointestinal Endoscopy (JSGE) recomended using of EMR only for HGD lesions, involving less than one-third of the circumference of the esophageal wall [179]. Regarding length of BE, recent observational studies reported good results when segments of BE more than 2 cm or flat mucosal lesions can be resected by CBE_EMR [170, 172, 178]. SRER is mostly limited to a 5-cm Barrett's segment [189]. The most important risk factors for recurrent disease after EMR without total eradication are following: piecemeal resection, long segment BE, no ablative therapy of the remaining BE after complete removal of HGD/IMC, and multifocal disease [170]. The main indications for curative endoscopic resection of early EAC included lesions limited to the mucosa, limited in size to 2 cm, well-to-moderately differentiated, no pathological lymph nodes, and no lymphovascular infiltration in the endoscopic resection specimen [187-190, 205, 206]. In *ESD*, a viscous fluid into the submucosal space is injected to provide a cushion under the lesion, followed by deeper resections into larger areas of submucosa using a special cutting device (knifes and snare) [174]. ESD has been used successfully for the treatment of large (> 1.5 cm) tumors of upper GI tract [207, 208]. No recurrence of EAC was observed in patients with BE [208]. One potential barrier to this approach is reflux-induced submucosal fibrosis in the distal esophagus [207]. Because of that stricture formation was observed in nearly half of cases [132]. The role of this method in long-segment BE with HGD is still limited, and is generally not widely recommended at this time [171, 172, 178].

Regarding all current data, EMR remains one of the preferred first-line endoscopic treatment for selected patients with early HGD and/or IMC because of its diagnostic/staging value and its established therapeutic role.EMR is characterized with high eradication rate of Barrett's dysplasia, but also with high rate of complications and recurrence. Because of that additional ablation is used to reach complite eliminate all dysplastic and non-dysplastic Barrett's epithelium, as well as complete reversion to normal squamous epithelium.

5.3.2. Endoscopic ablative therapies

Endoscopic ablative modalities used to eradicate BE include thermal energy application, argon plasma coagulation (APC), photodynamic therapy (PDT), radiofrequency ablation (RFA), and cryotherapy. In these modalities ablated epithelium is replaced by a neosquamous epithelium. Ablative therapies have an increasing role in the management of BE. In general, they are well tolerated. There are two major limitations related to ablative methods. First there is no possibility for histologic examination. The second problem is associated with the squamous overgrowth and risk of development of EAC beneath regenerated squamous epithelium after ablation, which may be due on the progression of buried Barrett's metaplasia or dysplasia [209]. Most of thermal energy application methods, as well as APC are unsuitable to treat BE with HGD or IMC alone. Despite that, they can be useful as an adjunct to EMR in the treatment of selected BE patients. Our data on 50 BE patients with LGD, treated by APC plus PPIs showed that de novo Barrett's metaplasia was observed in 23 patients, with islands of LGD in 12 cases at 10 years follow up. All of them were treated successfully by new endoscopy. No progression to HGD or EAC was found [210, 211]. No serious adverse events or strictures were observed.

For a long time of period *PDT* was the primary option for ablative therapy of early Barrett's cancer and HGD, as well as additional treatment to EMR [170, 171]. The principle of PDT based on light-sensitizing reaction which produces oxygen radicals and destrois targeted cells by inducing of cellular apoptosis. Porfimer sodium and 5-aminolevulinic acid (5-ALA) have been used for the relatively selective destruction of malignant and pre-malignant tissue.Several studies have demonstrated the efficacy of PDT in eradicating BE with dysplasia and IMC. Results of the major PDT studies have shown eradication rates of IM, LGD and HGD in a range of 44%-56%, 79%-100%, and 75%-100% respectively and suggest that PDT is an effective treatment modality for eradication of BE with HGD and IMC [212-218]. A retrospective study on 103 patients with LGD, HGD, and IMC, treated by porfimer PDT reported success rates of 92.9%, 77.5%, and 44.4% for each respective group after a mean follow-up of 50 months [215]. The initial response after 5-ALA PDT in patients with Barrett's dysplasia or early EAC has been range between 67% and 100% with a relatively high recurrence rate (30%) [216, 219]. Other study in which 5-ALA PDT was used after EMR, showed that it did not prevent recurrent disease, particularly when there were positive margins in the EMR specimen [220]. In a prospective study, 66 patients with HGD or IMC on BE after 5-ALA PDT were followed-up for a median of 37 months [216]. Complete response was observed in 97% of HGD group and 100% of IMC group. Disease-free survival of HGD patients was 89%, and 68% in IMC cases. The 5-year survival was 97% for HGD and 80% for IMC. There were no deaths related to Barrett's neoplasia. In a multicenter, randomized controlled trial, the long-term outcomes of porfimer sodium PDT plus twice-daily Omeprazole 20 mg (n = 138) versus PPI only (n=70) were evaluated [221, 222]. At 24 months, 77% of PDT+PPI treated patients had remission of Barrett's dysplasia versus 39% in the PPI group. At 5 years, there was no residual dysplasia in 59% of PDT-treated patients versus 14% of PPI group. Complete neosquamous mucosa was found in 52% of the patients in the PDT group but only in 7% in the control group. In addition, the cancer progression was prevented in 29% in PDT group v/s 15% in the PPI group. These data confirmed that PDT is an effective procedure for the eradication of BE with HGD and early EAC, but there are no randomized, controlled prospective trials which compared PDT and surgery. In Mayo study of BE patients with HGD who received PDT (*n* =129) or esophagectomy (*n* = 70), retrospective data were analysed [223]. No significant differences in mortality or long-term survival between different treatment groups were found. Overall mortality in the PDT group was 9% and in the surgery group was 8.5% over a median follow-up period of 59 months for the PDT group and 61 months for the surgery group. Although initial and long-term success for neoplasia eradication, several limitations for using of PDT as a primary choice for treatment of Barrett's neoplasia exist. The additional time required for the administration of the photosensitizers 2–3 days prior to endoscopic therapy, and the high price of PDT procedure are also pitfalls. The most important adverse effects are photosensitization, stricture formation, and the issue of buried glands that harbored neoplastic potential and decreased efficacy when compared with newer modalities [209, 212, 215, 223]. Post-procedure skin sunburn was reported in two-thirds of the patients [170, 172]. Other important side effects are acute chest pain, nausea and odynophagia. Symptomatic esophageal stricture formation was reported in average 30% of patients, and increased from 18% with one PDT session to 50% with two treatment sessions [215]. These strictures necessitate multiple endoscopic dilations and even esophageal stenting [169]. The significant risk factors associated with post-PDTstricture development include performance of EMR before PDT, history of prior esophageal stricture, and the number of photodynamic sessions (more than one in a single procedure) [223]. Adenocarcinoma arising from sub-squamous Barrett's esophagus glands after PDT was reported [209, 215]. However, the clinical significance of sub-squamous Barrett's glands is not fully defined. If PDT has been capable to effectively ablate lesions greater than 2mm in depth is discussed [224]. For this reason regular follow-up endoscopies with biopsies are very important. In one study including 349 patients with dysplasia or IMC were treated by EMR (80%) or PDT [225]. Only 13 patients were treated with a combination therapy of ER and PDT. Complete response was achieved in 96.6% of patients with endoscopic therapy. At 5-year follow up survival was 84% and there were no cancer-related deaths. Metachronous lesions occurred in 21.5% of the patients. After re-treatment, the long-term eradication was 95%. Other studies have shown similar success between EMR alone and EMR plus ablation therapy combining the diagnostic accuracy and therapeutic resection of EMR with adjuvant ablation to some degree [226, 227]. On the base of current data on efficacy and safety of PDT, this ablative modality remains an effective treatment for BE with HGD and IMC. There is a need to improve photosensitiser agents, dosimetry, and light parameters which should help minimize the associated complications. On the other hand the PDT use decrease in clinical practice in recent years. PDT was been replaced by newer ablative modalities with less risk of procedural complications as RFA and cryoablation.

RFA is one of the newer endoscopic treatment modalities. The ablation process includes direct thermal energy with the electrodes embedded in either the circumferential or focal device. The effect of RFA has been well studied in several trials in BE patients with or without dysplasia and IMC [228]. The safety and efficacy of RFA were first assessed on BE patients without dysplasia in the Ablation of intestinal metaplasia (AIM) study [217]. This multicenter trial showed a 70% complete remission of BE after circumferential RFA at 1 year follow-up. Stricture formation or buried BE was no found among 4306 biopsy specimens evaluated. The AIM-II trial (n=70) demonstrated complete eradication in 98% of patients treated with an additional mean of 1.5 circumferential RFA followed by 1.9 focal ablation procedures at 2.5-year follow-up [218]. Five-year outcomes from the AIM-II trial (n=50) showed complete remission in 92% of the patients [229]. Four (8%) patients had NDBE and were all re-treated successfully with focal ablation. In addition, no strictures, perforations, buried glands, dysplasia, or serious adverse events were reported. The results of these large clinical studies proved that NDBE can regress in response to RFA. The use of RFA for BE with dysplasia has also been evaluated in several additional studies and RFA has been shown to be efficacious. One study included 63 patients with LGD (n = 39) and HGD (n = 24) treated by circumferential or focal RFA [230]. At a median follow-up of 24 months, 79% and 89% of patients achieved complete remission of IM and dysplasia, respectively. Patients with LGD had a higher rate of response than patients with HGD for both eradication of IM (87% vs 67%) and dysplasia (95% vs 79%). In a multicenter randomized sham-controlled trial 127 BE patients with dysplasia (64 LGD and 63 HGD) received RFA (mean of 3.5 procedures/patient) or a sham procedure, as well as esomeprazole 40 mg twice daily [231]. At 12-month follow-up complete eradication of LGD occurred in 90.5% in the ablation group v/s 23% in controls, and 81% vs 19% for HGD and controls respectively. Complete eradication of IM was observed in 77% v/s 2% for RFA and control group respectively. There was less disease progression in patients in the ablation group (3.6% *vs* 16.3%) and fewer cancers developed (1.2% *vs* 9.3%). The rate of esophageal stricture in the RFA group was 6 %. All patients were successfully treated with endoscopic dilation (mean 2.6 sessions). This stricture rate is markedly lower than that reported for EMR. These data demonstrated a significant advantage for RFA in treatment of BE with HGD. In addition, after 3 years followed up, 98 % eradication of dysplasia and 91 % eradication of metaplasia were found. Although RFA appeared to be efficacious in clinical trials for both dysplastic and NDBE, it was unclear whether the results would be reproducible in community practice [172]. Regarding this, in one study were investigated 142 BE patients with HGD after circumferential RFA from 16 separate academic and community centers [232]. At 1 year follow-up, complete remission of HGD was observed in 90%, complete regression of LGD was found in 80%, and 54% of patients achieved complete eradication of BE. Only one stricture was observed as adverse event. The data of a multicenter practice registry from 4 community-based gastroenterology practices were also evaluated [233]. A total of 429 patients with confirmed IM with or without dysplasia were treated with circumferential RFA. Complete eradication of BE or regression of dysplasia were achieved in 72% and 89% of patients, respectively, at a median follow-up of 9 months (338 patients with ≥ 1 biopsy session after the initial treatment), as well as in 77% and 100%, respectively, with a median follow-up of 20 months (137 patients with ≥ 1 biopsy session ≥ 1 year after the initial treatment). No serious adverse events were reported, although esophageal strictures were observed in 2% (successfully treated by endoscopy). The observed safety and efficacy outcomes associated with RFA in this community practice study appeared to be comparable with those reported in clinical trials, supporting its wider applicability in community practice.

Several smaller trials have shown the possibility of combination of EMR of visible lesions with subsequent RFA for the treatment patients with dysplastic BE or EAC. The results of these studies showed that eradication rate of IM, any dysplasia, including also HGD was in

46%-100%, and 71%-100% respectively. [230, 232, 234-240]. In one study 44 patients with LGD, HGD, or IMC treated with RFA (31 patients had prior EMR for visible lesions before RFA) were evaluated [237]. Complete eradication of all dysplasia and IM was achieved in 98%. Post-ablation complications (all with prior EMR) included mucosal laceration and transient dysphagia ($n = 3$), and esophageal stricture (n = 4), which responded to endoscopic dilatation. No dysplasia recurred after a 21-months follow-up period. A more recent multicenter European trial reported results of 24 patients with BE and HGD or IMC who were treated with EMR for visible lesions and then serial RFA were applied [238]. The complete eradication rates of neoplasia, including those with EAC and IM were 100% and 95% respectively, after 22-months follow-up. No major adverse effects were observed. Regarding patients with BE segments >10 cm, one study reported complete response rates of 83% and 79 % for neoplasia and IM, respectively after focal EMR followed by RFA [241]. Both of these trials demonstrate neoplasia-free outcomes in their follow-up periods of 22 and 9 months, respectively. In a randomized control trial, CBE-EMR followed by serial focal EMR was compared with the focal EMR followed by RFA in BE up to 5 cm containing HGD or EAC [203]. Complete remission rates were similar between two groups (100% for CBE-EMR v/s 96% for EMR/RFA group). The most finding of this study is that CBE-EMR group showed higher rate of stenosis (88 % vs. 14 %). These results confirmed that RFA, applied after focal EMR of visible lesions can be effective therapy for the remaining Barrett's dysplastic epithelium, because RFA has associated with better safety profile. Most procedure-related side effects are mild, including fever, chest pain, superficial mucosal injury (non-transmural lacerations), nausea or sedation-related complications [217]. Esophageal function appears to be well preserved [242]. Stricture formation rate was up to 6%, much lower than the rate associated with EMR [234]. In combination with EMR complications are found more frequently [237, 238]. Nontransmural laceration associated with circumferential RFA following EMR was observed in 7% of patients, which occurred only at the level of the EMR. In contrast, no lacerations or stenosis occurred in patients treated with RFA alone [238]. Buried Barrett's glands have been evaluated in all RFA studies showing positive result in one of 5000 biopsies. Re-EMR specimens after ablation did not show any buried glands [237]. Neo-squamous epithelium on EMR specimens in a group of 22 post-RFA patients with baseline BE with IMC or HGD showed no evidence of persistent genetic abnormalities or buried BE glands [243].

RFA is characterized with very good control of the depth of ablative penetration [224]. Because of that many side effects are reduced. Now, RFA is seem to be the most efficacious modality to treats any stage of BE with a better safety profile than other ablation techniques (PDT) and EMR. RFA is also safely when combined with EMR for visible lesions. This combined endoscopic method is quickly integrated in routine clinical practice. RFA therapy for patients with NDBE and LGD seems to be capable to reverse to normal squamous epithelium for a long time (5 year) after procedure. In addition, RFA treatment reduces progression to EAC in patients with HGD. Because of that RFA has became one of the preferable method for the EET of BE with HGD and/or IMC.

Cryotherapy or CryoSpray Ablation therapy (CSA) is a relatively newer non contact ablation modality. Sprayed liquid nitrogen or carbon dioxide is applied onto the Barrett's mucosa, which produces tissue freeze-thaw cycles. Cryotherapy leads to intracellular disruption or tissue ischemia, with minimal damaging of extracellular matrix and fibrosis formation [169-172]. One prospective open-label cohort trial on 30 patients with BE and HGD or IMC undergoing CSA showed that 27 of the patients (90%) had pathological downgrading post-treatment [244]. Elimination of cancer or downgrading of HGD was achieved in 80% of IMC and 68% of HGD patients at a median of 1 year follow-up. The therapy was well tolerated, but one gastric perforation reported in a patient with Marfan syndrome in whom decompression during therapy was not performed. Of 6 patients who showed a complete response, 3 had recurrence of dysplasia or cancer in the gastric cardia.Recent trials demonstrate initial success with regression of HGD more than 90% for both liquid nitrogen or carbon dioxide cryotherapies [245-247]. A retrospective analysis of 60 patients with HGD treated by CSA (mean of 4 sessions) was done [245]. Complete eradication of HGD was observed in 97% (87% for all dysplasia) at a mean follow-up of 10.5 months. In 57% were found regression to squamous epithelium. Disease progression occurred in 1 patient. Overall, no serious adverse events occurred over the course of 333 sessions, with 3 strictures requiring endoscopic dilation. Other study reported that primary and additional treatment in refractory HGD or EAC with carbon dioxide resulted in a safe and effective ablation in more than 90% of the patients with a mean of six sessions [247]. In a four-center study of 23 patients (17 HGD, 4IMC, 3 early EAC), complete regression to HGD was found in 94% with HGD, and 100% with IMC and EAC [246]. Complete response to IM was observed in 53% with HGD, 75% with IMC, and 67% with cancer. No symptoms were reported in 48% of 323 procedures. Esophageal strictures developed in 3 patients, but all were successfully treated by dilation.In addition to early success with IMC, this therapy has also been considered as a treatment for patients with localized EAC that are not candidates for standard therapies. In a recent study it was demonstrated a 61.2 % complete local response [248]. The safety profile of cryotherapy appears to be good. CSA related adverse events include chest pain, dysphagia, odynophagia, sore throat, stenosis, and rarely perforation [244-246]. The overall incidence of stricture formation was 8 %. This rate is lower than the reported rates for EMR and PDT.

In summary, cryotherapy has become now as a potential alternative to the other endoscopic ablative modalities. According to present data, cryotherapy appears to be safe, well tolerated, and capable to ablate IM, dysplasia and early EAC. On the other hand, there is no evidence that cryotherapy leads to sustained reversion to normal squamous epithelium.The efficacy of this ablation method is lower when compared with RFA or PDT. There are no randomized trials comparing CSA with other endoscopic or nonendoscopic modalities. Further studies are needed also to assess long-term efficacy of cryotherapy, as well as its real clinical significance.

Two recent studies evaluated the cost-effectiveness of ablative therapy for BE [249, 250].One of them reported endoscopic ablation with continued surveillance is significantly more cost-effective than surveillance only [249]. A separate cost-effective analysis concluded that endoscopic ablation could be the preferred strategy for management of BE with HGD [250]. If ablation permanently eradicates ≥ 28% of LGD or 40% of NDBE, endoscopic ablation would be preferred to surveillance alone.

5.4. Surgical treatment

Until the past decade, esophagectomy for BE with HGD and IMC had been the traditional standard, because of the high rate of suspected risk of occult invasive carcinoma or recurrence [132, 184, 185, 251-253]. Surgery ensures accurate staging and adequate therapy including negative margins and lymph nodes extraction. Complete resection of the entire Barrett's segment is done in cases of unsuspected multifocal disease and to minimize the risk of metachronous lesion development in residual Barrett's [254]. Some studies reported significant morbidity and mortality associated with esophagectomy, with overall morbidity rates as high as 50% and mortality as high as 10% [255]. The immediate postoperative complications include pulmonary events, hemorrhage, anastomotic leak, infections, postoperative arrythmias and heart failure, and nerve palsy [132, 224]. The long-term complications are dysphagia, weight loss, GERD, esophageal strictures, cough and dumping which may impair health-related quality of life [256]. Reported mortality rates for esophagectomy usually were based on outcomes after surgery for cancer and not HGD. It is well known that patients with cancers are older, more morbid, and have more comorbidities than patients with HGD alone [257]. On the other hands the results from high-volume centers with greater surgical expertise have shown better outcomes [224]. The mortality rate from esophagectomy for cancer of 2%–3% was reported [258, 259]. In a Dutch study, based on the number of esophagectomies a year, hospitals were classified as low-volume centers (<10 resections a year), medium-volume centers (11–20 resections a year) and high-volume centers (>50 resections a year). Hospital mortality at these centers was 12.1%, 7.5% and 4.9%, respectively [260]. In another study a mortality rate of 1% after esophagectomy for HGD was found. Others data also confirmed that surgical resection of patients with HGD is associated with operative mortality of 0-2% and overall 5-year survival of 83%-88% (91% for HGD without invasion and 68% for those with invasion), and 10-year survival of 86% [261-264]. This result showed that regarding HGD and surgical experience, esophagectomy is a lower-risk surgery [257]. Recurrence rates of BE or EAC after esophagectomy have been assessed in a limited number of trials. In one study on BE patients with HGD or EAC, the 2-year surveillance of 85% was reported [175]. The cure rate for dysplasia or localized EAC was reported to be lower that 78% in another study [265]. These data raise questions about the need for continued endoscopic surveillance following surgical resection. Conventional approaches for esophagectomy are transhiatal and transthoracic resection. A randomized trial comparing of patients undergoing transhiatal esophagectomy (n=106) or transthoracic esophagectomy with lymphadenectomy (n=114) demonstrated a significantly lower rate of postoperative respiratory complications with the transhiatal approach (27% versus 57%), but greater survival was shown for the transthoracic approach at 5 years (39% versus 27%) [266]. One potential limitation of the transhiatal approach is the inability to retrieve lymph nodes required for nodal staging [267]. Minimally invasive esophagectomy avoids the thoracotomy and laparotomy has potential advantages over open esophagectomy because of a lower incidence of pulmonary complications, faster postoperative recovery, and decreased length of hospital stay [268, 269]. However, lymph node retrieval is largely inferior to the standards of open surgery. The morbidity and mortality of minimally invasive esophagectomy is not proven to be lower when compared with open esophagectomy at experienced centers [270]. Recommendations favoring minimally invasive esophagectomy over open esophagectomy cannot be made due to a lack of randomized trials comparing the two approaches. In patients with few comorbidities and an otherwise long life expectancy, a vagal-sparing esophagectomy can be considered to improve outcomes and quality of life. It was demonstrated lower infectious, respiratory, and anastomotic complications in patients with HGD or IMC undergoing this procedure compared with transhiatal esophagectomy. Quality of life advantages were also demonstrated because of the reduction of postvagotomy dumping and diarrhea, as well as a shorter hospital stay [271]. However, lymphadenectomy is not performed with this procedure. Regarding early cancer (IMC), esophagectomy with therapeutic lymphadenectomy is today reserved for more selected cases with evidence of submucosal invasion, lymph node metastasis, or unsuccessful endoscopic therapy, National Comprehensive Cancer Network (NCCN) recommended all modalities –EMR or ablation or esophagectomy [272], but European Society for Medical Oncology (ESMO) [273] pointed that surgery is the treatment of choice in early cancer. On the contrary, esophagectomy can be discussed in patients with high-risk features of HGD or IMC [274]. A patient's age, comorbidities, and willingness to undergo surgery should also be taken into account. According to the current AGA's guidelines for BE management "Esophagectomy in patients with HGD is an alternative; however, current evidence suggests that there is less morbidity with ablative therapy" The experts also enhance that patients with HGD or IMC "should be referred for evaluation by surgical centers that specialize in the treatment of foregut cancers and HGD" [151].

There are no prospective head-to-head randomized trials to compare EET versus surgery. However, when compared with esophagectomy, EET is less invasive, associated with low morbidity and mortality, and is more cost-effective in treating all types of BE. The reported outcomes of EET are superior to those of esophagectomy. Endoscopic procedures related mortality versus death from postoperative complications was 0% v/s 2.1% and the percent of patients free of carcinoma after EET v/s free of carcinoma after esophagectomy was 88% v/s 86% [191, 275]. Recurrence rates of EAC after EET were 12% and all were cured by further endoscopic therapy. In a long-term follow-up of 132 patients treated with EMR and 46 who underwent surgery, there was no difference in the 5-year survival rate between the surgically or endoscopically treated groups [276].

Now, EET with EMR, RFA or PDT is became a first chois of treatment for BE patients with confirmed HGD [151,169-172]. The key point to successful EET is appropriate selection of each patients. EET is also associated with complete reversion to normal squamous epithelium in NDBE or LGD. Despite that, there is no evidence EET is more cost-effective to reduce cancer risk than long-term endoscopic surveillance [14, 151, 234]. Regardless EET can be used for select BE patients with LGD who have high risk for progression to HGD and EAC [151].

6. Conclusions

All types of histologically proven esophageal columnar metaplasia, including gastric or specialized intestinal metaplasia should be included in the diagnosis of BE. But various definitions of BE still exist. Diagnosis and grading of dysplasia rely on careful endoscopic and histological examinations in a Barrett's segment, cofirmed by expert. There is different management strategy in BE with or without LGD and HGD because of the different prognostic profiles between them. There are no evidence regarding outcome of endoscopic surveillance but all professional organizations recommend this approach for all types of BE. When BE without evidence of dysplasia or cancer is found on biopsy, the management focuses on reflux control and risk of cancer development (periodic endoscopic surveillance, PPIs or fundoplication, and ASA for cardiovascular risk/disease). Patients with LGD might be managed similar to NDBE. Antireflux therapy (medical or surgical) and endoscopic surveillance to exclude HGD missed on prior biopsy or progression to EAC are recommended. There is a greater discrepancy regarding the management of BE with HGD. The options for management of these patients include intensive surveillance until EAC, EET with EMR, RFA, or PDT, and surgery. The EET and surveillance are both equal recommended as a first choice of treatment for patients with confirmed HGD on BE. An individualized approach based on risk startification and patient preference is also recommended, especially for LGD or HGD.

Author details

Borislav Vladimirov[1*], Radina Ivanova[2] and Ivan Terziev[3]

*Address all correspondence to: borislavvladimirov@yahoo.com

1 Clinic of Gastroenterology, University Hospital Tz. Joanna, Medical University, Sofia, Bulgaria

2 Laboratory of pathomorphology, University Hospital of Endocrinology, Medical University, Sofia, Bulgaria

3 Department of general and clinical pathology, University Hospital Tz. Joanna, Medical University, Sofia, Bulgaria

References

[1] Pohl H, Sirovich B, Welch HG. Esophageal adenocarcinoma incidence: are we reaching the peak? Cancer Epidemiol Biomarkers Prev. 2010;19(6):1468-70.

[2] Botterweck AA, Schouten LJ, Volovics A, Dorant E, van-Den-Brandt PA. Trends in incidence of adenocarcinoma of the oesophagus and gastric cardia in ten European countries. Int. J.Epidemiol. 2000;29(4): 645–54.

[3] Eloubeidi MA, Mason AC, Desmond RA, et al. Temporal trends (1973–1997) in survival of patients with esophageal adenocarcinoma in the United States: a glimmer of hope? Am J Gastroenterol. 2003;98(7):1627–1633.

[4] Lagergren J. Adenocarcinoma of oesophagus: what exactly is the size of the problem and who is at risk? Gut. 2005;54 (Suppl 1):i1-5.

[5] Bhat S, Coleman HG, Yousef F, Johnston BT, McManus DT, Gavin AT, Murray LJ. Risk of malignant progression in Barrett's esophagus patients: results from a large population-based study. J Natl Cancer Inst. 2011;103(13):1049-57.

[6] Wild CP, Hardie LJ. Reflux, Barrett's oesophagus and adenocarcinoma: burning questions. Nat Rev Cancer. 2003;3(9): 676-84.

[7] O'Connor JB, Falk GW, Richter JE. The incidence of adenocarcinoma and dysplasia in Barrett's esophagus: report on the Cleveland Clinic Barrett's Esophagus Registry. Am J Gastroenterol. 1999;94(8): 2037–2042.

[8] Drewitz DJ, Sampliner RE, Garewal HS. The incidence of adenocarcinoma in Barrett's esophagus: a prospective study of 170 patients followed 4.8 years. Am J Gastroenterol. 1997;92(2): 212-5.

[9] Sharma P, Falk GW, Weston AP, Reker D, Johnston M, Sampliner RE. Dysplasia and cancer in a large multicenter cohort of patients with Barrett's esophagus. Clin Gastroenterol Hepatol. 2006;4(5): 566-72.

[10] Schnell TG, Sontag SJ, Chejfec G, Aranha G, Metz A, O'Connell S, Seidel UJ, Sonnenberg A. Long-term nonsurgical management of Barrett's esophagus with high-grade dysplasia. Gastroenterology 2001;120(7):1607-19.

[11] Riddell RH, Odze RD. Definition of Barrett's esophagus: time for a rethink--is intestinal metaplasia dead? Am J Gastroenterol. 2009;104(10):2588-94.

[12] Dent J. Barrett's esophagus: A historical perspective, an update on core practicalities and predictions on future evolutions of management. J. Gastroenterol Hepatol. 2011;26(Suppl 1):11-30.

[13] Playford RJ. New British Society of Gastroenterology (BSG) guidelines for the diagnosis and management of Barrett's oesophagus. Gut. 2006 Apr;55(4): 442.

[14] Spechler SJ, Sharma P, Souza RF, Inadomi JM, Shaheen NJ, American Gastroenterological Association. American Gastroenterological Association technical review on the management of Barrett's esophagus. Gastroenterology. 2011;140(3): e18-52.

[15] Wang KK, Sampliner RE; Practice Parameters Committee of the American College of Gastroenterology. Updated guidelines 2008 for the diagnosis, surveillance and therapy of Barrett's esophagus. Am J Gastroenterol. 2008;103(3): 788-97.

[16] Crockett SD, Lippmann QK, Dellon ES, Shaheen NJ. Health-related quality of life in patients with Barrett's esophagus: a systematic review. Clin Gastroenterol Hepatol. 2009;7(6): 613-23.

[17] Shaheen NJ, Dulai GS, Ascher B, Mitchell KL, Schmitz SM. Effect of a new diagnosis of Barrett's esophagus on insurance status. Am J Gastroenterol. 2005;100(3): 577-80.

[18] Vakil N, van Zanten SV, Kahrilas P, Dent J, Jones R, Global Consensus Group. The Montréal definition and classification of gastroesophageal reflux disease: a global evidence-based consensus. Am. J. Gastroenterol. 2006; 101(8): 1900–20.

[19] Bellizzi AM, Odze RD. Histopathology of Barrett's esophagus: A review for the practicing gastroenterologist. Techniques in Gastrointestinal Endoscopy. 2010;12(2): 69-81.

[20] Oberg S, Johansson J, Wenner J, et al. Endoscopic surveillance of columnar-lined esophagus: Frequency of intestinal metaplasia detection and impact of antireflux surgery. Ann Surg. 2001;234(5): 619-626.

[21] Chandrasoma PT, Der R, Dalton P, et al. Distribution and significance of epithelial types in columnar-lined esophagus. Am J Surg Pathol. 2001;25(9): 1188-1193.

[22] Harrison R, Perry I, Haddadim W et al. Detection of intestinalmetaplasia in Barrett's esophagus: an observational comparator study suggests the need for a minimum of eight biopsies. Am. J. Gastroenterol. 2007; 102(6): 1154–61.

[23] Hahn HP, Blount PL, Ayub K, et al. Intestinal differentiation in metaplastic, nongoblet columnar epithelium in the esophagus. Am J Surg Pathol. 2009; 33(7):1006-1015.

[24] Liu W, Hahn H, Odze RD, et al. Metaplastic esophageal columnar epithelium without goblet cells shows DNA content abnormalities similar to goblet cell-containing epithelium. Am J Gastroenterol. 2009;104(4): 816-824.

[25] Gatenby PA, Ramus JR, Caygill CP, et al. Relevance of the detection of intestinal metaplasia in non-dysplastic columnar-lined oesophagus. Scand J Gastroenterol. 2008;43(5): 524-530.

[26] Kelty CJ, Gough MD, Van Wyk Q, et al. Barrett's oesophagus: Intestinal metaplasia is not essential for cancer risk. Scand J Gastroenterol. 2007; 42(11):1271-1274.

[27] Sharma P, Morales TG, Sampliner RE. Short segment Barrett's esophagus--the need for standardization of the definition and of endoscopic criteria. Am J Gastroenterol. 1998;93(7):1033-6.

[28] Sharma P, Dent J, Armstrong D et al. The development and validation of an endoscopic grading system for Barrett's esophagus: the Prague C&M Criteria. Gastroenterology. 2006;131(5): 1392–9.

[29] Lee YC, Cook MB, Bhatia S et al. Interobserver reliability in the endoscopic diagnosis and grading of Barrett's esophagus: an Asian multinational study. Endoscopy. 2010;42(9): 699–704.

[30] Reid BJ, Blount PL, Feng Z, Levine DS. Optimizing endoscopic biopsy detection of early cancers in Barrett's high-grade dysplasia. Am. J. Gastroenterol. 2000;95(11): 3089–96.

[31] Kariv R, Plesec TP, Goldblum JR et al. The Seattle protocol does not more reliably predict the detection of cancer at the time of esophagectomy than a less intensive surveillance protocol. Clin. Gastroenterol. Hepatol. 2009; 7(6): 653–8.

[32] Curvers WL, Bergman JJ. Multimodality imaging in Barrett's esophagus: looking longer, seeing better, and recognizing more. Gastroenterology. 2008;135(1): 297–312.

[33] Pech O. Declaration of bankruptcy for four-quadrant biopsies in Barrett's esophagus? Clin. Gastroenterol. Hepatol. 2009; 7(6): 610–2.

[34] Kara AM, Curves V, Bergman J. Advanced endoscopic imaging in Barrett's esophagus. Techniques in Gastrointestinal Endoscopy. 2010;12: 82-89.

[35] Wolfsen HC. New technologies for imaging of Barrett's esophagus. Surg Oncol Clin N Am. 2009;18(3):487-502.

[36] Fennerty, M.B. Tissue staining. Gastrointest Endosc Clin N Am. 1994;4(2): 297-311.

[37] Canto MI, Setrakian S, Willis JE, et al. Methylene blue staining of dysplastic and nondysplastic Barrett's esophagus: an in vivo and ex vivo study. Endoscopy. 2001;33(5): 391-400.

[38] Lim CH, Rotimi O, Dexter SP, et al. Randomized crossover study that used methylene blue or random 4-quadrant biopsy for the diagnosis of dysplasia in Barrett's esophagus. Gastrointest Endosc. 2006;64(2):195-9.

[39] Ragunath K, Krasner N, Raman VS, et al. Randomized, prospective cross-over trial comparing methylene blue-directed biopsy and conventional random biopsy for detecting intestinal metaplasia and dysplasia in Barrett's esophagus. Endoscopy. 2003;35(12): 998-1003.

[40] Wo JM, Ray MB, Mayfield-Stokes S, et al. Comparison of methylene blue-directed biopsies and conventional biopsies in the detection of intestinal metaplasia and dysplasia in Barrett's esophagus: a preliminary study. Gastrointest Endosc. 2001;54(3): 294-301.

[41] Ngamruengphong S, Sharma VK., Das A. Diagnostic yield of methylene blue chromoendoscopy for detecting specialized intestinal metaplasia and dysplasia in Barrett's esophagus: a meta-analysis. Gastrointest Endosc 2009; 69(6): 1021–1028.

[42] Olliver JR, Wild CP, Sahay P, et al. Chromoendoscopy with methylene blue and associated DNA damage in Barrett's oesophagus. Lancet. 2003;362(9381): 373-4.

[43] Sharma P, Weston AP, Topalovski M, Cherian R, Bhattacharyya A, Sampliner RE. Magnification chromoendoscopy for the detection of intestinal metaplasia and dysplasia in Barrett's oesophagus. Gut. 2003;52(1): 24-7.

[44] Vladimirov, B., A. Marinov, A., I. Terziev, R. Ivanova. Magnifying chromoendoscopy is useful for detection of Barrett's metaplasia and low-grade dysplasia recurrence af-

ter argon plasma coagulation (APC). 9th World Congress of OESO, Monaco, April 6-9, 2008, J Clin Gastroenterol 2008; 42(Suppl 1): S31.

[45] Kara MA, Ennahachi M, Fockens P, ten Kate FJ, Bergman JJ. Detection and classification of the mucosal and vascular patterns (mucosal morphology) in Barrett's esophagus by using narrow band imaging. Gastrointest Endosc. 2006;64(2): 155-66.

[46] Borisova, E.G. , Vladimirov, B. , Terziev, I. , Ivanova, R. , Avramov, L. 5-ALA/PpIX fluorescence detection of gastrointestinal neoplasia. Progress in Biomedical Optics and Imaging - Proceedings of SPIE, 2009;7368, art. no. 736824

[47] Borisova, E., Vladimirov, B, Avramov, L. 5-ALA/PpIX fluorescence detection of esophageal and stomach neoplasia: Effects of autofluorescence background from normal and inflammatory areas. Proceedings of SPIE - The International Society for Optical Engineering, 2008;7027, art. no. 70271A

[48] Kara MA, Peters FP, Ten Kate FJ, et al. Endoscopic video autofluorescence imaging may improve the detection of early neoplasia in patients with Barrett's esophagus. Gastrointest Endosc. 2005;61(6): 679-85.

[49] Kara MA, Peters FP, Fockens P, et al. Endoscopic video-autofluorescence imaging followed by narrow band imaging for detecting early neoplasia in Barrett's esophagus. Gastrointest Endosc. 2006;64(2): 176-85.

[50] Curvers WL, Singh R, Song LM, et al. Endoscopic tri-modal imaging for detection of early neoplasia in Barrett's oesophagus: a multi-centre feasibility study using high-resolution endoscopy, autofluorescence imaging and narrow band imaging incorporated in one endoscopy system. Gut. 2008;57(2):167-72.

[51] Curvers WL, van Vilsteren FG, Baak LC et al. Endoscopic trimodal imaging versus standard video endoscopy for detection of early Barrett's neoplasia: a multicenter, randomized, crossover study in general practice. Gastrointest Endosc. 2011;73(2): 195-203.

[52] Kiesslich, R., Gossner, L., Goetz, et al. In vivo histology of Barrett's esophagus and associated neoplasia by confocal laser endomicroscopy. Clin Gastroenterol Hepatol. 2006;4(8): 979-87.

[53] Pech O, May A, Günter E, Gossner L, Ell C. The impact of endoscopic ultrasound and computed tomography on the TNM staging of early cancer in Barrett's esophagus. Am. J. Gastroenterol. 2006; 101: 2223–9.

[54] Voltaggio L, Montgomery EA, Lam-Himlin D. A clinical and histopathologic focus on Barrett esophagus and Barrett-related dysplasia. Arch Pathol Lab Med. 2011;135(10): 1249-60.

[55] Glickman JN, Spechler SJ, Souza RF, Lunsford T, Lee E, Odze RD. Multilayered epithelium in mucosal biopsy specimens from the gastroesophageal junction region is a

histologic marker of gastroesophageal reflux disease. Am J Surg Pathol. 2009;33(6): 818–825.

[56] Takubo K, Sasajima K, Yamashita K, et al.Double muscularis mucosae in Barrett's esophagus. Hum Pathol. 1991; 22(11): 1158-1161.

[57] Abraham SC, Krasinskas AM, Correa AM, et al. Duplication of the muscularis mucosae in Barrett esophagus: An underrecognized feature and its implication for staging of adenocarcinoma. Am J Surg Pathol. 2007; 31 (11):1719-1725.

[58] Rice TW., Mendelin JE, Goldblum JR. Barrett's esophagus: pathologic considerations and implications for treatment. Semin Thorac Cardiovasc Surg. 2005;17(4): 292-300.

[59] Sharma P, Weston AP, Morales T, Topalovski M, Mayo MS, Sampliner RE. Relative risk of dysplasia for patients with intestinal metaplasia in the distal oesophagus and in the gastric cardia. Gut. 2000;46(1): 9–13.

[60] Ormsby AH, Goldblum JR, Rice TW, et al. Cytokeratin subsets can reliably distinguish Barrett's esophagus from intestinal metaplasia of the stomach. Hum Pathol. 1999;30(3): 288–294.

[61] Vladimirov B., R. Ivanova, I. Terziev. Cytokeratin 7 and 20 – markers for distinction of intestinal metaplasia subtypes of upper gastrointestinal tract. 9th World Congress of OESO, Monaco, April 6-9, 2008, J Clin Gastroenterol. 2008; 42(Suppl. 1): S29.

[62] Kurtkaya-Yapicier O, Gencosmanoglu R, Avsar E, Bakirci N, Tozun N, Sav A. The utility of cytokeratins 7 and 20 (CK7/20) immunohistochemistry in the distinction of short-segment Barrett esophagus from gastric intestinal metaplasia: is it reliable? BMC Clin Pathol. 2003;3(1): 5.

[63] Nurgalieva Z, Lowrey A, El-Serag HB. The use of cytokeratin stain to distinguish Barrett's esophagus from contiguous tissues: a systematic review. Dig Dis Sci. 2007;52(5): 1345-54.

[64] Mohammed IA, Streutker CJ, Riddell RH. Utilization of cytokeratins 7 and 20 does not differentiate between Barrett's esophagus and gastric cardiac intestinal metaplasia. Mod Pathol. 2002;15(6): 611–616.

[65] Schlemper RJ, Riddell RH, Kato Y, Borchard F, Cooper HS, Dawsey SM, et al. The Vienna classification of gastrointestinal epithelial neoplasia. Gut. 2000;47(2): 251–255.

[66] Vieth M, Langner C, Neumann H, Takubo K. Barrett's esophagus. Practical issues for daily routine diagnosis. Pathol Res Pract. 2012;208(5): 261-8.

[67] Hamilton SR, Aaltonen SA., editors. WHO Classification. Tumours of the Digestive System. IARC Press, Lyon: 2000.

[68] Bosman F, Carneiro F, Hruban R, Theise N., editors. WHO Classification of Tumours of the Digestive System. IARC Press, Lyon: 2010.

[69] Riddell RH, Goldman H, Ransohoff DF, et al. Dysplasia in inflammatory bowel disease: standardized classification with provisional clinical applications. Hum Pathol 1983;14(11): 931-968.

[70] Liu L, Hofstetter WL, Rashid A, et al. Significance of the depth of tumor invasion and lymph node metastasis in superficially invasive (T1) esophageal adenocarcinoma. Am J Surg Pathol. 2005;29(8): 1079-85.

[71] Reid BJ, Haggitt RC, Rubin CE, et al. Observer variation in the diagnosis of dysplasia in Barrett's esophagus. Hum Pathol. 1988;19(2):166-78.

[72] Alikhan M, Rex D, Khan A, Rahmani E, Cummings O, Ulbright TM. Variable pathologic interpretation of columnar lined esophagus by general pathologists in community practice. Gastrointest.Endosc. 1999; 50(1): 23–6.

[73] Montgomery E, Bronner MP, Goldblum JR, et al. Reproducibility of the diagnosis of dysplasia in Barrett esophagus: A reaffirmation. Hum Pathol. 2001;32(4):368-78.

[74] Curvers WL, Ten Kate FJ, Krishnadath KK et al. Low-grade dysplasia in Barrett's esophagus: overdiagnosed and underestimated. Am. J. Gastroenterol. 2010;105(7): 1523–30.

[75] Downs-Kelly E, Mendelin JE, Bennett AE et al. Poor interobserver agreement in the distinction of high-grade dysplasia and adenocarcinoma in pretreatment Barrett's esophagus biopsies. Am J Gastroenterol. 2008;103(9): 2333-40.

[76] Zhu W, Appleman HD, Greenson JK et al. A histologically defined subset of high-grade dysplasia in Barrett mucosa in predictive of associated carcinoma. Am. J. Clin. Pathol. 2009;132(1): 94–100.

[77] Montgomery E. Refining diagnostic criteria for high-grade dysplasia in Barrett esophagus. Am. J. Clin. Pathol. 2009; 132(1): 7–9.

[78] Biddlestone LR, Barham CP, Wilkinson SP, et al. The histopathology of treated Barrett's esophagus: Squamous reepithelialization after acid suppression and laser and photodynamic therapy. Am J Surg Pathol. 1998;22(2): 239-45.

[79] Hornick JL, Blount PL, Sanchez CA, et al. Biologic properties of columnar epithelium underneath reepithelialized squamous mucosa in Barrett's esophagus. Am J Surg Pathol. 2005;29(3): 372-80.

[80] Pouw RE, Gondrie JJ, Rygiel AM, et al. Properties of the neosquamous epithelium after radiofrequency ablation of Barrett's esophagus containing neoplasia. Am J Gastroenterol. 2009;104(6): 1366-73.

[81] Hornick JL, Mino-Kenudson M, Lauwers GY, et al. Buried Barrett's epithelium following photodynamic therapy shows reduced crypt proliferation and absence of DNA content abnormalities. Am J Gastroenterol. 2008;103(1): 38-47.

[82] Hage M, Siersema PD, Vissers KJ, et al. Genomic analysis of Barrett's esophagus after ablative therapy: Persistence of genetic alterations at tumor suppressor loci. Int J Cancer. 2006;118(1): 155-60.

[83] Mino-Kenudson M, Brugge WR, Puricelli WP, et al. Management of superficial Barrett's epithelium-related neoplasms by endoscopic mucosal resection: Clinicopathologic analysis of 27 cases. Am J Surg Pathol. 2005;29(5): 680-6.

[84] Larghi A, Lightdale CJ, Memeo L, et al. EUS followed by EMR for staging of high-grade dysplasia and early cancer in Barrett's esophagus. Gastrointest Endosc. 2005;62(1): 16-23.

[85] Mino-Kenudson M, Hull MJ, Brown I, et al. EMR for Barrett's esophagus-related superficial neoplasms offers better diagnostic reproducibility than mucosal biopsy. Gastrointest Endosc. 2007;66(4): 660-6.

[86] Prasad GA, Buttar NS, Wongkeesong LM, et al. Significance of neoplastic involvement of margins obtained by endoscopic mucosal resection in Barrett's esophagus. Am J Gastroenterol. 2007;102(11): 2380-2386.

[87] Vieth M, Ell C, Gossner L, et al. Histological analysis of endoscopic resection specimens from 326 patients with Barrett's esophagus and early neoplasia. Endoscopy. 2004;36(9): 776-781.

[88] Lauwers GY, Ban S, Mino M, et al. Endoscopic mucosal resection for gastric epithelial neoplasms: A study of 39 cases with emphasis on the evaluation of specimens and recommendations for optimal pathologic analysis. Mod Pathol. 2004;17(1): 2-8.

[89] Reid BJ, Levine DS, Longton G, et al. Predictors of progression to cancer in Barrett's esophagus: Baseline histology and flow cytometry identify low- and high-risk patient subsets. Am J Gastroenterol. 2000; 95(7): 1669-1676.

[90] Feith M, Stein HJ, Mueller J, Siewert JR. Malignant degeneration of Barrett's esophagus: the role of the Ki-67 proliferation fraction, expression of E-cadherin and p53. Dis Esophagus. 2004;17(4): 322-7.

[91] Lörinc E, Jakobsson B, Landberg G, Veress B. Ki67 and p53 immunohistochemistry reduces interobserver variation in assessment of Barrett's oesophagus. Histopathology. 2005;46(6): 642-8.

[92] Younes M, Lebovitz RM, Lechago LV, et al. p53 protein accumulation in Barrett's metaplasia, dysplasia, and carcinoma: A follow-up study. Gastroenterology. 1993;105(6): 1637-1642.

[93] Gimenez A, Minguela A, Parrilla P, et al. Flow cytometric DNA analysis and p53 protein expression show a good correlation with histologic findings in patients with Barrett's esophagus. Cancer. 1998;83(4): 641-651.

[94] Schulmann K, Sterian A, Berki A, et al. Inactivation of p16, RUNX3, and HPP1 occurs early in Barrett's-associated neoplastic progression and predicts progression risk. Oncogene. 2005;24(25): 4138-48.

[95] Merola E, Mattioli E, Minimo C et al. Immunohistochemical evaluation of pRb2/p130, VEGF, EZH2, p53, p16, p21waf-1, p27, and PCNA in Barrett's esophagus. J Cell Physiol. 2006;207(2): 512-9.

[96] Locke GR 3rd, Talley NJ, Fett SL, Zinsmeister AR, Melton LJ 3rd. Prevalence and clinical spectrum of gastroesophageal reflux: a population-based study in Olmsted County, Minnesota. Gastroenterology. 1997;112(5): 1448-56.

[97] Ronkainen J, Aro P, Storskrubb T et al. Prevalence of Barrett's esophagus in the general population: an endoscopic study. Gastroenterology. 2005;129(6): 1825-31.

[98] Spechler SJ. Barrett's esophagus. Semin Gastrointest Dis. 1996;7(2): 51–60.

[99] Cook MB., Wild CP, Forman D. A systematic review and meta-analysis of the sex ratio for Barrett's esophagus, erosive reflux disease, and nonerosive reflux disease. Am J Epidemiol. 2005;162(11): 1050-61.

[100] Abrams JA, Fields S, Lightdale CJ, Neugut AI. Racial and ethnic disparities in the prevalence of Barrett's esophagus among patients who undergo upper endoscopy. Clin Gastroenterol Hepatol. 2008;6(1): 30-4.

[101] Ward EM, Wolfsen HC, Achem SR, et al. Barrett's esophagus is common in older men and women undergoing screening colonoscopy regardless of reflux symptoms. Am J Gastroenterol. 2006;101(1):12–17.

[102] Lagergren J, Bergstrom R, Lindgren A, Nyren O. Symptomatic gastroesophageal reflux as a risk factor for esophageal adenocarcinoma. N Engl J Med. 1999;340(11): 825–831.

[103] Anderson LA, Murray LJ, Murphy SJ et al. Mortality in Barrett's oesophagus: results from a population based study. Gut. 2003;52(8): 1081-4.

[104] Schouten LJ, Steevens J, Huysentruyt CJ et al. Total cancer incidence and overall mortality are not increased among patients with Barrett's esophagus. Clin Gastroenterol Hepatol. 2011;9(9): 754-61.

[105] Boyer J, Laugier R, Chemali M et al. French Society of Digestive Endoscopy SFED guideline: monitoring of patients with Barrett's esophagus. Endoscopy. 2007;39(9): 840-2.

[106] Hirota WK, Zuckerman MJ, Adler DG et al. ASGE guideline: the role of endoscopy in the surveillance of premalignant conditions of the upper GI tract. Gastrointest Endosc. 2006;63(4): 570-80.

[107] Swain P. The future of wirelss capsule endoscopy. World J Gastroenterology 2008; 14(26): 4142-4145.

[108] Lin OS, Schrembre DB, Mergener K et al. Blinded comparison of esophageal capsule endoscopy for a diagnosis of barrett's esophagus in patients with chronic gastroesophageal reflux. Gastrointestinal Endoscopy 2007;65(4): 577-583.

[109] Bhardwaj A, Hollenbeak CS, Pooran N, Mathew A. A meta-analysis of the diagnostic accuracy of esophageal capsule endoscopy for Barrett's esophagus in patients with gastroesophageal reflux disease. Am J Gastroenterol. 2009;104(6): 1533-9.

[110] El-Serag HB, Naik AD. Surveillance in Barrett's esophagus: lessons from behavioral economics. Gastroenterology. 2009;137(3): 763–5.

[111] Lao-Sirieix P, Boussioutas A, Kadri SR et al. Non-endoscopic screening biomarkers for Barrett's oesophagus: from microarray analysis to the clinic. Gut. 2009;58(11): 1451–9.

[112] Kadri SR, Lao-Siriex P, O'Donovan M et al. Acceptability and accuracy of a non-endoscopic screening test for Barrett's oesophagus in primary care: cohort study. BMJ 2010; 341: c4372. doi: 11.1136/bmj.c4732.

[113] Sharma, P, Mcquaid K, Dent J et al. A critical review of the diagnosis and management of Barrett's esophagus: the AGA Chicago Workshop. Gastroenterology. 2004;127(1): 310-30

[114] Peters JH, Clark GW, Ireland AP, et al. Outcome of adenocarcinoma arising in Barrett's esophagus in endoscopically surveyed and nonsurveyed patients. J Thorac Cardiovasc Surg. 1994;108(5): 813-2.

[115] Fountoulakis A, Zafirellis KD, Dolan K et al. Effect of surveillance of Barrett's oesophagus on the clinical outcome of oesophageal cancer. Br J Surg. 2004;91(8): 997-1003.

[116] Corley DA, Levin TR, Habel LA et al. Surveillance and survival in Barrett's adenocarcinomas: a population-based study. Gastroenterology. 2002;122(3): 633-40.

[117] Sikkema M, De Jonge PJF, Steyerberg EW, Kuipers EJ. Risk of esophageal adenocarcinoma and mortality in patients with Barrett's esophagus: a systematic review and meta-analysis. Clin. Gastroenterol. Hepatol. 2010;8(3): 235–44.

[118] Kaltenbach T, Crockett S, Gerson LB. Are lifestyle measures effective in patients with gastroesophageal reflux disease? An evidence-based approach. Arch Intern Med. 2006;166(9): 965-71.

[119] Chiba N. Proton pump inhibitors in acute healing and maintenance of erosive or worse esophagitis: a systematic overview. Can J Gastroenterol. 1997;11(Suppl B): 66B–73B.

[120] Dent J, Bremner CJ, Collen MJ, Haggitt RC, Spechler SJ. Working party report to the World Congresses of Gastroenterology, Sydney 1990. Barrett's oesophagus. J. Gastroenterol. Hepatol. 1991; 6(1): 1–22.

[121] Khan M, Santana J, Donnellan C, Preston C, Moayyedi P. Medical treatments in the short term management of reflux oesophagitis. Cochrane Database Syst Rev. 2007;(2): CD003244.

[122] Abu-Sneineh A, Tam W, Schoeman M, et al. Effect of high-dose esomeprazole on gastric and oesophageal acid exposure and molecular markers in Barrett's oesophagus. Aliment. Pharmacol. Ther. 2010;32 (8): 1023–30.

[123] Gerson LB, Boparai V, Ullah N, Triadafilopoulos G. Oesophageal and gastric pH profiles in patients with gastro-oesophageal reflux disease and Barrett's oesophagus treated with proton pump inhibitors. Aliment Pharmacol Ther. 2004;20(6): 637-43.

[124] Fass R, Sampliner RE, Malagon IB, et al. Failure of oesophageal acid control in candidates for Barrett's oesophagus reversal on a very high dose of proton pump inhibitor. Aliment Pharmacol Ther. 2000;14(5): 597-602

[125] Basu KK, Bale R, West KP, de Caestecker JS. Persistent acid reflux and symptoms in patients with Barrett's oesophagus on proton-pump inhibitor therapy. Eur J Gastroenterol Hepatol. 2002;14(11): 1187-92.

[126] Mulholland MW, Reid BJ, Levine DS, Rubin CE. Elevated gastric acid secretion in patients with Barrett's metaplastic epithelium. Dig Dis Sci. 1989;34(9): 1329–34.

[127] Hirschowitz BI. Gastric acid and pepsin secretion in patients with Barrett's esophagus and appropriate controls. DigDis Sci. 1996;41(7): 1384–91.

[128] Milkes D, Gerson LB, Triadafilopoulos G. Complete elimination of reflux symptoms does not guarantee normalization of intraesophageal and intragastric pH in patients with gastroesophageal reflux disease (GERD). Am J Gastroenterol. 2004;99(6): 991-6.

[129] Yeh RW, Gerson LB, Triadafilopoulos G. Efficacy of esomeprazole in controlling reflux symptoms, intraesophageal, and intragastric pH in patients with Barrett's esophagus. Dis Esophagus. 2003;16(3): 193-8.

[130] Spechler SJ, Sharma P, Traxler B, Levine D, Falk GW. Gastric and esophageal pH in patients with Barrett's esophagus treated with three esomeprazole dosages: a randomized, double-blind, crossover trial. Am J Gastroenterol. 2006;101(9): 1964-71.

[131] Gerson LB, Mitra S, Bleker WF, Yeung P. Control of Intra-oesophageal pH in Patients With Barrett's Oesophagus on Omeprazole-sodium Bicarbonate Therapy. Aliment Pharmacol Ther. 2012;35(7): 803-9.

[132] Konda VJ, Dalal K. Optimal management of Barrett's esophagus: pharmacologic, endoscopic, and surgical interventions. Ther Clin Risk Manag. 2011; 7:447-58.

[133] Lanas A. Potent gastric acid inhibition in the management of Barrett's esophagus. Drugs. 2005;65(Suppl. 1): 75–82.

[134] Cooper BT, Chapman W, Neumann CS, Gearty JC. Continuous treatment of Barrett's oesophagus patients with proton pump inhibitors up to 13 years: observations on regression and cancer incidence. Aliment Pharmacol Ther 2006; 23(6): 727–33.

[135] Bhardwaj A, McGarrity TJ, Stairs DB, Mani H. Barrett's Esophagus: Emerging Knowledge and Management Strategies. Patholog Res Int. 2012; 2012:814146. doi: 10.1155/2012/814146.

[136] Sampliner RE. Reduction of acid exposure and regression of Barrett's esophagus. Dig Dis. 2000;18(4): 203–207.

[137] Weston AP, Badr AS, Hassanein RS. Prospective multivariate analysis of factors predictive of complete regression of Barrett's esophagus. Am J Gastroenterol. 1999;94(12): 3420–3426.

[138] García Rodríguez LA, Lagergren J, Lindblad M. Gastric acid suppression and risk of oesophageal and gastric adenocarcinoma: a nested case control study in the UK. Gut. 2006; 55(11):1538-44.

[139] Souza RF, Shewmake K, Terada LS, Spechler SJ. Acid exposure activates the mitogen-activated protein kinase pathways in Barrett's esophagus. Gastroenterology. 2002;122(2): 299-307.

[140] Sirieix PS, O'Donovan M, Brown J, Save V, Coleman N, Fitzgerald RC. Surface expression of minichromosome maintenance proteins provides a novel method for detecting patients at risk for developing adenocarcinoma in Barrett's esophagus. Clin Cancer Res. 2003;9(7): 2560–6.

[141] Kedika RR, Souza RF, Spechler SJ. Potential anti-inflammatory effects of proton pump inhibitors: a review and discussion of the clinical implications. Dig Dis Sci. 2009;54(11): 2312–7.

[142] Abu-Sneineh A, Tam W, Schoeman M, Fraser R, Ruszkiewicz AR, Smith E, Drew PA, Dent J, Holloway RH.Gastric and Oesophageal Acid Exposure and Molecular Markers in Barrett's Oesophagus. Aliment Pharmacol Ther. 2010; 32(8): 1023-30.

[143] Spechler SJ, Fitzgerald RC, Prasad GA, Wang KK. History, molecular mechanisms, and endoscopic treatment of Barrett's esophagus. Gastroenterology. 2010;138(3): 854-69.

[144] Chang EY, Morris CD, Seltman AK, O'Rourke RW, Chan BK, Hunter JG, Jobe BA. The effect of antireflux surgery on esophageal carcinogenesis in patients with Barrett esophagus. Ann. Surg. 2007;246(1): 11–21.

[145] Lagergren J, Ye W, Lagergren P, Lu Y. The risk of esophageal adenocarcinoma after antireflux surgery. Gastroenterology. 2010;138(4): 1297–301.

[146] El-Serag HB, Aguirre TV, Davis S, Kuebeler M, Bhattacharyya A, Sampliner RE. Proton pump inhibitors are associated with reduced incidence of dysplasia in Barrett's esophagus. Am J Gastroenterol. 2004;99(10): 1877–83.

[147] Hillman LC, Chiragakis L, Shadbolt B, Kaye GL, Clarke AC. Effect of proton pump inhibitors on markers of risk for high-grade dysplasia and oesophageal cancer in Barrett's oesophagus. AlimentPharmacol Ther. 2008;27(4): 321–6.

[148] Hillman LC, Chiragakis L, Shadbolt B, Kaye GL, Clarke AC. Proton-pump inhibitor therapy and the development of dysplasia in patients with Barrett's oesophagus. Med J Aust 2004;180(8): 387–91.

[149] Gatenby PA, Ramus JR, Caygill CP, Charlett A, Winslet MC, Watson A. Treatment modality and risk of development of dysplasia and adenocarcinoma in columnar-lined esophagus. Dis Esophagus. 2009;22(2): 133–142.

[150] Nguyen DM, El-Serag HB, Henderson L, Stein D, Bhattacharyya A, Sampliner RE. Medication usage and the risk of neoplasia in patients with Barrett's esophagus. Clin Gastroenterol Hepatol. 2009;7(12): 1299–1304.

[151] Spechler SJ, Sharma P, Souza RF, Inadomi JM, Shaheen NJ. American Gastroenterological Association medical position statement on the management of Barrett's esophagus. Gastroenterology. 2011;140(3):1084–1091.

[152] Zehetner J, DeMeester SR, Ayazi S, et al. Long-term follow-up after anti-reflux surgery in patients with Barrett's esophagus. J Gastrointest Surg. 2010;14(10): 1483–1491.

[153] Lagergren J, Viklund P. Is esophageal adenocarcinoma occurring late after antireflux surgery due to persistent postoperative reflux? World J Surg. 2007;31(3): 465–469.

[154] Lagergren J, Ye W, Lagergren P, Lu Y. The risk of esophageal adenocarcinoma after antireflux surgery. Gastroenterology 2010;138(4): 1297–301.

[155] Parrilla P, Martínez de Haro LF, Ortiz A, Munitiz V, Serrano A,Torres G. Barrett's esophagus without esophageal stricture does not increase the rate of failure of Nissen fundoplication. Ann. Surg. 2003;237(4): 488–93.

[156] Anderson LA, Johnston BT, Watson RGP, et al. Nonsteroidal anti-inflammatory drugs and the esophageal inflammation-metaplasia-adenocarcinoma sequence. Cancer Res. 2006;66(9): 4975–82.

[157] Thrift AP, Pandeya N, Smith KJ, Green AC, Webb PM, Whiteman DC. The use of nonsteroidal anti-inflammatory drugs and the risk of Barrett's oesophagus. Aliment Pharmacol Ther. 2011;34(10): 1235-44.

[158] Duan L, Wu AH, Sullivan-Halley J, Bernstein L.Nonsteroidal anti-inflammatory drugs and risk of esophageal and gastric adenocarcinomas in Los Angeles County. Cancer Epidemiol Biomarkers Prev. 2008;17(1): 126–34.

[159] Sadeghi S, Bain CJ, Pandeya N, Webb PM, Green AC, Whiteman DC; Australian Cancer Study.Aspirin, nonsteroidal anti-inflammatory drugs, and the risks of cancers of the esophagus. Cancer Epidemiol Biomarkers Prev. 2008;17(5): 1169–78.

[160] Ilyas S, DeMars CJ, Buttar NS. Chemoprevention in Barrett's esophagus. J. Gastroint-est. Cancer 2007; 38(1): 1–9.

[161] Nguyen DM, Richardson P, El-Serag HB. Medications (NSAIDs, statins, proton pump inhibitors) and the risk of esophageal adenocarcinoma in patients with Barrett's esophagus. Gastroenterology. 2010;138(7): 2260–6.

[162] Gatenby PA, Ramus JR, Caygill CP, Winslet MC, Watson A.Aspirin is not chemoprotective for Barrett's adenocarcinoma of the oesophagus in multicentre cohort. Eur. J. Cancer Prev. 2009;18(5): 381–4.

[163] Corley DA, Kerlikowske K, Verma J, Buffler P. Protective association of aspirin/NSAIDs and esophageal cancer: a systematic review and meta-analysis. Gastroenterology 2003; 124(1): 47–56.

[164] Kastelein F, Spaander MC, Biermann K, Steyerberg EW, Kuipers EJ, Bruno MJ; Probar-study Group. Nonsteroidal anti-inflammatory drugs and statins have chemopreventative effects in patients with Barrett's esophagus. Gastroenterology. 2011;141(6): 2000-8.

[165] Vaughan TL, Dong LM, Blount PL, et al. Non-steroidal anti-inflammatory drugs and risk of neoplastic progression in Barrett's oesophagus: A prospective study. Lancet Oncol. 2005;6(12): 945–952.

[166] Heath EI, Canto MI, Piantadosi S, et al. Secondary chemoprevention of Barrett's esophagus with celecoxib: Results of a randomized trial.J Natl Cancer Inst. 2007;99(7): 545–557.

[167] Ogunwobi OO, Beales IL.Statins inhibit proliferation and induce apoptosis in Barrett's esophageal adenocarcinoma cells. Am J Gastroenterol. 2008;103(4): 825-37.

[168] Konturek PC, Burnat G, Hahn EG. Inhibition of Barret's adenocarcinoma cell growth by simvastatin: involvement of COX-2 and apoptosis-related proteins. J Physiol Pharmacol. 2007;58(Suppl 3):141-8.

[169] Chennat J, Waxman I. Endoscopic treatment of Barrett's esophagus: From metaplasia to intramucosal carcinoma. World J Gastroenterol. 2010;16(30): 3780-3785.

[170] Bisschops R. Optimal Endoluminal Treatment of Barrett's Esophagus: Integrating Novel Strategies into Clinical Practice. Expert Rev Gastroenterol Hepatol. 2010;4(3): 319-333.

[171] Konda VJ, Waxman I. Endotherapy for Barrett's esophagus. Am J Gastroenterol. 2012;107(6): 827-33.

[172] Hudson M, Lin CL, Habr F.Current state of endoscopic therapies in Barrett's esophagus and esophageal cancer. Hosp Pract (Minneap). 2011;39(1):170-80.

[173] ASGE TECHNOLOGY COMMITTEE, Kantsevoy SV, Adler DG, Conway JD, Diehl DL, Farraye FA, Kwon R, Mamula P, Rodriguez S, Shah RJ, Wong Kee Song LM, Tierney WM. Endoscopic mucosal resection and endoscopic submucosal dissection. Gastrointest Endosc. 2008; 68(1): 11-18.

[174] Wang KK, Prasad G, Tian J. Endoscopic mucosal resection and endoscopic submucosal dissection in esophageal and gastric cancers. Curr Opin Gastroenterol. 2010;26(5): 453–458.

[175] Chennat J, Konda VJ, Waxman I. Endotherapy for Barrett's esophagus: which, how, when, and who? Gastrointest Endosc Clin N Am. 2011;21(1): 119–133.

[176] May A , Gossner L , Behrens A et al. A prospective randomized trial of two diff erent endoscopic resection techniques for early stage cancer of the esophagus. Gastrointest Endosc. 2003; 58(2): 167–175.

[177] Abrams JA , Fedi P , Vakiani E et al. Depth of resection using two diff erent endoscopic mucosal resection techniques. Endoscopy. 2008;40(5): 395 – 9.

[178] Garud SS, Keilin S, Cai Q, Willingham FF. Diagnosis and management of Barrett's esophagus for the endoscopist. Therap Adv Gastroenterol. 2010;3(4): 227-38.

[179] Ell C, May A, Gossner L, Pech O, Günter E, Mayer G, Henrich R, Vieth M, Müller H, Seitz G, Stolte M. Endoscopic mucosal resection of early cancer and high-grade dysplasia in Barrett's esophagus. Gastroenterology. 2000;118(4): 670-7.

[180] Pech O, Behrens A, May A, et al. Long-term results and risk factor analysis for recurrence after curative endoscopic therapy in 349 patients with high-grade intraepithelial neoplasia and mucosal adenocarcinoma in Barrett's oesophagus. Gut. 2008;57(9): 1200–1206.

[181] May A, Gossner L, Pech O, Müller H, Vieth M, Stolte M, Ell C. Intraepithelial high-grade neoplasia and early adenocarcinoma in short-segment Barrett's esophagus (SSBE): curative treatment using local endoscopic treatment techniques. Endoscopy 2002; 34(8): 604-610.

[182] Pech O, May A, Gossner L, Ell C. Barrett's esophagus: endoscopic resection. Gastrointest Endosc Clin N Am 2003; 13(3): 505-512.

[183] Mino-Kenudson M, Brugge WR, Puricelli WP, Nakatsuka LN, Nishioka NS, Zukerberg LR, Misdraji J, Lauwers GY. Management of superficial Barrett's epithelium-related neoplasms by endoscopic mucosal resection: clinicopathologic analysis of 27 cases. Am J Surg Pathol. 2005; 29(5): 680-686.

[184] Tschanz ER. Do 40% of patients resected for Barrett esophagus with high-grade dysplasia have unsuspected adenocarcinoma? Arch Pathol Lab Med. 2005;129(2):177–180.

[185] Wang VS, Hornick JL, Sepulveda J, Mauer R, Poneros JM. Low prevalence of submucosal invasive carcinoma at esophagectomy for high-grade dysplasia or intramucosal adenocarcinoma in Barrett's esophagus: a 20 year experience. Gastrointest Endosc. 2009;69(4): 777–783.

[186] Pech O, Behrens A, May A et al. Long-term results and risk factor analysis for recurrence after curative endoscopic therapy in 349 patients with high-grade intraepithelial neoplasia and mucosal adenocarcinoma in Barrett's oesophagus. Gut. 2008;57(9): 1200-6.

[187] Peters FP, Brakenhoff KP, Curvers WL et al. Endoscopic cap resection for treatment of early Barrett's neoplasia is safe: a prospective analysis of acute and early complications in 216 procedures. Dis Esophagus. 2007;20(6):510-5.

[188] Peters FP, Kara MA, Curvers WL et al. Multiband mucosectomy for endoscopic resection of Barrett's esophagus: feasibility study with matched historical controls. Eur J Gastroenterol Hepatol. 2007;19(4): 311-5.

[189] Peters FP, Kara MA, Rosmolen WD et al. Stepwise radical endoscopic resection is effective for complete removal of Barrett's esophagus with early neoplasia: a prospective study. Am J Gastroenterol. 2006;101(7): 1449-57.

[190] Peters FP, Kara MA, Rosmolen WD et al. Endoscopic treatment of high-grade dysplasia and early stage cancer in Barrett's esophagus. Gastrointest Endosc. 2005;61(4): 506-14.

[191] Ell C, May A, Pech O et al. Curative endoscopic resection of early esophageal adenocarcinomas (Barrett's cancer). Gastrointest Endosc. 2007;65(1): 3-10.

[192] Behrens A, May A, Gossner L et al. Curative treatment for high-grade intraepithelial neoplasia in Barrett's esophagus. Endoscopy. 2005;37(10): 999-1005.

[193] Conio M, Repici A, Cestari R et al. Endoscopic mucosal resection for high-grade dysplasia and intramucosal carcinoma in Barrett's esophagus: an Italian experience. World J Gastroenterol. 2005;11(42): 6650-5.

[194] Seewald S, Akaraviputh T, Seitz U et al. Circumferential EMR and complete removal of Barrett's epithelium: a new approach to management of Barrett's esophagus containing high-grade intraepithelial neoplasia and intramucosal carcinoma. Gastrointest Endosc. 2003;57(7): 854-9.

[195] Giovannini M, Bories E, Pesenti C et al. Circumferential endoscopic mucosal resection in Barrett's esophagus with high-grade intraepithelial neoplasia or mucosal cancer: preliminary results in 21 patients. Endoscopy. 2004;36(9):782-7.

[196] Lopes CV, Hela M, Pesenti C et al. Circumferential endoscopic resection of Barrett's esophagus with high-grade dysplasia or early adenocarcinoma. Surg Endosc. 2007;21(5): 820-4.

[197] Pouw RE, Peters FP, Sempoux C, Piessevaux H, Deprez PH. Stepwise radical endoscopic resection for Barrett's esophagus with early neoplasia: report on a Brussels' cohort. Endoscopy. 2008;40(11): 892-8.

[198] Chennat J, Konda VJ, Ross AS et al. Complete Barrett's eradication endoscopic mucosal resection: an effective treatment modality for high-grade dysplasia and intramucosal carcinoma – an American single-center experience. Am J Gastroenterol. 2009;104(11): 2684-92.

[199] Pech O, May A, Rabenstein T, Ell C. Endoscopic resection of early oesophageal cancer. Gut. 2007;56(11):1625-34.

[200] Pouw RE , Seewald S , Gondrie JJ et al. Stepwise radical endoscopic resection for eradication of Barrett's oesophagus with early neoplasia in a cohort of 169 patients. Gut. 2010;59(9): 1169-77.

[201] Tang SJ, Tang L, Jazrawi SF. Circumferential endoscopic mucosal resection of a 14-cm Barrett's dysplasia with the Duette mucosectomy device (with videos). Gastrointest. Endosc. 2008; 68(4): 786–789.

[202] Peters FP, Krishnadath KK, Rygiel AM et al. Stepwise radical endoscopic resection of the complete Barrett's esophagus with early neoplasia successfully eradicates pre-existing genetic abnormalities. Am J Gastroenterol. 2007;102(9): 1853-61.

[203] van Vilsteren FG , Pouw RE , Seewald S et al. Stepwise radical endoscopic resection versus radiofrequency ablation for Barrett's oesophagus with high-grade dysplasia or early cancer: a multicentre randomised trial. Gut 2011;60(6): 765-73.

[204] Yoshida M, Hanashi T, Momma K, Yamada Y, Sakaki N, Koike M et al. Endoscopic mucosal resection for radical treatment of esophageal cancer. Gan To Kagaku Ryoho. 1995;22(7): 847-54.

[205] Manner H, May A, Pech O et al. Early Barrett's carcinoma with "low-risk" submucosal invasion: long-term results of endoscopic resection with a curative intent. Am. J. Gastroenterol. 2008;103(10): 2589–2597.

[206] Buskens CJ, Westerterp M, Lagarde SM et al. Prediction of appropriateness of local endoscopic treatment for high-grade dysplasia and early adenocarcinoma by EUS and histopathologic features. Gastrointest. Endosc.2004; 60(5): 703–710.

[207] Seewald S, Ang TL, Gotoda T, Soehendra N. Total endoscopic resection of Barrett esophagus. Endoscopy. 2008;40(12): 1016–1020.

[208] Yoshinaga S, Gotoda T, Kusano C, Oda I, Nakamura K, Takayanagi R.Clinical impact of endoscopic submucosal dissection for superficial adenocarcinoma located at the esophagogastric junction. Gastrointest Endosc. 2008;67(2): 202–209.

[209] Van Laethem JL , Peny MO , Salmon I et al. Intramucosal adenocarcinoma arising under squamous re-epithelialisation of Barrett's oesophagus. Gut. 2000;46(4): 574 – 7.

[210] Vladimirov, B., L. Dinkov, M. Donov, I. Terziev, N. Grigorov, R. Mitova, J. Churchev, E. Astrukov. Endoscopic APC therapy of Barrett. 8th UEGW, Brussels, 25-30 November, 2000, Endoscopy. 2000; 32(Suppl.1): E32 (P90E).

[211] Vladimirov, B., .L. Dinkov, .M. Donov, .I. Terziev, .N. Grigorov, .R. Mitova, .J. Churchev. Endoscopic Argon plasma coagulation plus PPI versus PPI only in patients with low-grade dysplasia of Barrett's esophagus. 10th UEGW, Geneva 19-24 October, 2002, Gut 2002; 51(Suppl III): A26.

[212] Gross SA, Wolfsen HC. The role of photodynamic therapy in the esophagus. Gastrointest Endosc Clin N Am. 2010; 20(1): 35-53.

[213] Ackroyd R, Kelty CJ, Brown NJ, Stephenson TJ, Stoddard CJ, Reed MW. Eradication of dysplastic Barrett's oesophagus using photodynamic therapy: long-term follow-up. Endoscopy. 2003;35(6): 496-501.

[214] Overholt BF, Panjehpour M, Haydek JM. Photodynamic therapy for Barrett's esophagus: follow-up in 100 patients. Gastrointest Endosc. 1999;49(1): 1-7.

[215] Overholt BF, Panjehpour M, Halberg DL. Photodynamic therapy for Barrett's esophagus with dysplasia and/or early stage carcinoma: long-term results. Gastrointest Endosc. 2003;58(2): 183-8.

[216] Pech O, Gossner L, May A et al. Long-term results of photodynamic therapy with 5-aminolevulinic acid for superficial Barrett's cancer and high-grade intraepithelial neoplasia. Gastrointest Endosc. 2005;62(1): 24-30.

[217] Sharma VK, Wang KK, Overholt BF et al. Balloon-based, circumferential, endoscopic radiofrequency ablation of Barrett's esophagus: 1-year follow-up of 100 patients (with video). Gastrointest Endosc. 2007;65(2): 185-95.

[218] Fleischer D, Overholt B, Sharma VK et al. Endoscopic ablation of Barrett's esophagus: a multicenter study with 2.5-year follow-up. Gastrointest Endosc. 2008;68(5): 867-76.

[219] Hage M, Siersema PD, van Dekken H et al. 5-aminolevulinic acid photo-dynamic therapy versus argon plasma coagulation for ablation of Barrett's oesophagus: a randomised trial. Gut. 2004;53(6): 785-90.

[220] Peters F, Kara M, Rosmolen W et al. Poor results of 5-aminolevulinic acid-photodynamic therapy for residual high-grade dysplasia and early cancer in Barrett esophagus after endoscopic resection. Endoscopy. 2005;37(5): 418-24.

[221] Overholt BF, Lightdale CJ, Wang KK et al. Photodynamic therapy with porfimer sodium for ablation of high-grade dysplasia in Barrett's esophagus: international, partially blinded, randomized Phase III trial. Gastrointest Endosc. 2005;62(4): 488-98.

[222] Overholt BF, Wang KK, Burdick JS, Lightdale CJ, Kimmey M, Nava HR, Sivak MV Jr, Nishioka N, Barr H, Marcon N,Pedrosa M, Bronner MP, Grace M, Depot M. International Photodynamic Group for High-Grade Dysplasia in Barrett's Esophagus. Five-year efficacy and safety of photodynamic therapy with Photofrin in Barrett's high-grade dysplasia. Gastrointest Endosc. 2007;66(3): 460–468.

[223] Prasad GA, Wang KK, Buttar NS, Wongkeesong LM, Krishnadath KK, Nichols FC 3rd, Lutzke LS, Borkenhagen LS. Long-term survival following endoscopic and surgical treatment of high-grade dysplasia in Barrett's esophagus. Gastroenterology. 2007;132(4): 1226-1233.

[224] Anwar SA , Kanthan SK, Riaz AA. Current Management of Barrett's Oesophagus. BJMP 2009; 2(4): 8-14.

[225] Wolfsen HC, Hemminger LL, Raimondo M, Woodward TA. Photodynamic therapy and endoscopic mucosal resection for Barrett's dysplasia and early esophageal adenocarcinoma. South Med J. 2004;97(9): 827–830.

[226] Lovat LB, Jamieson NF, Novelli MR, et al. Photodynamic therapy with m-tetrahydroxyphenyl chlorin for high-grade dysplasia and early cancer in Barrett's columnar lined esophagus. Gastrointest Endosc. 2005;62(4): 617–623.

[227] Pacifico RJ, Wang KK, Wongkeesong LM, Buttar NS, Lutzke LS. Combined endoscopic mucosal resection and photodynamic therapy versus esophagectomy for management of early adenocarcinoma in Barrett's esophagus. Clin Gastroneterol Hepatol. 2003;1(4): 252–257.

[228] Ganz RA, Utley DS, Stern RA, Jackson J, Batts KP, Termin P. Complete ablation of esophageal epithelium with a balloon-based bipolar electrode: a phase evaluation in the porcine and in the human esophagus. Gastrointest Endosc. 2004;60(6): 1002–1010.

[229] Fleischer DE, Overholt BF, Sharma VK, et al. Endoscopic ablation of Barrett's esophagus: a multicenter study with 2.5 year follow-up. Gastrointest Endosc. 2008;68(5): 867–876.

[230] Sharma VK, Jae Kim H, Das A, Wells CD, Nguyen CC, Fleischer DE. Circumferential and focal ablation of Barrett's esophagus containing dysplasia. Am J Gastroenterol. 2009;104(2): 310–317.

[231] Shaheen NJ, Overholt BF, Sampliner RE et al. Durability of radiofrequency ablation in Barrett's esophagus with dysplasia. Gastroenterology. 2011;141(2): 460-8.

[232] Ganz RA, Overholt BF, Sharma VK, et al; U.S. Multicenter Registry. Circumferential ablation of Barrett's esophagus that contains high-grade dysplasia: a U.S. multicenter registry. Gastrointest Endosc. 2008;68(1): 35–40.

[233] Lyday WD, Corbett FS, Kuperman DA, et al. Radiofrequency ablation of Barrett's esophagus: outcomes of 429 patients from a multicenter community practice registry. Endoscopy. 2010;42(4): 272–278.

[234] Shaheen NJ, Sharma P, Overholt BF et al. Radiofrequency ablation in Barrett's esophagus with dysplasia. N. Engl. J. Med. 2009;360(22): 2277–2288.

[235] Gondrie JJ, Pouw RE, Sondermeijer CM et al. Effective treatment of early Barrett's neoplasia with stepwise circumferential and focal ablation using the HALO system. Endoscopy. 2008;40(5): 370–379.

[236] Gondrie JJ, Pouw RE, Sondermeijer CM et al. Stepwise circumferential and focal ablation of Barrett's esophagus with high-grade dysplasia: results of the first prospective series of 11 patients. Endoscopy. 2008;40(5): 359–369.

[237] Pouw RE, Gondrie JJ, Sondermeijer CM et al. Eradication of Barrett esophagus with early neoplasia by radiofrequency ablation, with or without endoscopic resection. J. Gastrointest. Surg. 2008;12(10): 1627–1637.

[238] Pouw RE, Wirths K, Eisendrath P et al. Efficacy of radiofrequency ablation combined with endoscopic resection for Barrett's esophagus with early neoplasia. Clin. Gastroenterol. Hepatol. 2010;8(1): 23–29.

[239] Roorda AK, Marcus SN, Triadafilopoulos G. Early experience with radiofrequency energy ablation therapy for Barrett's esophagus with and without dysplasia. Dis. Esophagus. 2007;20(6): 516–522.

[240] Hernandez JC, Reicher S, Chung D et al. Pilot series of radiofrequency ablation of Barrett's esophagus with or without neoplasia. Endoscopy. 2008;40(5): 388–392.

[241] Herrero LA , van Vilsteren FG , Pouw RE et al. Endoscopic radiofrequency ablation combined with endoscopic resection for early neoplasia in Barrett's esophagus longer than 10 cm. Gastrointest Endosc.2011;73(4): 682-90.

[242] Beaumont H, Gondrie JJ, McMahon BP et al. Stepwise radiofrequency ablation of Barrett's esophagus preserves esophageal inner diameter, compliance, and motility. Endoscopy. 2009;41(1): 2–8.

[243] Pouw RE, Gondrie JJ, Rygiel AM, Sondermeijer CM, et al. Properties of the neosquamous epithelium after radiofrequency ablation of Barrett's esophagus containing neoplasia. Am J Gastroenterol. 2009;104(6): 1366-1373.

[244] Dumot JA, Vargo JJ 2nd, Falk GW, Frey L, Lopez R, Rice TW. An open-label, prospective trial of cryospray ablation for Barrett's esophagus high-grade dysplasia and early esophageal cancer in high-risk patients. Gastrointest Endosc. 2009;70(4): 635–644.

[245] Shaheen NJ, Greenwald BD, Peery AF, et al. Safety and efficacy of endoscopic spray cryotherapy for Barrett's esophagus with high-grade dysplasia. Gastrointest Endosc. 2010;71(4): 680–685.

[246] Greenwald BD, Dumot JA, Horwhat JD, Lightdale CJ, Abrams JA. Safety, tolerability, and efficacy of endoscopic low-pressure liquid nitrogen spray cryotherapy in the esophagus. Dis Esophagus. 2010;23(1):13-9.

[247] Canto M, Gorospe EC, Shin EJ et al. Carbon dioxide (CO2) cryotherapy is a safe and effective treatment of Barrett's esophagus with HGD/intramucosal carcinoma. Gastrointest. Endosc. 2009; 69: AB341.

[248] Greenwald BD, Dumot JA, Abrams JA et al. Endoscopic spray cryotherapy for esophageal cancer: safety and efficacy. Gastrointest Endosc. 2010;71(4): 686 – 93.

[249] Das A, Wells C, Kim HJ, Fleischer DE, Crowell MD, Sharma VK. An economic analysis of endoscopic ablative therapy for management of nondysplastic Barrett's esophagus. Endoscopy. 2009;41(5):400–408.

[250] Inadomi JM, Somsouk M, Madanick RD, Thomas JP, Shaheen NJ. A cost-utility analysis of ablative therapy for Barrett's esopahgus. Gastoenterology. 2009;136(7): 2101–2114.

[251] Ferguson MK, Naunheim KS. Resection for Barrett's mucosa with high-grade dysplasia: implications for prophylactic photodynamic therapy. J Thorac Cardiovasc Surg 1997;114(5):824-829.

[252] Pellegrini CA, Pohl D. High-grade dysplasia in Barrett's esophagus: surveillance or operation? J Gastrointest Surg. 2000; 4(2): 131-134.

[253] Pech O, Behrens A, May A, et al. Long-term results and risk factor analysis for recurrence after curative endoscopic therapy in 349 patients with high-grade intraepithelial neoplasia and mucosal adenocarcinoma in Barrett's oesophagus. Gut. 2008; 57(9): 1200-1206.

[254] Bozio G, Baulieux J, Mabrut JY. The role of surgery in the management of Barrett's esophagus (from dysplasia to cancer). J Visc Surg. 2011;148(1): 19–26.

[255] Bailey SH, Bull DA, Harpole DH, et al. Outcomes after esophagectomy: A ten-year prospective cohort. Ann Thorac Surg. 2003;75(1): 217–222.

[256] Viklund, P.,Wengstrom, Y., Rouvelas, I., Lindblad, M. and Lagergren, J. Quality of life and persisting symptoms after oesophageal cancer surgery. Eur J Cancer. 2006;42(10): 1407–1414.

[257] Fernando HC, Murthy SC, Hofstetter W, et al. The Society of Thoracic Surgeons practice guideline series: Guidelines for the management of Barrett's esophagus with high-grade dysplasia. Ann Thorac Surg. 2009;87(6): 1993–2002.

[258] Birkmeyer JD, Stukel TA, Siewers AE, Goodney PP, Wennberg DE, Lucas FL. Surgeon volume and operative mortality in the United States. N Engl J Med. 2003;349(22): 2117–2127.

[259] Law S. Esophagectomy without mortality: What can surgeons do? J Gastrointest Surg. 2010;14 (Suppl 1): S101–S107.

[260] van Lanschot JJ, Hulscher JB, Buskens CJ, et al. Hospital volume and hospital mortality for esophagectomy. Cancer. 2001;91(8):1574-8.

[261] Rice TW. Pro: Esophagectomy is the treatment of choice for high-grade dysplasia in Barrett's esophagus. Am J Gastroenterol. 2006;101(10): 2177–2179.

[262] Reed MF, Tolis G Jr, Edil BH, et al. Surgical treatment of esophageal high-grade dysplasia. Ann Thorac Surg. 2005;79(4): 1110–1115.

[263] Tseng EE, Wu TT, Yeo CJ, Heitmiller RF. Barrett's esophagus with high grade dysplasia: Surgical results and long-term outcome – anupdate. J Gastrointest Surg. 2003;7(2): 164–170.

[264] Headrick JR, Nichols FC 3rd, Miller DL, et al. High-grade esophageal dysplasia: Long-term survival and quality of life after esophagectomy. Ann Thorac Surg. 2002;73(6): 1697–1702.

[265] Wolfsen HC, Hemminger LL, DeVault KR. Recurrent Barrett's esophagus and adenocarcinoma after esophagectomy. BMC Gastroenterol.2004;4: 18.

[266] Hulscher JB, van Sandick JW, de Boer AG, et al. Extended transthoracic resection compared with limited transhiatal resection for adenocarcinoma of the esophagus. N Engl J Med. 2002;347(21): 1662–1669.

[267] Wolff CS, Castillo SF, Larson DR, et al. Ivor Lewis approach is superior to transhiatal approach in retrieval of lymph nodes at esophagectomy.Dis Esophagus. 2008;21(4): 328–333.

[268] Biere SS, Cuesta MA, van der Peet DL. Minimally invasive versus open esophagectomy for cancer: A systematic review and metaanalysis.Minerva Chir. 2009;64(2): 121–133.

[269] Biere SS, Maas KW, Bonavina L, et al. Traditional invasive vs minimally invasive esophagectomy: a multi-center, randomized trial (TIME-trial). BMC Surg. 2011;11: 2.

[270] Decker G, Coosemans W, De Leyn P, et al. Minimally invasive esophagectomy for cancer. Eur J Cardiothorac Surg. 2009;35(1): 13–20.

[271] Peyre CG, DeMeester SR, Rizzetto C, et al. Vagal-sparing esophagectomy: The ideal operation for intramucosal adenocarcinoma and Barrett with high-grade dysplasia. Ann Surg. 2007;246(4): 665–671.

[272] Ajani JA., Barthel JS., Bekaii-Saab T. et al. Esophageal Cancer. J Natl Compr Canc Netw. 2008;6(9):818-49.

[273] Stahl M, Oliveira J, ESMO Guidelines Working Group. Esophageal cancer: ESMO clinical recommendations for diagnosis, treatment and follow-up. Ann Oncol. 2009;20(Suppl 4): 32-3.

[274] Konda VJ, Ferguson MK. Esophageal resection for high-grade dysplasia and intramucosal carcinoma: When and how? World J Gastroenterol. 2010;16(30): 3786–3792.

[275] Prasad GA, Wu TT, Wigle DA, Buttar NS et al. Endoscopic and surgical treatment of mucosal (T1a) esophageal adenocarcinoma in Barrett's esophagus. Gastroenterology 2009;137(3): 815–823.

[276] Schembre DB, Huang JL, Lin OS et al. Treatment of Barrett's esophagus with early neoplasia: a comparison of endoscopic therapy and esophagectomy. Gastrointest. Endosc.2008; 67(4): 595–601.

Clinical Outcome of Endoscopic Submucosal Dissection for 352 Lesions of Superficial Gastric Neoplasms in 284 Patients

Yasutoshi Ochiai, Shin Arai, Masamitsu Nakao,
Makoto Nishimura, Takashi Shono, Kouichi Nonaka,
Osamu Togawa, Keiko Ishikawa and Hiroto Kita

Additional information is available at the end of the chapter

http://dx.doi.org/10.5772/52521

1. Introduction

One of the most significant topics for therapeutic endoscopy in recent years is the development of new therapeutic strategies for gastric neoplasms, called endoscopic submucosal dissection (ESD)[1]-[7]. This technique was developed to allow resection of difficult lesions with characteristics such as large size, irregular shape, coexisting ulcer findings or difficult location that could not be resected en bloc using conventional endoscopic mucosal resection (EMR). One of the most important benefits of this procedure is to obtain accurate histological diagnosis. Additional benefits of ESD include that it is minimally invasive in nature and allows preservation of the entire stomach, resulting in the improved postoperative quality of life[8], [9]. Therefore, ESD is widely accepted as a standard treatment strategy for gastric neoplasm.

In this study, we conducted consecutive gastric ESD for superficial gastric neoplasms, and compared the results between under 64 years old (non elderly group; NEG) and over 65 years old (elderly group; EG) to evaluate the safety, efficacy and long-term outcomes, especially in the elderly people. We defined over 65 years old as EG according to a definition of World Health Organization (WHO).

Design: Retrospective, non-randomized, controlled clinical study

2. Patients and methods

Between April 2007 and March 2010, a total of 284 patients with superficial gastric neoplasm were treated with ESD at our institution. The resected specimens were evaluated histopathologically in all cases. Using a database, outcomes were compared between NEG and EG, retrospectively, including resected specimen size, tumor size, en-bloc resection rate, complete en-bloc resection rate, mean procedure time, hospital days after ESD, histopathological findings, complications and 1 and 3-year overall survival rate. After the initial treatment, all cases were observed (mean period: 796.5 days, range: 6-1812 days), and the local recurrence rate and overall survival period of the each group were analyzed. Data were collected and analyzed.

2.1. Preoperative diagnosis

The indication for ESD was determined from the endoscopic feature of the lesions, including white light observation, chromoendoscopy. Magnifying endoscopy with narrow band imaging (NBI) were also used, whenever necessary, in order to recognize the demarcated line between normal mucosa and lesion and to estimate the depth of the lesion[10]. Endoscopic ultrasonography (EUS) was also performed for the assessment of the invasion depth and/or presence of ulceration in cases in which submucosal invasion or ulceration is suspected. Contrast-enhanced computed tomography (CECT) was performed for preoperative detection of distant and/or lymph node metastases.

2.2. ESD technique

The ESD technique has been precisely described elsewhere[11]-[13]. In brief, ESD procedures were performed by using video endoscopes (GIF-Q260J; Olympus Optical Co, Ltd, Tokyo, Japan). A tip-transparent hood was attached to the top of the endoscope (Figure 1). A high-frequency power supply VIO300D (ERBE Elektromedizin, Germany) was used. Either flush knife (KD-2618 JN-15; Fujinon, Tokyo, Japan) (Figure 2a), dual knife (KD-650; Olympus, Tokyo, Japan) (Figure 2b), or flex knife (KD-630L; Olympus, Tokyo, Japan) (Figure 2c) was used as the electrosurgical knife for circumferential mucosal cutting around the tumor with a sufficient safety margin and also submucosal dissection beneath the lesion. Hook knife (KD-620LR; Olympus) (Figure 2d) was used if necessary. Sodium hyaluronate 0.4% (Mucoup; Johnson & Johnson, Tokyo, Japan), mixed with a small amount of indigo carmine dye and epinephrine, was used as the material for local injection into submucosal layer. By mixing a small amount of indigo carmine dye and epinephrine into sodium hyaluronate solution, visualization of the submucosal layer to be dissected was much easier, and bleeding during the procedure was also diminished. The resected specimen was removed and evaluated histopathologically. Hemostatic forceps (HDB2422W; Pentax, Tokyo, Japan) (Figure 2e) were used to control bleeding during the procedure or for ablation of visible vessels on the mucosal defect after resection. One day after the ESD, a second-look endoscopy was performed, along with preventive hemostasis, as needed. ESD was usually carried out under conscious sedation using midazolam and pethidine hydrochloride. The patients were preselected and treated under general anesthesia in cases that the treatment time was expected to exceed 2 hours.

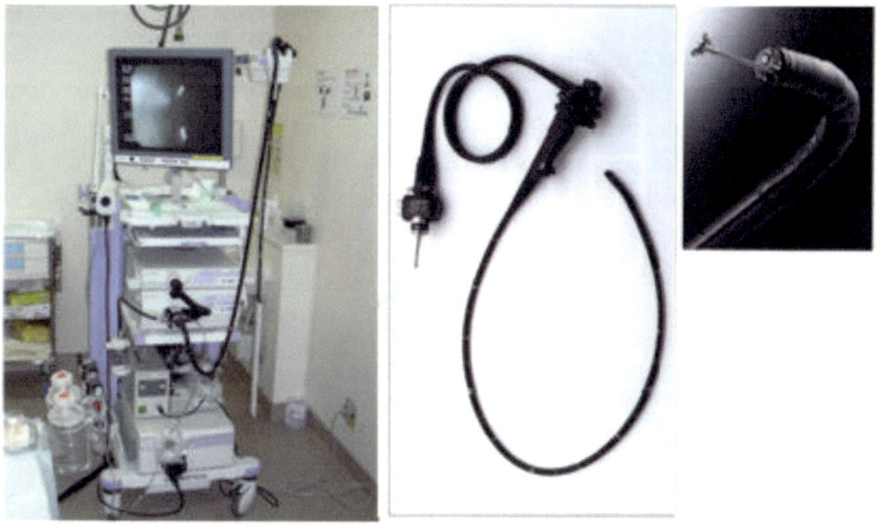

Figure 1. Endoscopy system

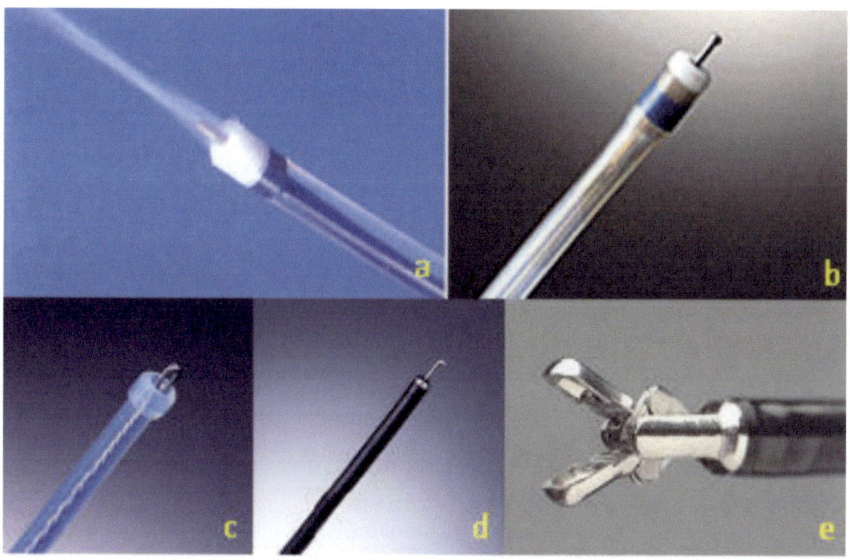

Figure 2. a. flush knife, b. dual knife, c. flex knife, d. fook knife, e. hemostatic forceps

2.3. Histological assessment

The resected specimen was cut into 2-mm slices after fixation in formalin. Histological type, size, depth of invasion, lateral and vertical margins, and lymphatic-vascular invasion were evaluated in each slice according to the Japanese Classification of Gastric Carcinoma[14].

2.4. Definition of complete and incomplete resection

It is usually easier to histologically evaluate the status of the resected specimen when the lesion is resected in one-piece. The quality of resection was also assessed by the status of the resected specimen: when the tumor was resected as a single piece and also when the margin was definitely free of tumorous glands, resection was considered to be complete. Multifragment resections were defined as incomplete when tumorous glands were histologically present at its edge, even if the lesion was completely removed by the endoscopical evaluation.

2.5. Definition of curative and non-curative resection

Gotoda et al studied surgically resected specimens from early gastric cancer (EGC) patients and assessed the rate of cases with EGC without lymph node metastasis, upon the following four indication criteria [15]; (1) differentiated intramucosal cancer without ulceration, regardless of size, (2) differentiated intramucosal cancer with ulceration, 30mm or less in size, (3) differentiated minute submucosal penetrative cancer (SM1), 30mm or less in size, (4) undifferentiated intramucosal cancer without ulceration, 20mm or less in size(Figures 3 to 8) [16]. If the lesion belongs to one of the four indication criteria with non-lymphatic and/or vascular involvement and the resected specimen was regarded as complete resection, the treatment was defined as curative resection. The remaining ones were defined as non-curative resection. In cases that the resected specimen was diagnosed histologically as possible node-positive cancer, additional gastrectomy with lymphadenectomy was considered.

2.6. Complications

Postoperative bleeding was defined as hematemesis or melena requiring an endoscopic hemostatic procedure after ESD. Perforation during the procedure was sutured by clipping and confirmed by detection of free air on plain radiography[17].

2.7. Follow up care

All the patients who underwent ESD were regularly observed with endoscopic examinations to check for local recurrence and/or a 2nd primary lesion as well as CTs to evaluate the existence of distant or lymph node metastases once or twice a year. In cases that underwent surgical procedure after the endoscopic resection, the patients were observed in the same way.

2.8. Statistical analysis

Comparisons between groups were performed using the χ^2 test and Mann-Whitney test for categorical variables. A P value $<.05$ was considered statistically significant. The overall survival rate was assessed by Kaplan–Meier analysis. All analyses were performed on a personal computer using SAS JMP version 8.0.1 (SAS Institute Inc. USA).

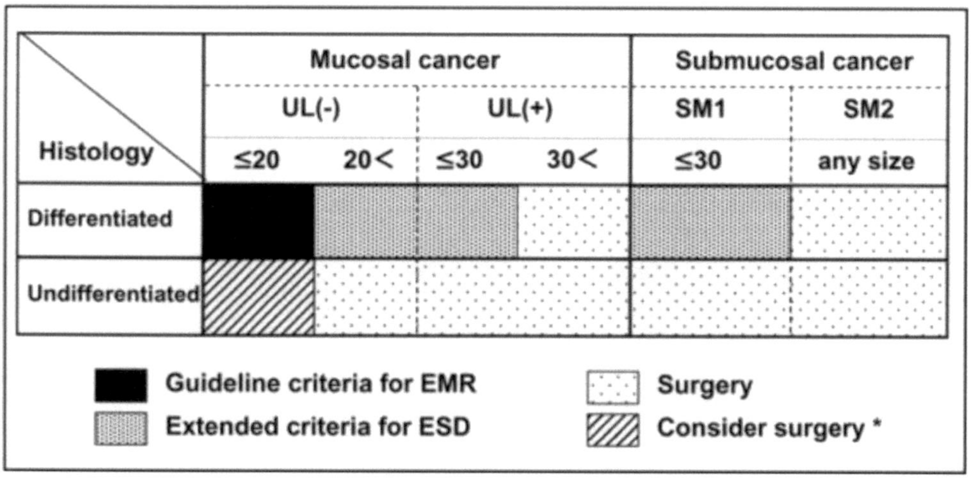

Figure 3. Extended criteria for endoscopic resection. Tumor size is shown in millimeters.UL; ulcerative findings,SM;sub-mucosal

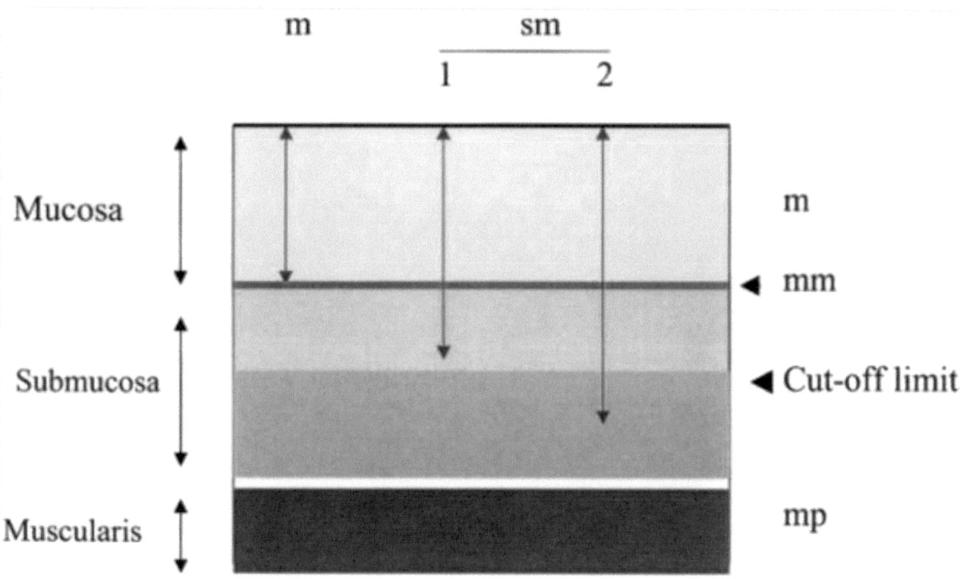

Figure 4. Depth of invasion of the submucosa in the columnar epithelium.Depth of invasion of the submucosa in the columnar epithelium assessed in the specimen obtained after surgery. Depth of submucosal invasion is divided into two groups: superficial (sm1) and deep (sm2) with respect to a cutoff limit determined on a micrometric scale (500 μ in the stomach).

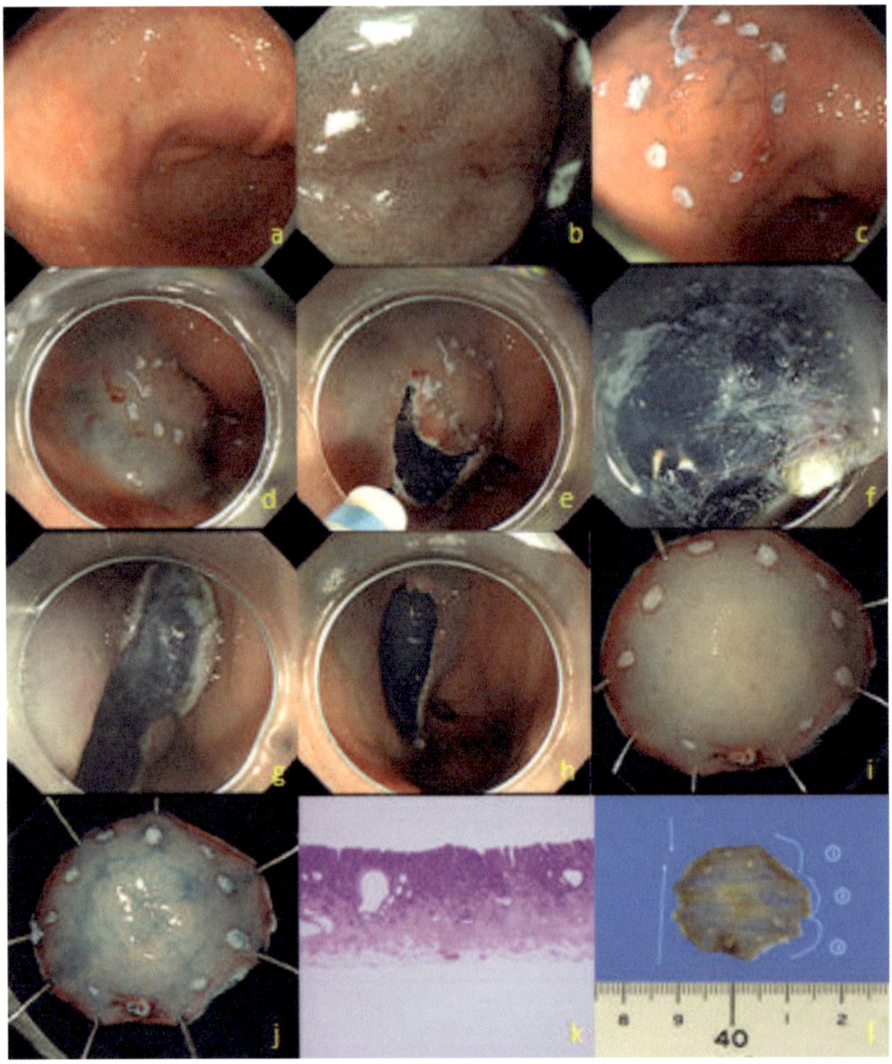

Figure 5. A case meet withguidline criteria. (a) Conventional endoscopic view revealed 0- II a, located in the lower part of the stomach. (b) Magnifying endoscopy with NBI.(c) After indigo carmine dye spraying. The border was well demarcated.(d) After injection of sodium hyaluronate. (e)to(g) Mucosal incision and dissection.(h) Gastric ulcer after ESD.(i) Resected specimen.(j) Resected specimen after indigo carmine dye spraying.(k) (l) Histopathological assessment of the resected specimen. 0- II a, 24 × 20 mm, intramucosal carcinoma, well-differentiated type. Tumor size was 5 mm.

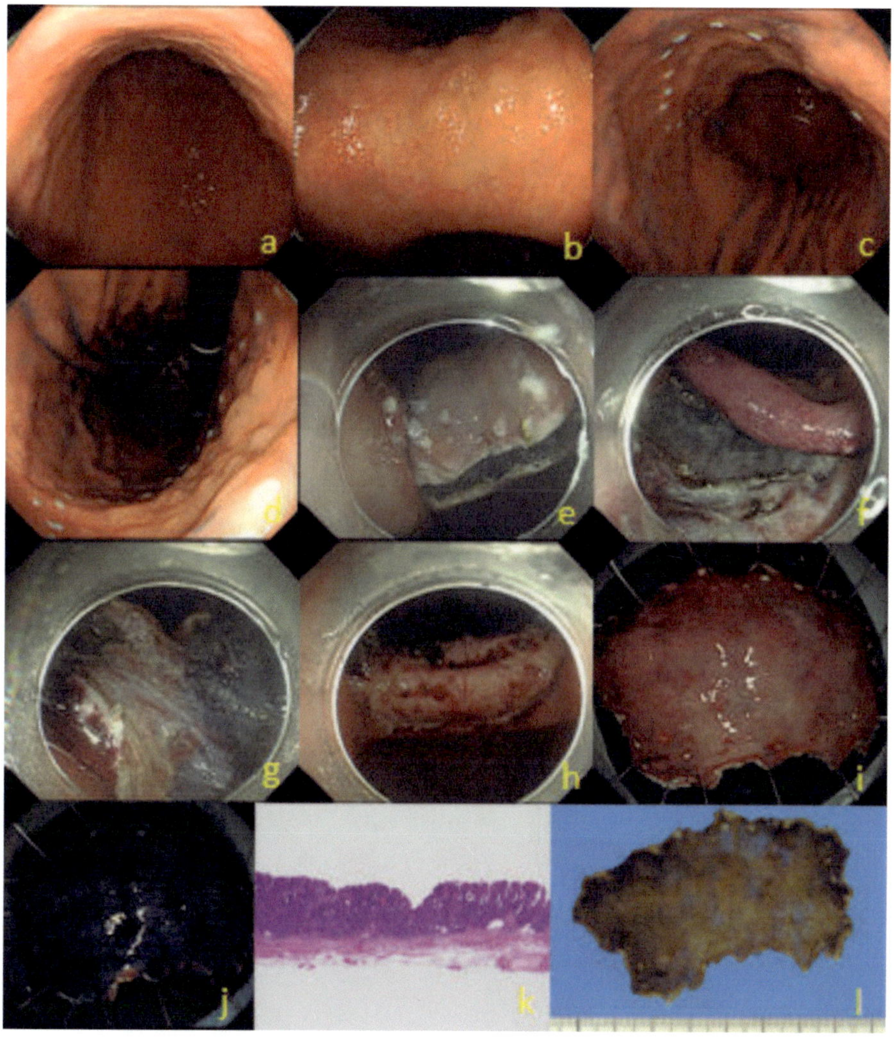

Figure 6. A case meet with extended criteria (20mm<). (a)(b) Conventional endoscopic view revealed 0- II a, located in the lower part of the stomach. (c)(d) After marking.(e)~(g) Mucosal incision and dissection.(h) Gastric ulcer after ESD.(i) Resected specimen.(j) Resected specimen after indigo carmine dye spraying.(k) (l) Histopathological assessment of the resected specimen. 0- II a, 75 × 45 mm, intramucosal carcinoma, well-differentiated type. Tumor size was 63 mm.

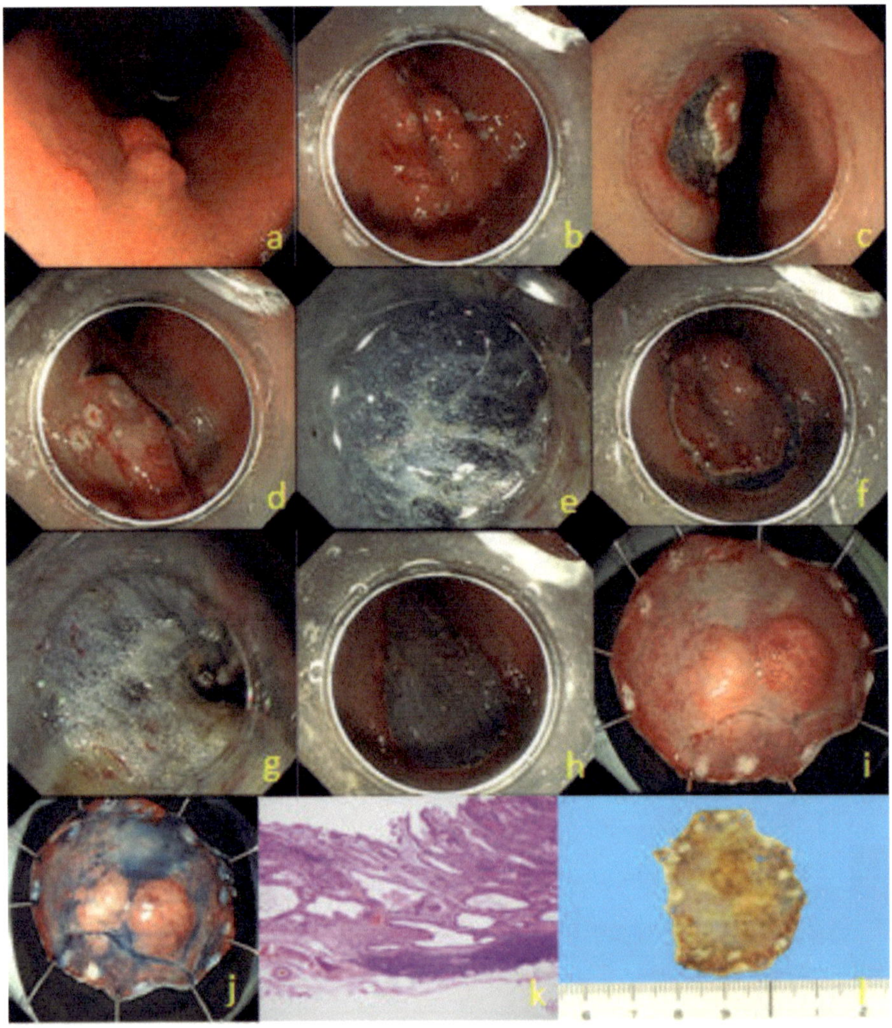

Figure 7. A case meet with extended criteria (sm invasion). (a) Conventional endoscopic view revealed 0-II a, located in the middle part of the stomach. (b) After marking.(c)~(g) Mucosal incision and dissection.(h) Gastric ulcer after ESD. (i) Resected specimen.(j) Resected specimen after indigo carmine dye spraying.(k) (l) Histopathological assessment of the resected specimen.0- II a, 35 x 32 mm, intramucosal carcinoma, well-differentiated type. Tumor size was 19 mm. One point with submucosal invasion is observed.

http://dx.doi.org/10.5772/52521

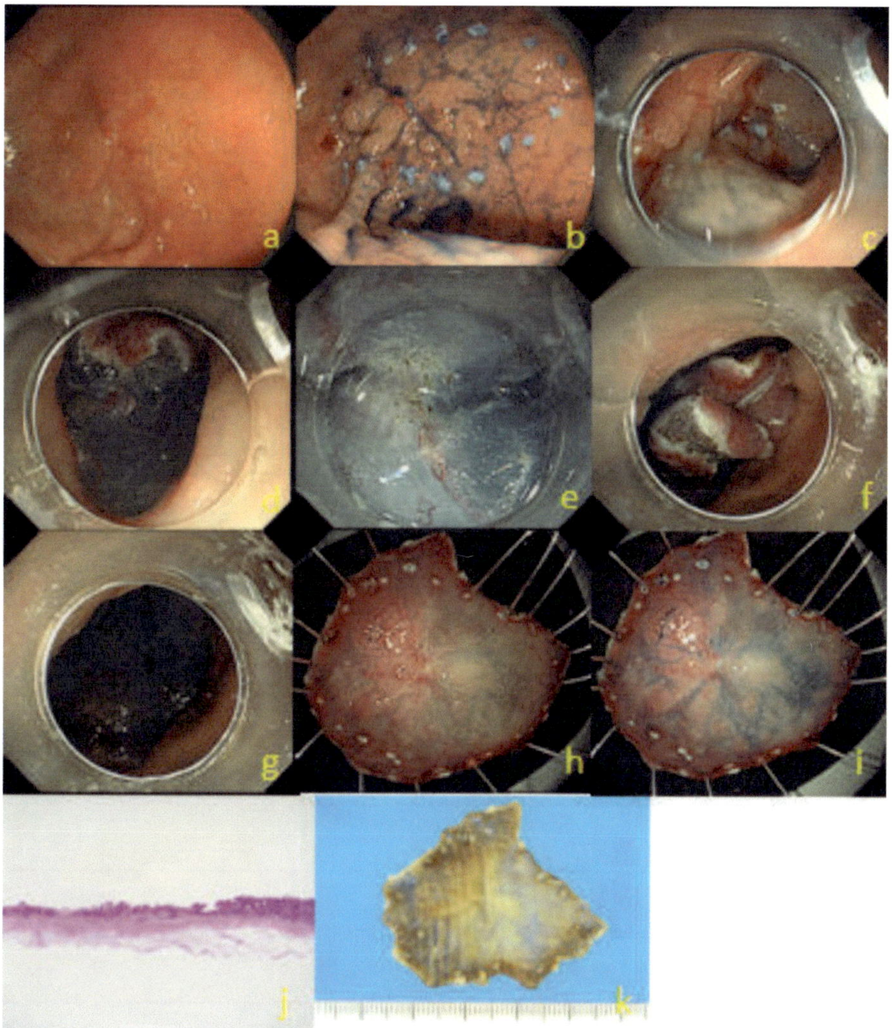

Figure 8. A case meet with extended criteria (Ul+)(a) Conventional endoscopic view revealed 0- II c with ulcer finding, located in the lower part of the stomach. (b) After indigo carmine dye spraying and marking.(c)After injection of sodium hyaluronate. (d)~(f) Mucosal incision and dissection. Fibrosis was recognized.(g) Gastric ulcer after ESD.(h) Resected specimen.(i) Resected specimen after indigo carmine dye spraying.(k) (l) Histopathological assessment of the resected specimen.0-II a, 45 × 35 mm, intramucosal carcinoma, well-differentiated type. Tumor size was 30 mm.Considerable fibrosis was recognized under thelesion.

3. Results

3.1. Patient characteristics and short-term outcome

The demographic data of the patients is shown in Table 1. 72 patients were categorized as NEG (61 males, mean age: 59.4, range: 45-64) and 212 patients were EG (164 males, mean age: 73.5, range: 65-87), showing that major patients were elderly and male. Underlying disease was found as follows; liver cirrhosis in 2 and 3, chronic renal failure requiring hemodialysis in 0 and 4, diabetes in 3 and 13 in NEG and EG, respectively. Cancer was additionally found in the other parts of the body 3 and 16 cases in NEG and EG, respectively. Antithrombotic therapy was taken in 5 and 29 in NEG and EG.

	Total	NEG	EG	p-value
	(n=284)	(n=284)	(n=284)	
Age(years)	69.9	59.4	73.5	<0.0001
range	45~87	45~64	65~87	
Gender(male/female)	225/59	61/11	164/48	NS
Background				
Underlying disease				
Liver cirrhosis	5(1.8%)	2	3	NS
Hemodialysis	5(1.8%)	0	4	NS
Diabetes	16(5.6%)	3	13	NS
Double cancer	19(6.7%)	3	16	NS
Antithrombotic therapy	34(12%)	5	29	NS

Table 1. Patient characteristics

Clinical and histological data was shown in Table 2. Histopathologically, there were 66 cases of adnocarcinoma and 15 adenomas in NEG, and 250 adnocarcinoma cases and 21 adenomas in EG. Tumors were located less in the upper part of stomach. Tumor was confined to mucosa in most cases. The rate of the cases with ulceration was higher in EG. Tumor size was more than 20 mm in most cases. Gross type was many depressed and elevated type in most cases (Figure 9).

	total	NEG	EG
	(n=352)	(n=81)	(n=271)
Histological type			
carcinoma	316	66	250
D/UD	313/3	64/2	249/1
adenoma	36	15	21
Tumor location			
U	61	17	44
M	131	35	96
L	160	29	131
Depth			
M	292	66	226
SM1	31	7	24
SM massive	29	8	21
Ulceration	61	18	43
Tumor size			
20mm≧	260	61	199
20mm<	92	20	72
Gross type			
Depressed	152	33	119
Flat	20	5	15
Elevated	180	43	137

Table 2. Clinical and histological data. D; differentiated carcinoma,UD; undifferentiated carcinoma

Short term outcomes are shown in Table 3. The mean size of the resected specimen was 36 mm in diameter (range: 10-60 mm) in NEG, and 35 mm in diameter (range: 12-110 mm) in EG (P=NS). The mean size of the tumor was 15 mm in diameter (range: 2-39 mm) in NEG, and 17 mm in diameter (range: 1-94 mm) in EG (P=NS). The en-bloc resection rates were 96.2% and 98.9% in NEG and EG, respectively (P=NS). The complete en-bloc resection rate were 90.1% and 89.7% in NEG and EG (P=NS). The curative resection rate were 81.4% and 87.8% in NEG and EG(P=NS).

	total	NEG	EG	p-value
	(n=352)	(n=81)	(n=271)	
Tumor size(mm)	16±11.6	15±8.3	17±12.4	NS
range	(1~94)	(2~39)	(1~94)	
resected specimen size(mm)	35±15.5	36±11.8	35±16.8	NS
range	(10~110)	(10~60)	(12~110)	NS
En block resection rate(%)	98.2(346/352)	96.2(73/81)	98.9(243/271)	NS
Complete en block resection rate(%)	89.7 (316/352)	90.1 (73/81)	89.7 (243/271)	NS
Curative resection rate(%)	86.36(304/352)	81.48(66/81)	87.82(238/271)	NS
Procedure time(min)	83.02	92.84	80.08	NS
Complication				
Perforation(%)	0.85(3/352)	1.23(1/81)	0.74(2/271)	NS
Postoperative bleeding(%)	1.42(5/352)	3.70(3/81)	0.74(2/271)	NS
Hospital days after ESD(day)	6.577(2~19)	6.432(2~14)	6.620(3~19)	NS

Table 3. Short term outcomes

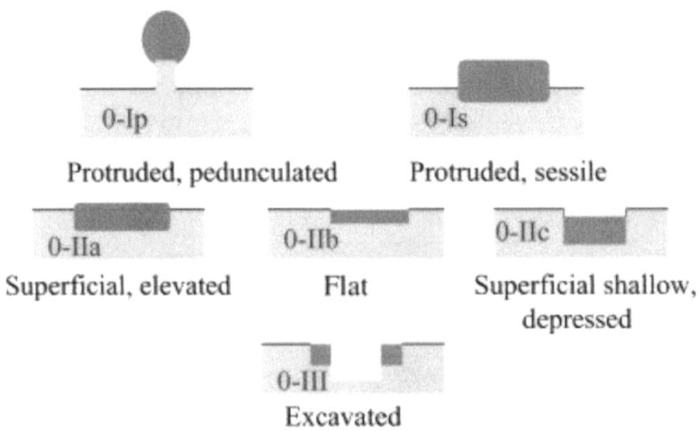

Figure 9. Schematic representation of the major variants of type 0 neoplastic lesions of the digestive tract.Schematic representation of the major variants of *type 0* neoplastic lesions of the digestive tract: polypoid*(Ip and Is)*, non-polypoid *(IIa, IIb, and II c)*, non-polypoid and excavated *(III)*. Terminology as proposed in a consensus macroscopic description of superficial neoplastic lesions

Of 15 cases that were judged as non-curative resection in NEG, 8 cases were additionally treated with surgical resection, while 7cases, including 1 adenoma, were followed up without surgical resection. In EG, of 33 cases judged as non-curative resection, 20 cases were additionally treated with surgical resection, while 13 cases, all adenocarcinoma, were followed up without surgical resection.

http://dx.doi.org/10.5772/52521

The mean procedure time was 92 min in NEG and 80 min in EG (P=0.045). The hospital days after ESD was 6.4 days (range: 2-14) in NEG and 6.6 days (range: 3-19) in EG (P=NS). There were 4 cases of complications in NEG (1 cases of perforation and 3 cases of delayed bleeding), and 4 cases in EG (2 cases of perforation and 2 cases of delayed bleeding) (P=NS). All cases with perforation were managed and controlled conservatively.

3.2. Long-term outcomes

Four patients in NEG and 7 patients in EG died from irrelevant diseases during the follow up period. No patient in either group died from any associated complications of the endoscopic treatment or progression of gastric neoplasm. No cases of local recurrence or distant metastasis were observed during follow-up in each group. During the follow-up periods of median 843 days in NEG (range 14–1812 days) and 775 days in EG (range 6–1789 days), the 1–year overall survival rates were 100% and 99% in NEG and EG, respectively. The 3-year overall survival rates were 89% and 94% in NEG and EG, respectively (Figures 10,11, Table4).

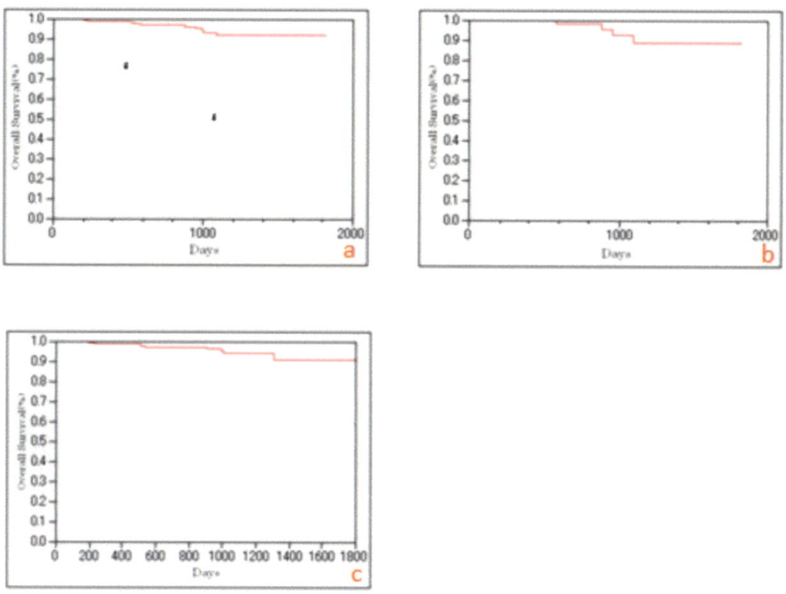

Figure 10. Overall survival (a) Overall survival(total), (b) Overall survival in NEG, (c) Overall Survival in EG

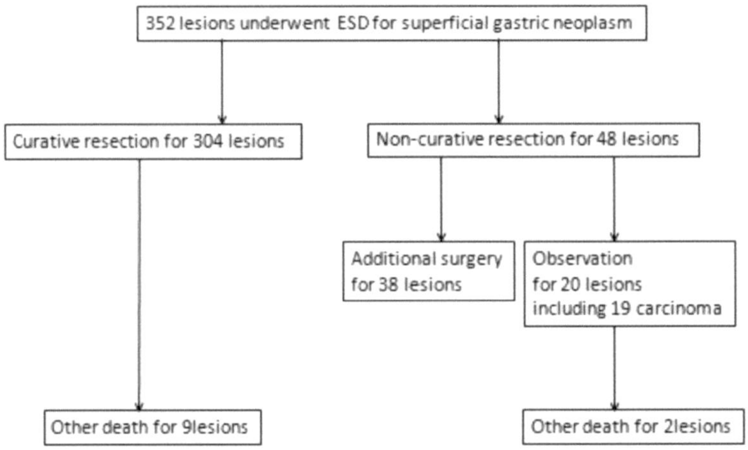

Figure 11. Flow diagram in this study

	total	NEG	EG	p-value
	(n=352)	(n=81)	(n=271)	
Madian follow-up	796.5	843	775	NS
Local recurrencerate(%)	0 (0/352)	0 (0/81)	0 (0/271)	NS
distant metastasis rate(%)	0 (0/352)	0 (0/81)	0 (0/271)	NS
the 1–year overall survival rates (%)	99	100	99	
the3–year overall survival rates (%)	92	89	94	

Table 4. Long term outcomes

3.3. Limitations

A single-center, retrospective analysis.

4. Discussion

It is a great advancement that ESD has been introduced into endoscopic therapy of early gastric cancer (EGC). However, in the present status, ESD requires difficult skills that can be obtained only after intensive training. With less trained skills, there is a high risk of hemorrhage, perforation, etc., which hampers the wide prevalence of this technique. Since it also takes a longer time to perform ESD than other endoscopic treatments, this method would be better regarded as an endoscopic surgery. In order to acquire complete curability by EMR, it is necessary to meet two conditions: "a tumor is resected in one piece without residual tumor" and "there is no metastasis." Introduction of ESD into the therapeutics for EGCs practically met the former condition. Therefore, the latter condition, the possibility of metastasis, is an important factor to determine the indication. At the present time, the possibility of lymph node metastasis is judged from pathological features of the primary lesion, and the indication is considered as standard for such lesions that have practically no probability of metastasis. However, there are many EGCs without metastasis even if lesions do not meet the ongoing criteria of indication for endoscopic therapy that has been described in the previous section. Indication of EMR could be extended if another index is established, that indicates the probability of lymph node metastasis more precisely. Introduction of molecular biological techniques or sentinel node navigation may bring about a new standard of determination of EGCs without metastasis that have not been predicted by conventional diagnostic methods. In the future, we would be able to extend the indication of EMR without impairing complete curability by establishing a reliable prediction factor on lymph node metastasis.

The criteria of indication of endoscopic therapy for EGCs described in this chapter has been set based on the data analyzing the outcomes of the therapeutic efforts for EGCs that have been done in Japan thus far. However, most reports, evaluating the risk of lymph node metastases, have been based on the pathological examinations of surgically resected specimens, which contain some problems. For example, surgical specimens were sectioned at 5 mm intervals to prepare pathological specimens in most cases. Therefore, there was a possibility that submucosal invasion might have been unrecognized between the sections examined. Micro metastases might be missed by routine pathological examinations of the surgically resected lymph nodes, which could influence the prognosis as reported.To evaluate the validity of endoscopic therapy of EGCs, particularly of ESD that enables extended indication, we need to verify it based on the follow-up data of long-term prognosis after the therapies. There are differences between Japanese and western classification systems used to define the pathology of early forms of GI cancers. These differences have made it difficult for western endoscopists to extrapolate the outcomes of EMR reported in Japanese studies to their own practices.Efforts are ongoing among pathologists to correlate the two classifications.

Early gastric cancer cases included in the indication of endoscopic resection are those with high surgical curability, and the achievement of an equivalent outcome by endoscopic treatment is an absolute requirement. However, ESD is frequently selected for elderly patients because surgery for them is high-risk[18]. Since our hospital is a specializedinstitution comprised of Cancer, Heart Disease, Stroke, and Emergency and Critical Care Centers, many elderly patients are at high-risk, and course observation without additional treatment is selected even after non-curable resection in many cases.

In many reports on the investigation of surgery for elderly gastric cancerpatients, the prevalence of preoperative complications was high. In our study, the prevalence of underlying diseases, such as those requiring hemodialysis, diabetes, and double cancers, and antithrombotic therapy was high in the elderly group, although no significant difference was detected.

However, the short- and long-termoutcomes were favorable, and no significant differences were noted between the 2 groups[18]. A significant difference was observed only in the treatment time, but it may have been due to the fact that trainees performed treatment under supervision by experts in many patients in the non-elderly group because they had no risk factor.

It would be beneficial for patients if this type of reliable endoscopic therapy that is less invasive than surgery would prevail. Thus, it is certainly warranted to develop and improve safer and more reliable maneuvers as well as to establish a training program to teach correct maneuvers. In addition, from the medico economical aspect, a new concept of endoscopic surgery should be taken into consideration so that the technique, labor and benefit to patients are recognized with an appropriate reimbursement.

5. Conclusion

On the basis of our results, ESD was safe and effective even in the elderly people. ESD is a feasible method for the treatment of superficial gastric neoplasm. The long-term outcomes following ESD are promising. This method has a potential to spread our indications and to reduce the need for surgery in patients with early gastric cancer.

Nomenclature (where applicable)-

Endoscopic submucosal dissection; ESD, endoscopic mucosal resection; EMR, elderly group; EG, non elderly group; NEG, World Health Organization; WHO, narrow band imaging; NBI, endoscopic ultrasonography; EUS, contrast-enhanced computed tomography; CECT, early gastric cancer; EGC, ulcerative findings; UL, submucosal; SM, early gastric cancer; EGC

Author details

Yasutoshi Ochiai, Shin Arai, Masamitsu Nakao, Makoto Nishimura, Takashi Shono, Kouichi Nonaka, Osamu Togawa, Keiko Ishikawa and Hiroto Kita

International Medical Center, Saitama Medical University, Japan

References

[1] Gotoda T. A large endoscopic resection by endoscopic submucosal dissection procedure for early gastric cancer. ClinGastroenterolHepatol 2005;3:S71-3.

[2] Hosokawa K, Yoshida S. [Recent advances in endoscopic mucosal resection for early gastric cancer]. Gan To Kagaku Ryoho 1998;25:476-83.

[3] Miyamoto S, Muto M, Hamamoto Y, Boku N, Ohtsu A, Baba S, Yoshida M, Ohkuwa M, Hosokawa K, Tajiri H, Yoshida S. A new technique for endoscopic mucosal resection with an insulated-tip electrosurgical knife improves the completeness of resection of intramucosal gastric neoplasms. GastrointestEndosc 2002;55:576-81.

[4] Ohkuwa M, Hosokawa K, Boku N, Ohtu A, Tajiri H, Yoshida S. New endoscopic treatment for intramucosal gastric tumors using an insulated-tip diathermic knife. Endoscopy 2001;33:221-6.

[5] Oyama T, Tomori A, Hotta K, Morita S, Kominato K, Tanaka M, Miyata Y. Endoscopic submucosal dissection of early esophageal cancer. ClinGastroenterolHepatol 2005;3:S67-70.

[6] Yamamoto H, Sekine Y, Higashizawa T, Kihira K, Kaneko Y, Hosoya Y, Ido K, Saito K, Sugano K. Successful en bloc resection of a large superficial gastric cancer by using sodium hyaluronate and electrocautery incision forceps. GastrointestEndosc 2001;54:629-32.

[7] Yahagi N, Fujishiro M, Kakushima N, Kobayashi K, Hashimoto T, Oka M, Iguchi M, Enomoto S, Ichinose M, Niwa H, Omata M. Endoscopic submucosal dissection for early gastric cancer using the tip of an electrosurgical snare (thin type). Digestive Endoscopy 2004;16:34-38.

[8] Chung IK, Lee JH, Lee SH, Kim SJ, Cho JY, Cho WY, Hwangbo Y, Keum BR, Park JJ, Chun HJ, Kim HJ, Kim JJ, Ji SR, Seol SY. Therapeutic outcomes in 1000 cases of endoscopic submucosal dissection for early gastric neoplasms: Korean ESD Study Group multicenter study. GastrointestEndosc 2009;69:1228-35.

[9] Isomoto H, Yamaguchi N. Endoscopic submucosal dissection in the era of proton pump inhibitors. J ClinBiochemNutr 2009;44:205-11.

[10] Ochiai Y, Arai S, Nakao M, Shono T, Kita H. Diagnosis of boundary in early gastric cancer. World J GastrointestEndosc 2012;4:75-9.

[11] Kita H, Yamamoto H, Miyata T, Sunada K, Iwamoto M, Yano T, Yoshizawa M, Hanatsuka K, Arashiro M, Omata T, Sugano K. Endoscopic submucosal dissection using sodium hyaluronate, a new technique for en bloc resection of a large superficial tumor in the colon. Inflammopharmacology 2007;15:129-31.

[12] Yamamoto H, Kawata H, Sunada K, Satoh K, Kaneko Y, Ido K, Sugano K. Success rate of curative endoscopic mucosal resection with circumferential mucosal incision assisted by submucosal injection of sodium hyaluronate. GastrointestEndosc 2002;56:507-12.

[13] Yamamoto H, Kita H. Endoscopic therapy of early gastric cancer. Best Pract Res ClinGastroenterol 2005;19:909-26.

[14] Japanese classification of gastric carcinoma--2nd English edition--response assessment of chemotherapy and radiotherapy for gastric carcinoma: clinical criteria. Gastric Cancer 2001;4:1-8.

[15] Gotoda T, Yanagisawa A, Sasako M, Ono H, Nakanishi Y, Shimoda T, Kato Y. Incidence of lymph node metastasis from early gastric cancer: estimation with a large number of cases at two large centers. Gastric Cancer 2000;3:219-225.

[16] The Paris endoscopic classification of superficial neoplastic lesions: esophagus, stomach, and colon: November 30 to December 1, 2002. GastrointestEndosc 2003;58:S3-43.

[17] Hoteya S, Iizuka T, Kikuchi D, Yahagi N. Benefits of endoscopic submucosal dissection according to size and location of gastric neoplasm, compared with conventional mucosal resection. J GastroenterolHepatol 2009;24:1102-6.

[18] Kusano C, Iwasaki M, Kaltenbach T, Conlin A, Oda I, Gotoda T. Should elderly patients undergo additional surgery after non-curative endoscopic resection for early gastric cancer? Long-term comparative outcomes. Am J Gastroenterol 2011;106:1064-9.

Chapter 10

The Current Role of Endoscopic Stenting in Upper Gastrointestinal Surgery

Pok Eng Hong and Chin Kin Fah

Additional information is available at the end of the chapter

http://dx.doi.org/10.5772/52631

1. Introduction

Stenting is well established in the non-operative management of many sites, including, vascular system, biliary tree and tracheobronchial tree. Within the upper gastrointestinal tract, stenting is most frequently employed in oesophagus, but currently the role of stenting in stomach and duodenal has widely gained acceptance.

The first stent widely used in the esophagus was constructed from silicon rubber tube (Silastic, Dow Corning. Midland, MI). In 1959, Celestine described the use of plastic endoprosthesis introduced through laparotomy via an open gastrostomy to palliate the esophageal stricture but it was associated with high complication as high as 45%.[1] In 1970s, Atkinson introduced an endoscopically placed plastic endoprosthesis[2], which became popular over the years as it is associated with fewer complications despite smaller internal diameter. (Figure 1)

However, the invention of the self- expanding metal stent (SEMS) (Figure 2) marked the new era of modern esophageal stenting as it is associated with higher success rate, fewer complications and ease of insertion. The first description of the endoscopic placement of an expanding metallic spiral stent was made by Frimberger in 1983.[3] There are currently at least eight different types of metallic stent on the market, covered and uncovered, some of which have anti-reflux valves.

The use of endoscopic stent has an increasing role in upper gastrointestinal tract diseases as it offers immediate relief of obstruction and immediate coverage for anastomotic leak in a minimally invasive approach. Recently various self-expanding metal or plastic stents have been developed for palliation of malignant obstruction of the gastrointestinal tracts. The major impact of these newer stents relates to the ease of insertion due to smaller delivery system with fewer complications and self –expandable property. However, the physician's perception of ease of placement has major influence in choosing the type of stent to be used.[4]

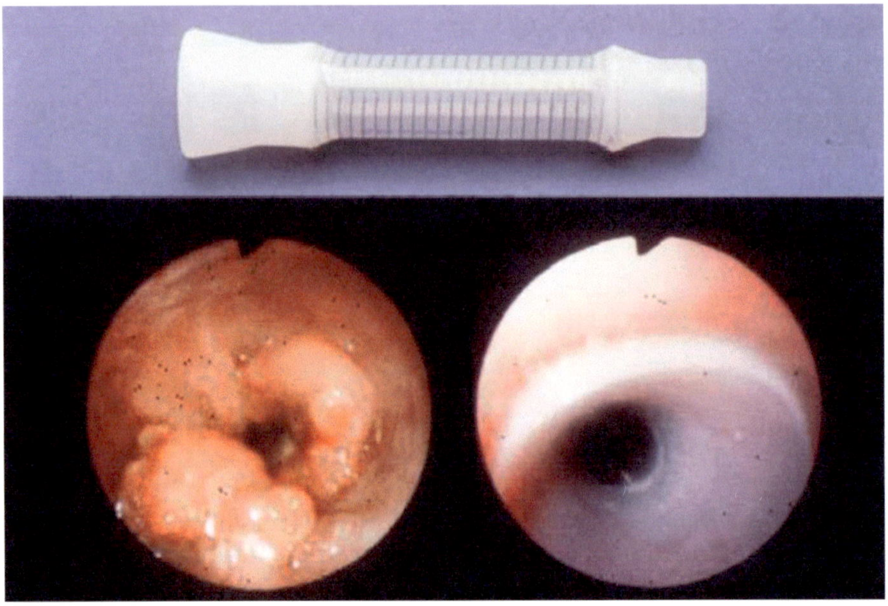

Figure 1. A Plastic stent which is successfully place endoscopically through the esophageal cancer

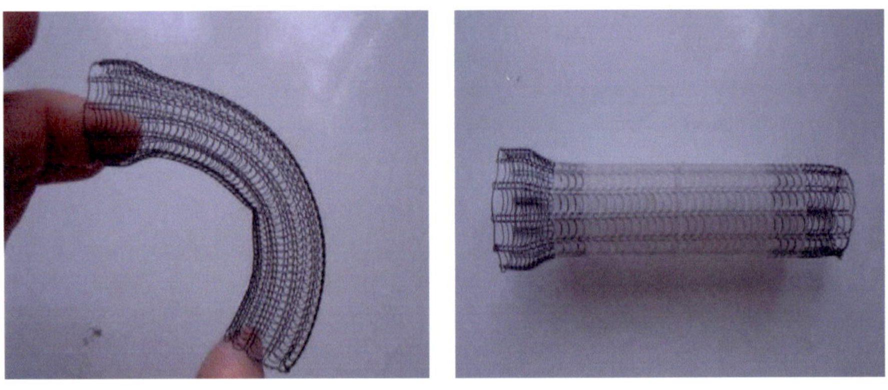

Figure 2. A retrievable self-expanding metallic stent

This review mainly focuses on the current status of self-expanding stent placement in esophageal and gastric disease, as well as considering the suitable candidate, side-effect, potential complications in relation to our experience of endoscopic stenting in various upper gastrointestinal tract disease, particularly in the management of post-operative complication.

http://dx.doi.org/10.5772/52631

2. Current availability stents and theirs indication

The stents are broadly classified into metallic and plastic stent. Metallic stents are made from nitinol (nickel-titanium alloy) or stainless steel and all are self-expanding metallic stents (SEMS). Although the metal used in this stent are made to be inert, resistant to erosion and non-allergenic but when the stent coils embedded into the mucosa, they still could trigger mild inflammatory reaction with fibrosis formation that reduce the risk of migration but it makes its removal difficult. The nitinol stent has thermal shape memory feature that enables it to expand at body temperature and adapts to the shape of a particular lesion. The initial type of metallic stent was uncovered but because of issues of tumour in-growth through the stent and tissue reaction, thus the current available stent is fully or partially covered. Current design of covered stent incorporates features such as partly uncovered portion, proximal flaring, placing the covering material on inside, to reduce the migration rate. The materials used for covered stent are silicone or plastic. However, the risk of stent migration is higher in the covered stent especially in high risk area such as distal esophagus. The covered stent is useful in benign lesion as it is easier to remove once the stricture expands. Stents are available in a wide variety of lengths and diameters. The most commonly available used stents are usually the 10-12cm long, 18- 21 mm diameter, covered SEMS. Besides, the availability of proximal release stent allows the stenting of very high esophageal lesion much easier with precise positioning under endoscopic guidance without flouroscopy[5] (Figure 3)

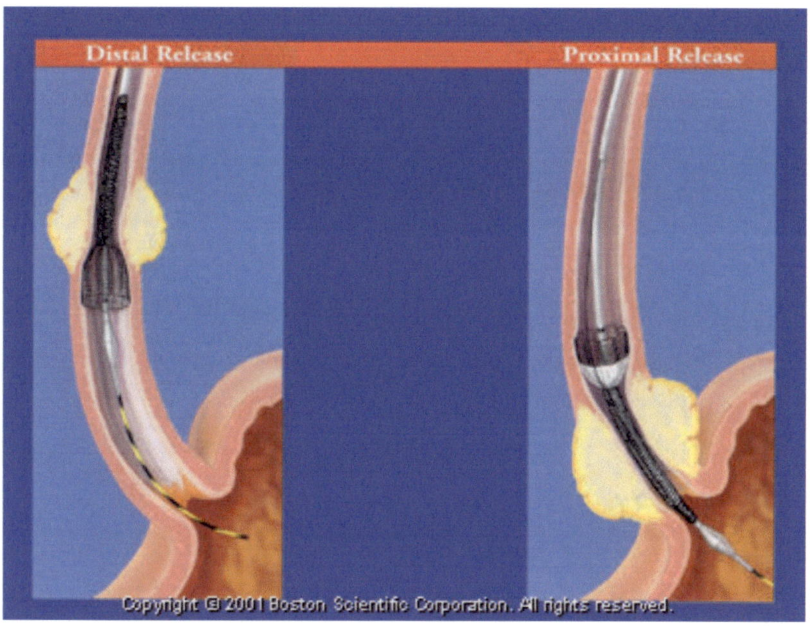

Figure 3. Two types of stent release mechanism

The self-expanding plastic stent (SEPS) is the latest development of stent design and it is indicated for esophageal stenosis such as refractory benign strictures and malignant esophageal stricture. Polyflex esophageal stent (Boston Scientific, USA) is the only stent on the market which is indicated for benign esophageal stricture and can be placed temporary up to 9 months according to manufacture guideline. However, the utility of this device is constrained by the requirement of a relatively large (12-14 mm) rigid introducer, manual assembly and the necessity of fluoroscopic guidance using a wire for appropriate positioning.

The important type of stents that are available on the market are given in Table 1

Name	**Manufacturer**	**Material**	Diameter (mm)	Length (mm)	**Delivery system size (mm)**	**Special features**
Polyflex	Boston Scientific, USA	Polyester, silicone covered	16-21	90-150	12.0-14.0	Need manual assembly prior to stent placement. Indicated for benign esophageal stricture
Niti-S	Taewoong Medical, Korea	Nitinol wire, silicone covered	16-20	60-150	5.8-6.5	Fully covered. Proximal/ distal release available. Retrievable if misplaced. Proximal lasso. Antireflux variant available
Ultraflex™	Boston Scientific, USA	Nitinol wire, polyurethane covered	18-23	100-150	6	Partially covered at mid-portion. Ideal for upper 1/3 esophagus. Little expansile force. Not intended to be repositioned of removed once deployed. Large proximal flares
Z-stent ®	Wilson-Cook Medical,USA	Stainless steel, polyurethane covered	18	80-140	10	Non-shortening partially covered stent. Preloaded on a Z-speed introduction system
Bonastent™	Standard Sci-Tech, Korea	Nitinol wire, silicone covered	18	60-150	5	Fully covered. Repositionable if misplaced less than 50% of its length. Small delivery diameter (5 mm) Proximal and distal lasso,.Antireflux variant available
Choo stent ™	M.I.Tech, Korea	Nitinol wire, silicone covered	18	60-170	6	Retrievable if misplaced. Proximal and distal lasso. Antireflux variant available
Alimaxx-ES™	Merit Medical system, USA	Nitinol wire, polyurethane covered	12-14	70-120	7.4	Fully covered. Antimigration struts. Proximal suture knot for removal

Table 1. Commercially available covered esophageal stents

3. Indications and contraindications for stent placement

3.1. Indications

The aim for stenting is the palliation of malignant dysphagia in esophageal or gastric cancer in patients whom are not candidate for surgical resection due to extensive local or metastatic disease or poor functional status. Trecheo-esophageal fistula due to locally advanced cancer which leads to recurrent aspiration pneumonia is a good indication as studies has shown the used of covered stent may increase survival as compared to other therapies.[6]

The used of covered stent in benign esophageal lesions such as leak or perforation especially in high risk patients too precarious for major operation, has gain increasing acceptance in upper GI surgery.[7] In this selected group of patient, the choice of stent is utmost important as the stent must be left long enough for the leak to heal but without complication of difficult removal later on. The new designed fully covered stent such as SEMS (Nitinol coved stent) and SEPS (Polyflex) are particular suitable in this situation. Most stents are left for 2 to 3 months for the perforation to heal.

The use of stent in benign esophegeal stricture has also gain popularity in recent years.[8] Those refractory esophageal strictures with failure of serial dilatation probably are the best candidate in this indication.[9] Placement of fully covered retrievable stent after dilation as non-permanent dilator and remove it after 1 to 2 months after the fibrosis has stabilised.

There are no real contraindications for stenting due to improvement of the stent design. Traditionally, it is not advisable to stent in high esophageal lesion due to risk of aspiration, pain or risk of tracheal compression. However, with the availability of new design and proximal release stent which allow accurate endoscopic placement make the treatment of this lesion a possibility.[10] In patient with advanced esophageal cancer with very short of expectancy (< 4 weeks) should probably not considered a candidate for stenting.

3.2. Complications of stent placement

Informed consent should be obtained prior to stent placement especially the information regarding the expected benefit, risk and possible short and long term complications should be properly conveyed to patients

The use of stenting has been shown to improve quality of life indices.[11, 12] The improvement of dysphagia has been the objective of the esophegeal stenting. The dysphagia score is used to assess the degree of dysphagia. (Table 2)[13] Most published series showed the overall immediate technical success rate in 100%, with improvement of dysphagia score approaching 90%.[12] The ability of oral intake to allow gastronomic pleasure is also another benefit, which not only improve the quality of life but possibly the nutrition status of the patient.

Minor procedure complications which lead to morbidity were seen up to 40% in various series.[14, 15] Intra-procedure complications such as aspiration, sedation risk, malposition of the stent, bleeding and perforation could occur. Early complications may include chest pain, bleeding or tracheal compression. Late complications such as stent migration, tumour overgrowth or ingrowth[16-18], delayed perforation, food bolus impaction, fistula formation may occur. However, fistula and perforation due to stent insertion are uncommon. Early chest pain occur in most patient, but prolonged pain only occur in fewer than 13% of patients.[18] Pain is most severe with high stricture and when large diameter of stent is used.[19] The migration rate for those uncovered stent is less than 3% in esophagus, but increases to 6% if placed across the cardia.[13, 17] The migration rate of covered stent is generally up to 30%, especially when positioned across cardia.[17, 18, 20] The migrated stent should be retrieved endoscopically as it may cause small bowel obstruction or perforation.[21]

Dysphagia score	Degree of dysphagia
0	No dysphagia
1	Able to swallow some solid food only
2	Able to swallow semi-solid only
3	Able to swallow liquids only
4	Complete dysphagia

Table 2. The dysphagia score

4. Technique of insertion

Before placement of the stent, a barium swallow should be obtained to delineate the site and length of the esophageal stricture. The stent could be deployed under endoscopic visualization, fluoroscopic guidance with the aid of guide wire and sometime require pre-dilatation of the lesion. It is especially helpful to have a nurse who experienced in complex endoscopic procedure to facilitate the success of stent deployment. Esophageal dilation is usually done before stent insertion but it is not a pre-requisite for successful stent deployment. The precise requirement of dilatation generally depends on the type of stent to be used, dilatation to no more than 12mm is recommended, which will facilitate introduction of the delivery system and allow rapid expansion of the stent. However, most people advocate do not pre-dilate the stricture as the stricture itself with hold the stent to reduce the risk of migration.

During procedure, the patient lies in left lateral position, Xylocaine spray is applied to the pharynx, the patient is sedated with an intravenous agent such as midazolam and analgesia is provided such as fentanyl. If the endoscope is managed to transverse the lesion, the proximal and distal border of the lesion are marked using radio-opaque markers, endoclips or contrast such as lipoidal agent. The stent is introduced over the guide wire until the marking on the stent are placed within 2cm of more margins proximal and distal to the lesion. Final adjustment is made under fluoroscopic guidance to ensure that the stent adequately covers the Lesion's marking. By slowly retracting the outer sheath of the delivery system while maintaining the position of the inner shaft, the stent is deployed under fluoroscopic guidance. It is important that the inner shaft of the delivery system is held stationary against the body while deployment and not allowed to move, as any movement may cause malposition of the stent. Endoscopic visualization of the stent placemen also could be performed, especially with the aid of transnasal endoscopy which allows direct visual control of the esophageal stent placement without fluoroscopy.[22] After full deployment of stent and the expansion of the stent is verified fluoroscopically, the olive tip and the delivery system should be removed with care to prevent the dislodgment of the stent. For those stent that is placed too distally, a strong forcep could be used to hold the proximal lasso and the traction of it allow the stent narrows and be positioned more proximally. (Figure 4) Immediately after the procedure, non-ionic contrast medium is introduced through the catheter to look for any procedural related complications, especially esophageal perforation and to ascertain the stent patency. Endoscopy also can be done to ascertain the position of the stent but the endoscope should not be passed through the stent to prevent dislodgment of the stent. Chest x-ray should be carried out later to verify the position of the stent to look for sign of perforation.

Patient should stayed overnight for post-procedure monitoring. Some patients might complain of chest discomfort or chest pain which could be relieved with simple analgesia. Occasionally the pain is so severe which needs stent removal.

Patient with stent must modify their diet to prevent food impaction that lead to stent occlusion. Diet should be introduced as tolerated. Patient with stent placed without anti-reflux valve should be started on a high dose proton pump inhibitor indefinitely to prevent gastroesophageal reflux. Stent occlusion due to food impaction could be dislodged endoscopically but those occlusion arises due to tumour overgrowth necessitate co-axial stenting on previous stent or laser ablation.

Technical points to consider

- Covered stent should be used for tumour with high risk of fistula formation and to prevent in-growth of tumour through the metal mesh.
- Stents with antireflux valve should be considered if position across the gastroesophageal junction due to disabling gastroesophageal reflux.[20, 23]
- The proximal margin of the stent could be hold to mucosal tissue using endoclips to prevent stent migration.[24][25](Figure 5)
- The partially migrated stent could be fixed with another covered stent, placed coaxially overlapping the upper portion of the migrated stent.
- Those SEMS that is difficult to be removed due to tissue in-growth through the uncovered portion, a covered SEPS could be inserted overlapping the SEMS to press the tissue out of the stent mesh and causing pressure necrosis. Both of the stent could be removed few days later.[26, 27]

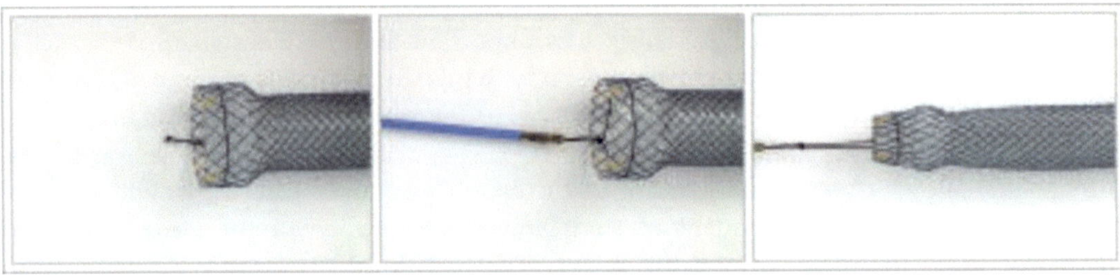

Figure 4. The proximal lasso could be retracted with strong grasper resulting narrowing of the stent body for easier removal.

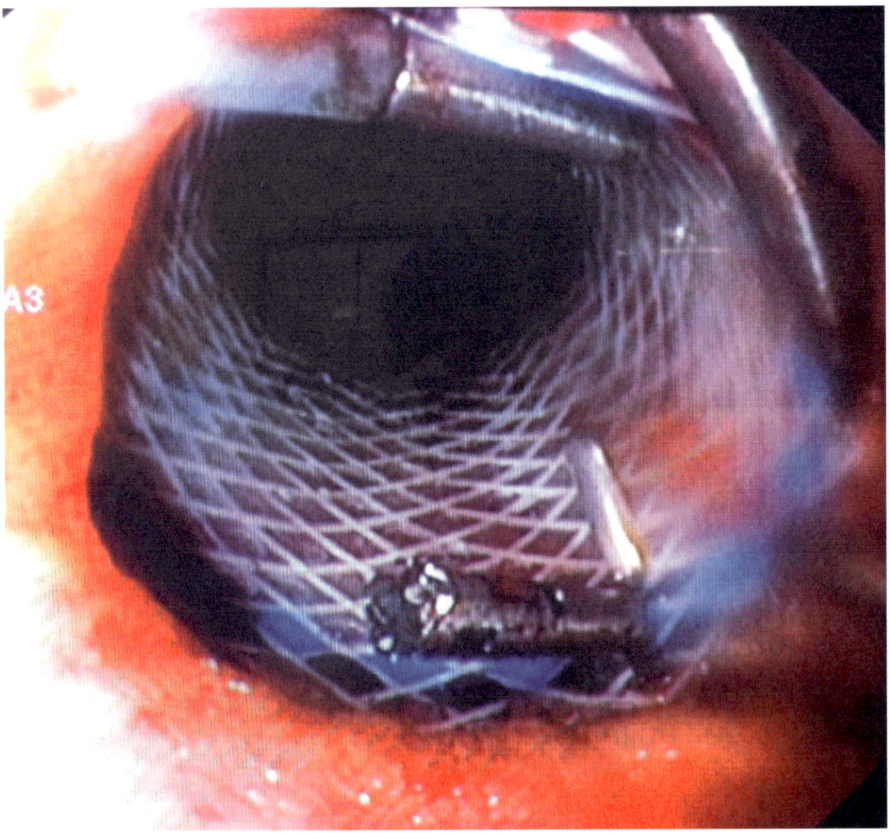

Figure 5. Use of endoclips to hold the proximal margin of stent to prevent stent migration.

5. Specific use of stent in upper gastrointestinal disease

The role of stenting in upper GI disease can be broadly dived into:

Esophagus:

1. Stents used in esophageal malignancy
2. Stents used in benign esophageal lesion such as stricture or perforation
3. Stents used in post-operative complication

Stomach:

1. Stents used in gastric outlet obstruction
2. Stents used in bariatric surgery

6. Esophageal stenting in malignancy

Most patients with upper GI cancer especially esophageal cancers presented late with locally advanced or metastatic disease, which preclude them form surgical resection.[28] Patients may have no symptoms until the diameter of the esophageal lumen has been reduced by 50% resulting in late presentation and poor prognosis.[29] However, the problem of dysphagia, vomiting and malnutrition will severely impair the quality of life of these patients. A variety of endoscopic treatment modalities such as thermal ablation, brachytherapy, photodynamic therapy, chemical injection, argon beam therapy and endoluminal stenting have been utilized with these objectives in mind, with options determined by the location and size of the tumour, as well as the patient's expected prognosis.[29] The use self-expanding stent in this kind of patients as a form of palliation,[30] instead of surgical bypass, is particular helpful in relieving the obstruction while allow them to eat, manage their oropharyngeal secretions, reduce aspiration risk, and improve the nutrition status.

The esophageal stenting in malignancy can broadly divided into two situation:

1. Palliation in advanced cancer
2. Temporary stenting for patient undergoing neoadjuvant therapy

Palliation in advanced cancer

SEMS placement is a safe and effective technique with good symptom palliation in advanced esophageal cancer.[17] Case series showed that the dysphagia score improved faster, 85% within 2 week as compare to radiotherapy which the onset of palliation was slower, with only 50% of patients palliated at 2 weeks.[31] Successful stent placements are achieved in up to 98% cases.[32] In palliation of malignant esophagorespiratory fistula or perforation, covered metallic stent have a clinical success rate of 95-100%.[33, 34] (Figure 6) Sometime, fistulas close to the upper esophageal sphincter may be closed with placement of parallel covered metallic stents in the esophagus and trachea.[35] The quality of life also reported to improve after palliative esophageal stenting. [12] Another major problem of esophageal stenting in advanced cancer is the tumour overgrowth which leads to recurrent dysphagia in patient who is survives long enough.[16, 36] This can be easily intervened with co-axial stent as overlapping stent. [36](Figure 7)

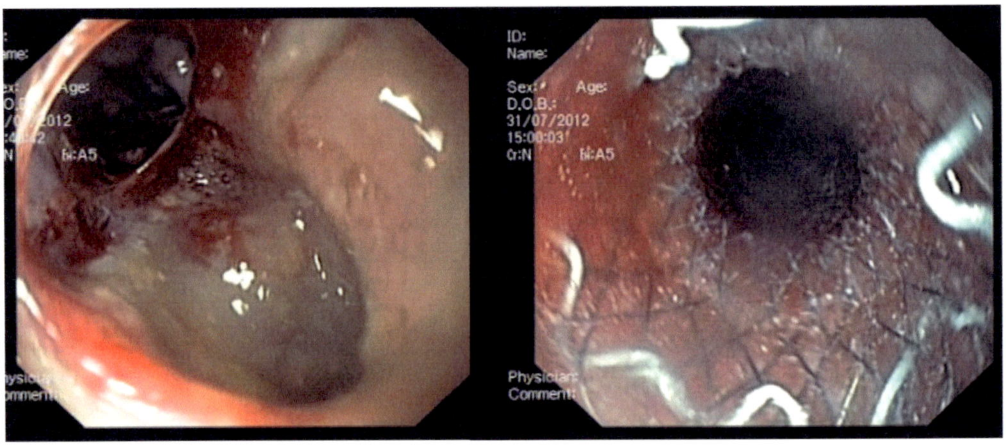

Figure 6. A locally advanced esophageal cancer with tracheoesophageal fistula presented with recurrent aspiration pneumonia and treated successfully with a covered esophageal stent for symptomatic relief.

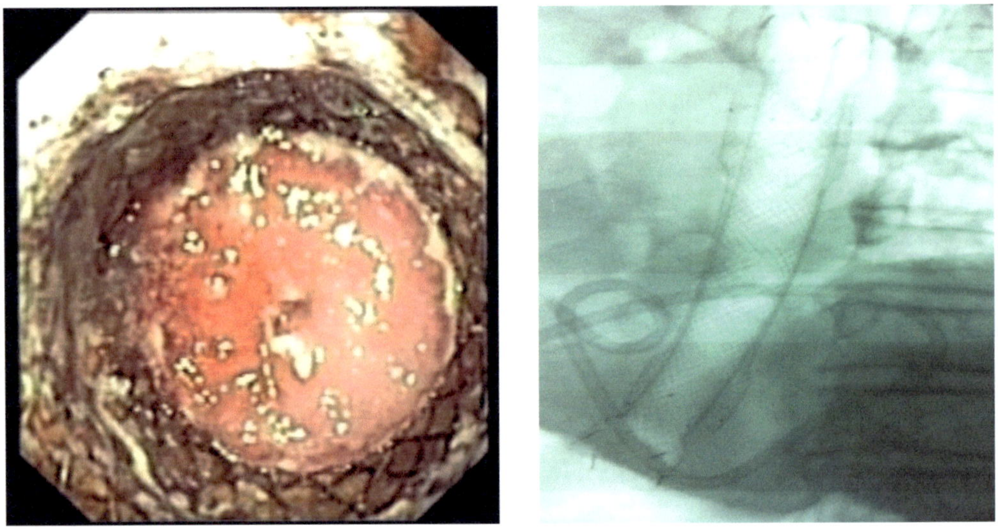

Figure 7. Tumour over growth at the distal end of the covered stent which was treated with another co-axial covered stent across the previous old stent to relieve the obstruction.

Temporary stenting before neoadjuvant therapy

Due to malignancy induced cachexia and dysphagia, nutrition compromise is extremely common for those patients undergoing neoadjuvant chemotherapy or radiotherapy, which result in poorer outcome after surgery. The insertion of stent in this setting has been reported to have higher stent related complication such as migration or perforation and also difficulty of surgery later on. However, with the advent of fully covered SEMS with much reduced complication rate has led to renew interest in this indication.

The use of stenting in neoadjuvant setting results in improvement of dysphagia score and nutrition has been reported in several studies.[37-39] Although it is safe with effective palliation of symptom with minimal complication, the migration does occur up to 48% especially in esophageal stenting across the gastroesophageal stenting.[40] However, the migration of stent is usually indicating a positive response to neoadjuvant therapy and the stent could easily be retrieved prior to surgery.[38] The fully covered SEMS do not appear to compromise surgical resection. [40]There is no increased risk of peri-operative complication due to stent in all these series.

7. Benign esophageal strictures

Benign esophageal stricture in the esophagus can be due to a variety of causes such as reflux esophagitis, corrosive ingestion, post-radiation exposure, etc. The initial treatment of choice is serial dilatations. However, up to 30-40% of these strictures will recur and require repeated dilatation or even surgery.[41, 42] It is particularly important to differentiate between esophageal strictures that are simple (focal, straight strictures with a diameter that allows endoscope to passage) and those that are more complex (long, >2 cm, tortuous strictures with a narrow diameter).[9] These complex strictures are considered refractory when they cannot be dilated to an adequate diameter. The concept of using esophageal stent as a non-permanent dilator provides an alternative treatment of esophageal stricture instead of surgery.[43] The use of non-removable metal stents in benign esophageal stricture has been complicated by hyperplastic tissue reaction, tissue ingrowth, stricture formation and erosion into the surrounding organ. Therefore, removable fully covered self-expanding metal stent is recommended although the problem of tissue reaction or stent migrations also occur with these devises.[44]. The suggested stent of choice to be used in benign esophageal stricture is Polyflex stent (Boston Scientific, USA) as it causes less tissue reaction. This is the only SEPS available in the market and is approved for refractory benign stricture and treatment of trachea-esophageal fistula. This is self-expanding plastic stent made of polyester mesh that is fully covered with a silicone membrane with proximal flare to prevent migration. A systemic review showed the Polyflex is moderate effective, achieving dilatation free remission in 52% cases and achieves lower success rate when dealing with upper esophageal stricture.[8] This could due to more complex anatomy in upper esophagus which prevents effective remodelling of the stricture by SEPS. A recent meta-analysis showed that the efficacy of self-expanding covered stent placement in benign refractory strictures is only 46.2 % and associated with migration rate of 26.4 %.[45] Our early experience with this stent has been quite positive for the management of recurrent and refractory benign stricture. (Figure 8 and 9)

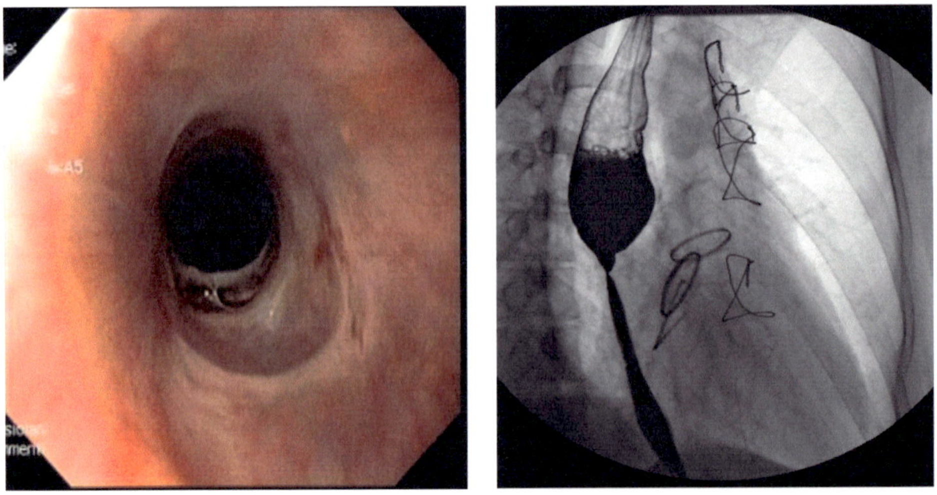

Figure 8. A 35 years old lady developed a short segment benign esophageal stricture at mid esophagus after cardiac surgery for closure of VSD and heart valve replacement. Multiple oesophageal dilatation had failed to relieve the obstruction. A polyflex stent was inserted temporary as non-permanent dilator with good symptomatic relief.

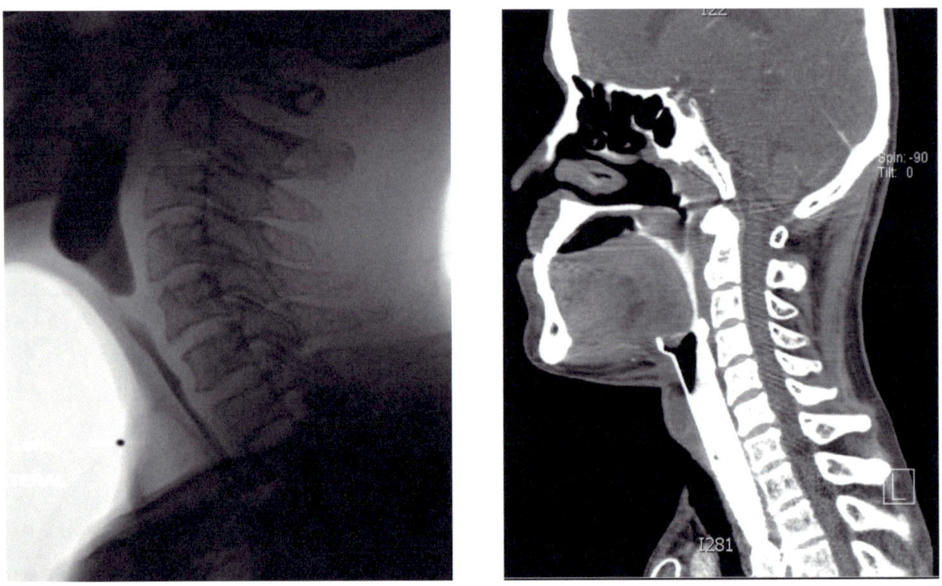

Figure 9. A high pharyngoesophageal stricture after laryngopharyngectomy treated with a proximal release fully covered Nitinol stent (TaewoongNiti-S, Korea) under endoscopic control.

8. Post-operative complication

Anastomotic leak in upper GI surgery is a serious complication especially when the leak is within the thoracic cavity with septic consequences. The sites of leak most commonly encountered are gastroesophageal or gastrojejunostomy or esophagojejunostomy anastomosis. Early intervention from the subtle clinical clues is the key to successful management. Traditionally, the management has most often consisted of re-operation for repair and drainage, prolonged hospitalisation and sometime necessitate resection of diversion which requires subsequent restorative surgery.

The use of endoluminal stenting for esophageal leak instead of surgical intervention has been reported with good outcome.[46, 47] In a large series, up to 77.6% of patients with post-operative leak responded to stenting with a median duration of SEMS treatment of 83 days and the stent should be removed after 6 weeks.[48]Polyflex of SEPS type has also been used with good success rate.[49]

The role of endoluminal stenting in Peri-operative setting could be considered in situations such as:

1. Those patients with an anastomotic leak that are diagnosed late in the course and in whom operative closure is not feasible.

2. Those patients with an anastomotic leak with medical condition who are too precarious for surgical intervention.

3. Those patients with chronic fistula due to anastomotic failure.

However, It has been shown that those anastomotic leak located in cervical esophagus, gastroesophageal junction, esophageal injury longer than 6 cm or an anastomotic leak associated with a more distal conduit leak tend to be not treated effectively with stenting. Therefore, traditional operative repair suggested to be used as initial therapy.[50]

In our practice, the authors found that the fully covered retrievable stent and with large diameter up to 21-23mm should be used for effective sealing of the defect. There is a problem of peri-stent leak especially from the jejunal limb in some cases. However, it is usually a contained leak which could be drained percutaneously under image guidance. (Figure 10) Sometime, another stent has to be inserted across the previous stent for effective sealing. The SEPS is preferred to be used as it causes less tissue reaction and ease to be removed later. The inserted stent should be removed within 2 months and sometime we left it permanently in patient with advanced cancer. Similarly, post-operative anastomotic stricture could also be managed effectively with stent. Leakage at the anastomosis and stapler anastomosis were found to be the risk factors for the development of strictures.[51, 52] Improvement in quality of life and relief of dysphagia could be achieved when dilatation of the stricture fails. In conclusion, endoluminal stenting is a minimally invasive therapy of anastomotic complication which is a safe and effective. It results in rapid leak occlusion and avoids morbidity of re-operative repair.

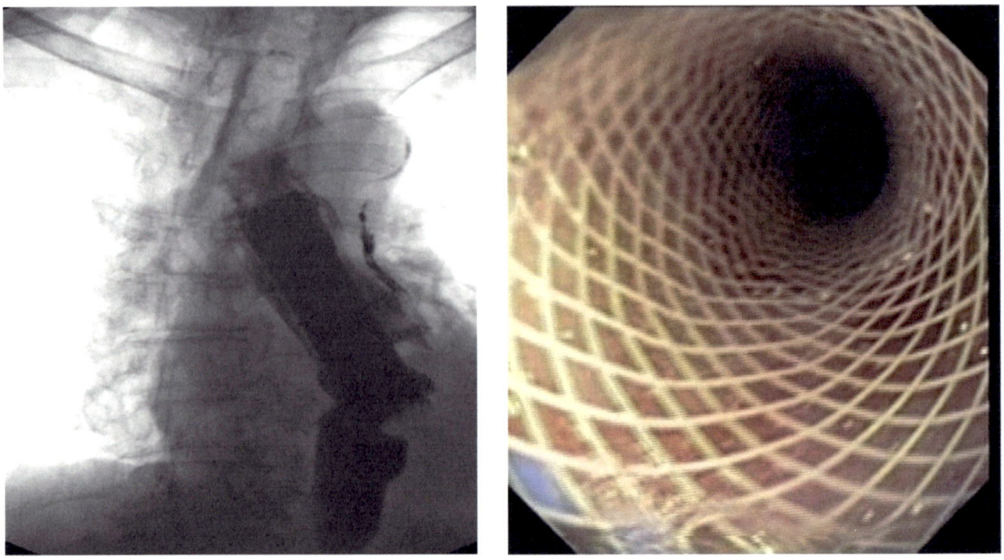

Figure 10. Post esophagectomy anastomotic leak. Two leak points at the anastomotic site located at both lateral corner of the staple line. A fully covered Polyflex stent, measured 21 mm diameter and 90 mm length inserted. The leak was successfully contained and a percutaneously drain was inserted into the chest cavity for external drainage.

9. Esophageal perforation

Esophageal perforation is most commonly iatrogenic induced but occasionally it occurs spontaneously such as in Boerhaeve's syndrome. It carries a dismal prognosis due to mediastinitis and severe sepsis. Esophageal stenting has been shown to be effective in managing the leak as a less morbid intervention if compared with surgery.[48, 53] Several case series showed an effective healing leak rate up to 90%.[48, 54] The key to success outcome is prompt recognition of leak with rapid esophageal stenting immediately after the perforation and adequate debridement and lavage of the thoracic cavity. (Figure 11)

10. Stents used in gastric outlet obstruction

The usual causes of gastric outlet obstruction are due to tumour in gastric antrum, duodenal stricture, or obstruction secondary to direct invasion or extrinsic compression from pancreatic carcinoma. The aim in palliation in patients with malignant gastric outlet obstruction is to reestablish oral intake by restoring gastrointestinal continuity. Gastric outlet obstruction was traditionally treated with surgical gastroenterostomy and stenting is usually reserved for patients who are not fit for surgery.

Prolong nasojejunal tube feeding or percutaneous jejunostomy to provide nutrition is not an ideal palliation treatment in those patients not fit for surgical bypass as the tube will cause significant discomfort in these terminal ill patients. Therefore, internal stenting of the lesion will offer the best method of palliation for these patients, apart from relieve of obstruction but also able them to resume oral intake. (Figure 12) Stents can be successfully deployed in the majority of patients.[55] Stent placement appears to lead to a shorter time to symptomatic improvement, shorter time to resumption of an oral diet, and shorter hospital stays as compared with surgical options.[56] However, surgical bypass results in better long-term outcomes as compared to internal stenting. A recent randomised controlled trial showed that despite slow initial symptom improvement, gastrojejunostomy is associated with better long-term results and is therefore the treatment of choice in patients with a life expectancy of 2 months or longer.[57] Currently, the metallic uncovered stents are commonly used to prevent the risk of migration.

Another interesting use of stent in locally advanced gastric cancer such as linitis plastica type which may cause gastroesophageal and gastric outlet obstruction. The placement of an extra long, covered stent traversing the cardioesophageal junction up to duodenum will provide symptomatic relief (Figure 13). The stent not only provides some degree of peroral intake but is able to relieve of the gastric outlet obstruction probably due to peri-stent flow.

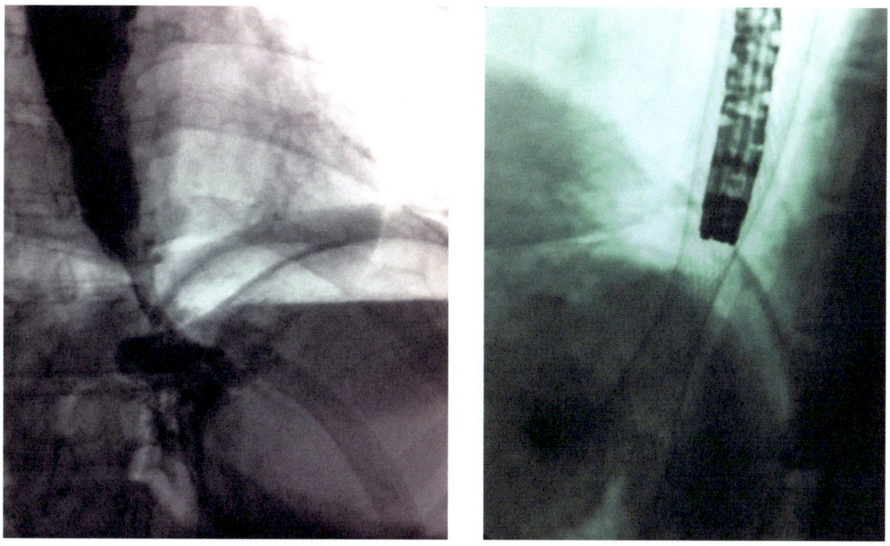

Figure 11. Lower esophageal perforation occurred after endoscopic dilatation and the defect was immediately stented under fluoroscopic control.

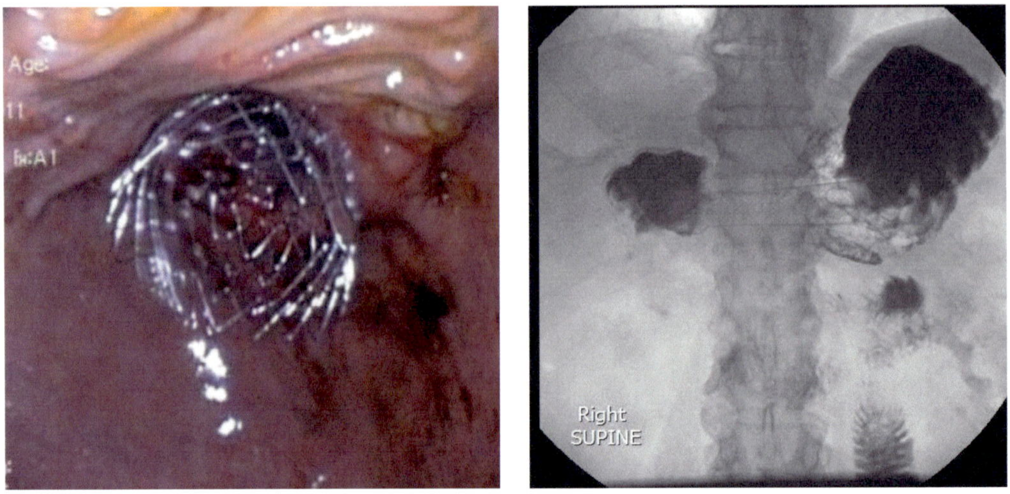

Figure 12. Barium meal showed good of barium trough the through the pyloric obstruction after internal stenting.

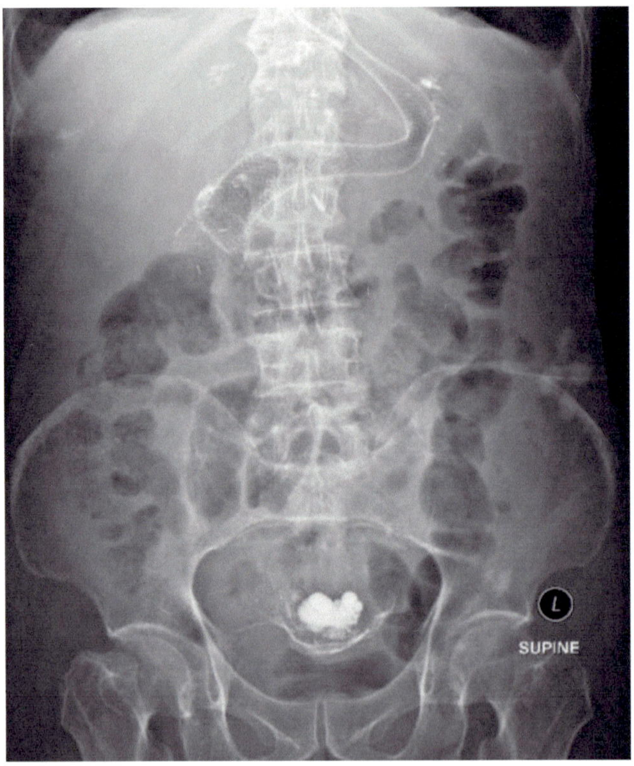

Figure 13. An extra long 23cm, fully covered Nitinol stent (Taewoong Niti-S, Korea) deployed crossing the gastroesophageal junction and pylorus in a' linitis plastic type' gastric cancer to bypass the obstruction.

11. Bariatric surgery

Bariatric surgery has become an effective solution to treat morbid obesity. Laparoscopic adjustable gastric banding and laparoscopic Roux-en-Y gastric bypass carry a mortality rate of 0.1% and 0.5%, respectively. [58] Therefore, surgery on this high risk group of patients can be dangerous especially leak occur and carry a high risk of mortality if not detected and treated expediently. The leak usually arises from stapler line failures due to surgical technique, ischaemia and patient comorbid conditions. In sleeve gastrectomy, the leak site is usually found in the upper sleeve near the gastroesopheal junction.[59] Recently, the placement of long endoluninal stent have been demonstrated to be safe and effective to exclude the leak site, allowing oral intake and speeding healing.[59, 60]

The recent development of bariatric surgery is the placement of the EndoBarrier duodenal jejunal bypass liner which appears to be a promising, safe and effective method for facilitating weight loss.[61] The EndoBarrier is a plastic flexible tube which is endoscopically placed in the duodenal bulb, directly behind the pylorus. It extends from the duodenum to the proximal jejunum. Recent studies have demonstrated significant weight reduction in comparison to control-diet patients.[62] However, the lack of long term result and small samples size studies call for a need for longer randomised controlled trial before its widespread use.[63]

12. Which stent to use

All the stent are equally effective in achieving symptomatic palliation in malignant dysphagia. The type of stent chosen is usually based on subjective physician's preference. However, the stents vary in features such as the ease of insertion, removability, migration and occlusion rates. Covered and uncovered stents have different functional characteristics and stent type must be selected on an individual basis. A recent meta-analysis suggests that SEMS are superior to SEPS in terms of stent insertion-related mortality, morbidity, and quality of palliation.[4] The uncovered variety is disadvantaged by high rate of tumour in-growth.[4] The currently available SEPS, Polyflex is cumbersome to use due to its larger introduced system and higher rate of migration. However, the SEPS is equally effective in relieving dysphagia and useful in case of tissue ingrowth/overgrowth after SEMS placement.[64]

13. Conclusion

Stenting in upper gastrointestinal disease is now fully established in the management advanced cancer and complication due to surgery such as stricture or anastomotic leak. It offers a minimally invasive approach to address obstructive symptom and improve quality of life of patients. In difficult cases, a multi-disciplinary team approach involving surgeon, gastroenterologist and radiologist is the corner stone of successful endoscopic palliative therapy.

Continuous innovation of new stent will lead to higher technical and clinical success rates of endoscopic stenting, while reducing complication rates. Therefore, stenting will become much simpler and more convenient to use for physician but also more comfortable for the patients. Future development in stenting includes biodegradable stents for benign disease to reduce stent related complication [65] and radioactive [66]or drug-eluting[67] stents for malignant disease which will decrease tumour growth and sustain the stent patency.

Acknowledgements

The authors wish to thanks Professor Dato' Dr K L Goh, Head of Gastroenterology and Hepatology, University of Malaya for letting us to use some of his personal photo collection in preparation of this manuscript.

Author details

Pok Eng Hong and Chin Kin Fah*

*Address all correspondence to: mdskfc@gmail.com

Department of Surgery, Medical Faculty, University of Malaya, Kuala Lumpur, Malaysia

References

[1] Celestin, L.R., Permanent intubation in inoperable cancer of the oesophagus and cardia: a new tube.Annals of the Royal College of Surgeons of England, (1959). , 165-170.

[2] Atkinson, M. and R. Ferguson, Fibreoptic endoscopic palliative intubation of inoperable oesophagogastric neoplasms. British Medical Journal, 1977. 1(6056): p. 266-7.

[3] Frimberger, E., Expanding spiral--a new type of prosthesis for the palliative treatment of malignant esophageal stenoses.Endoscopy, (1983). Suppl 1: , 213-214.

[4] Yakoub, D., et al., (2008). Evidence-based choice of esophageal stent for the palliative management of malignant dysphagia.World J Surg,. 32(9): , 1996-2009.

[5] Lazaraki, G., et al., Malignant esophageal dysphagia palliation using insertion of a covered Ultraflex stent without fluoroscopy: a prospective observational study.Surg Endosc, (2011). , 628-635.

[6] Rodriguez, A.N. and J.P. Diaz-Jimenez, Malignant respiratory-digestive fistulas.Curr Opin Pulm Med, (2010). , 329-333.

[7] Blackmon, S.H., et al., Utility of removable esophageal covered self-expanding metal stents for leak and fistula management.Ann Thorac Surg, (2010). discussion 936-7., 931-936.

[8] Repici, A., et al., Systematic review: the role of self-expanding plastic stents for benign oesophageal strictures.Aliment Pharmacol Ther, (2010). , 1268-1275.

[9] Siersema, P.D., Treatment options for esophageal strictures.Nat Clin Pract Gastroenterol Hepatol, (2008). , 142-152.

[10] Xinopoulos, D., et al., Self-expanding plastic stents for inoperable malignant strictures of the cervical esophagus.Dis Esophagus, (2009). , 354-360.

[11] Diamantis, G., et al., Quality of life in patients with esophageal stenting for the palliation of malignant dysphagia.World J Gastroenterol, (2011). , 144-150.

[12] Madhusudhan, C., et al., Palliative stenting for relief of dysphagia in patients with inoperable esophageal cancer: impact on quality of life.Dis Esophagus, (2009). , 331-336.

[13] Adam, A., et al., Palliation of inoperable esophageal carcinoma: a prospective randomized trial of laser therapy and stent placement.Radiology, (1997). , 344-348.

[14] Wenger, U., et al., A nationwide study of the use of self-expanding stents in patients with esophageal cancer in Sweden. Endoscopy, 2005. 37(4): p. 329-34.

[15] Tong, D.K., S. Law, and K.H. Wong, The use of self-expanding metallic stents (SEMS) is effective in symptom palliation from recurrent tumor after esophagogastrectomy for cancer. Dis Esophagus, 2010. 23(8): p. 660-5.

[16] Mayoral, W., et al., Nonmalignant obstruction is a common problem with metal stents in the treatment of esophageal cancer.Gastrointestinal Endoscopy, (2000). , 556-559.

[17] Cwikiel, W., et al., Malignant dysphagia: palliation with esophageal stents--long-term results in 100 patients.Radiology, (1998). , 513-518.

[18] Acunas, B., et al., Palliation of malignant esophageal strictures with self-expanding nitinol stents: drawbacks and complications.Radiology, (1996). , 648-652.

[19] Song, H.Y., et al., Covered, expandable esophageal metallic stent tubes: experiences in 119 patients.Radiology, (1994). , 689-695.

[20] Kocher, M., et al., Esophageal stent with antireflux valve for tumors involving the cardia: work in progress.J Vasc Interv Radiol, (1998). , 1007-1010.

[21] Zhang, W., W.J. Meng, and Z.G. Zhou, Multiple perforations of the jejunum caused by a migrated esophageal stent.Endoscopy, (2011). , E145-E146.

[22] Borgulya, M., C. Ell, and J. Pohl, Transnasal endoscopy for direct visual control of esophageal stent placement without fluoroscopy. Endoscopy, 2012. 44(4): p. 422-424.

[23] Power, C., et al., Superiority of anti-reflux stent compared with conventional stents in the palliative management of patients with cancer of the lower esophagus and esophago-gastric junction: results of a randomized clinical trial.Dis Esophagus, (2007). , 466-470.

[24] Park, S.Y., et al., [The usefulness of clip application in preventing migration of self-expandable metal stent in patients with malignant gastrointestinal obstruction].Korean J Gastroenterol, (2007). , 4-9.

[25] Kim, I.D., et al., Prevention of covered enteral stent migration in patients with malignant gastric outlet obstruction: a pilot study of anchoring with endoscopic clips.Scand J Gastroenterol, (2010). , 100-105.

[26] Langer, F.B., et al., Solving the problem of difficult stent removal due to tissue ingrowth in partially uncovered esophageal self-expanding metal stents.Ann Thorac Surg, (2010). , 1691-1692.

[27] Hirdes, M.M., et al., The Stent-in-Stent Technique Is Effective and Safe for Removal of Embedded Esophageal Stents.Gastrointestinal Endoscopy, (2010). , Ab315-Ab316.

[28] Mason, R., Palliation, of., & oesophageal, cancer. Surg Oncol, (2001). , 123-126.

[29] Kubba, A.K. and N. Krasner, An update in the palliative management of malignant dysphagia. Eur J Surg Oncol, 2000. 26(2): p. 116-29.

[30] Sreedharan, A., et al., Interventions for dysphagia in oesophageal cancer.Cochrane Database Syst Rev, (2009). , CD005048.

[31] Hanna, W.C., et al., What is the optimal management of dysphagia in metastatic esophageal cancer? Curr Oncol,. (2012). e60-e66.

[32] Burstow, M., et al., Outcome of palliative esophageal stenting for malignant dysphagia: a retrospective analysis.Dis Esophagus, (2009). , 519-525.

[33] Ross, W.A., et al., Evolving role of self-expanding metal stents in the treatment of malignant dysphagia and fistulas.Gastrointest Endosc, (2007). , 70-76.

[34] McGrath, J.P., et al., Expandable metal stents in the palliation of malignant dysphagia and oesophageal-respiratory fistulae.Ir Med J, (2001). , 270-272.

[35] Oida, T., et al., (2011). Double Stents: Airway Stenting after Esophageal-Stent Implantation for Esophageal Cancer.Hepato-Gastroenterology, 58(112): , 1985-1988.

[36] Conio, M., et al., Self-expanding plastic stent to palliate symptomatic tissue in/overgrowth after self-expanding metal stent placement for esophageal cancer.Dis Esophagus, (2010). , 590-596.

[37] Brown, R.E., et al., A prospective phase II evaluation of esophageal stenting for neoadjuvant therapy for esophageal cancer: optimal performance and surgical safety. J Am Coll Surg, 2011. 212(4): p. 582-8; discussion 588-9.

[38] Siddiqui, A.A., et al., Placement of fully covered self-expandable metal stents in patients with locally advanced esophageal cancer before neoadjuvant therapy.Gastrointest Endosc, (2012). , 44-51.

[39] Lopes, T.L. and M.A. Eloubeidi, A pilot study of fully covered self-expandable metal stents prior to neoadjuvant therapy for locally advanced esophageal cancer. Dis Esophagus, 2010. 23(4): p. 309-15.

[40] Pellen, M.G., et al., Safety and efficacy of self-expanding removable metal esophageal stents during neoadjuvant chemotherapy for resectable esophageal cancer.Dis Esophagus, (2012). , 48-53.

[41] Spechler, S.J., et al., American Gastroenterological Association medical position statement on the management of Barrett's esophagus.Gastroenterology, (2011). , 1084-1091.

[42] Patterson, D.J., et al., Natural history of benign esophageal stricture treated by dilatation.Gastroenterology, (1983). , 346-350.

[43] Dua, K.S., et al., Removable Self-Expanding Plastic Esophageal Stent as a Continuous, Non-Permanent Dilator in Treating Refractory Benign Esophageal Strictures: A Prospective Two-Center Study. American Journal of Gastroenterology, 2008. 103(12): p. 2988-2994.

[44] Bakken, J.C., et al., Use of a fully covered self-expandable metal stent for the treatment of benign esophageal diseases.Gastrointestinal Endoscopy, (2010). , 712-720.

[45] Thomas, T., et al., Esophageal stents for benign refractory strictures: a meta-analysis.Endoscopy, (2011). , 386-393.

[46] van Boeckel, P.G., et al., Systematic review: temporary stent placement for benign rupture or anastomotic leak of the oesophagus.Aliment Pharmacol Ther, (2011). , 1292-1301.

[47] Nguyen, N.T., et al., (2011). Management of Gastrointestinal Leaks After Minimally Invasive Esophagectomy: Conventional Treatments vs.Endoscopic Stenting. Journal of Gastrointestinal Surgery, 15(11): , 1952-1960.

[48] van Heel, N.C., et al., Short-term esophageal stenting in the management of benign perforations.Am J Gastroenterol, (2010). , 1515-1520.

[49] Fernandez,A., et al., Self-expanding plastic stents for the treatment of post-operative esophago-jejuno anastomosis leak. A case series study. Rev Esp Enferm Dig, (2010). , 704-710.

[50] Freeman, R.K., et al., Analysis of Unsuccessful Esophageal Stent Placements for Esophageal Perforation, Fistula, or Anastomotic Leak.Ann Thorac Surg, (2012).

[51] Ikeya, T., et al., Endoscopic balloon dilation for benign esophageal anastomotic stricture: factors influencing its effectiveness.Hepatogastroenterology, (1999). , 959-966.

[52] Honkoop, P., et al., Benign anastomotic strictures after transhiatal esophagectomy and cervical esophagogastrostomy: risk factors and management.J Thorac Cardiovasc Surg, (1996). discussion 1147-8., 1141-1146.

[53] Swinnen, J., et al., Self-expandable metal stents for the treatment of benign upper GI leaks and perforations.Gastrointest Endosc, (2011). , 890-899.

[54] Johnsson, E., L. Lundell, and B. Liedman, Sealing of esophageal perforation or ruptures with expandable metallic stents: a prospective controlled study on treatment efficacy and limitations. Dis Esophagus, 2005. 18(4): p. 262-6.

[55] Shaw, J.M., et al., Self-expanding metal stents as an alternative to surgical bypass for malignant gastric outlet obstruction.Br J Surg, (2010). , 872-876.

[56] Zheng, B., et al., Endoscopic stenting versus gastrojejunostomy for palliation of malignant gastric outlet obstruction.Dig Endosc, (2012). , 71-78.

[57] Jeurnink, S.M., et al., Surgical gastrojejunostomy or endoscopic stent placement for the palliation of malignant gastric outlet obstruction (SUSTENT study): a multicenter randomized trial.Gastrointest Endosc, (2010). , 490-499.

[58] Morino, M., et al., Mortality after bariatric surgery: analysis of 13,871 morbidly obese patients from a national registry.Ann Surg, (2007). discussion 1007-9., 1002-1007.

[59] Sakran, N., et al., Gastric leaks after sleeve gastrectomy: a multicenter experience with 2,834 patients.Surg Endosc, (2012).

[60] Puli, S.R., I.S. Spofford, and C.C. Thompson, Use of self-expandable stents in the treatment of bariatric surgery leaks: a systematic review and meta-analysis.Gastrointest Endosc, (2012). , 287-293.

[61] Verdam, F.J., et al., [EndoBarrier for counteracting obesity and metabolic syndrome].Ned Tijdschr Geneeskd, (2012). , A3844.

[62] Schouten, R., et al., A multicenter, randomized efficacy study of the EndoBarrier Gastrointestinal Liner for presurgical weight loss prior to bariatric surgery. Ann Surg, 2010. 251(2): p. 236-43.

[63] Mathus-Vliegen, E.M., [Endobarrier: a unique but still premature concept]. Ned Tijdschr Geneeskd, 2012. 156(13): p. A4590.

[64] Conio, M., et al., Self-expanding plastic stent to palliate symptomatic tissue in/overgrowth after self-expanding metal stent placement for esophageal cancer.Diseases of the Esophagus, (2010). , 590-596.

[65] Cerna, M., et al., Covered Biodegradable Stent: New Therapeutic Option for the Management of Esophageal Perforation or Anastomotic Leak.Cardiovascular and Interventional Radiology, (2011). , 1267-1271.

[66] Guo, J.H., et al., Self-expandable esophageal stent loaded with I-125 seeds: Initial experience in patients with advanced esophageal cancer.Radiology, (2008). , 574-581.

[67] Park, C.G., et al., Polymeric nanofiber coated esophageal stent for sustained delivery of an anticancer drug.Macromolecular Research, (2011). , 1210-1216.

Section 3

Lower Gastrointestinal Tract

Chapter 11

Ileoscopy; How and Why to Do It

Arjuna P. De Silva

Additional information is available at the end of the chapter

http://dx.doi.org/10.5772/52628

1. Introduction

Colonoscopy is a widely practiced procedure. Ileal intubation is widely regarded as the gold standard for evidence of complete colonoscopy[1]. However, this is not routinely attempted because of perceived technical difficulty, excess time thought to be added to the procedure or the low diagnostic yield that it was thought to provide [2]. However, there is mounting clinical evidence that ileoscopy is of clinical benefit [3]. It also important to remember that if ileoscopy is not routinely practiced, performing an ileoscopy may become difficult even when there is a definite clinical indication for doing so, such as, when Crohn's disease or ileal tuberculosis is suspected.

Currently the position employed to intubate ileum is with the patient in the left lateral position and entering the valve at the 6 o' clock position [4]. However, we have sometimes encountered difficulty when performing ileoscopy in this position leading to extra time being taken during busy endoscopy lists. During such difficult procedures we found that placing the patient in the prone position facilitated ileal intubation.

The available evidence for routine ileoscopy during colonoscopy is controversial. Some studies have demonstrated a benefit of ileoscopy in selected patients. These include patients with diarrhoea, inflammatory bowel disease (IBD), suspected ileocecal tuberculosis (TB), right lower quadrant pain and hematochezia[5,6,7,89,10]. Most studies on place of routine ileoscopy during colonoscopy were done in Western populations and only a few studies conducted among Asians [6, 8].

Relatively low prevalence of Crohn's disease (CD) [8, 10] high prevalence of gastrointestinal infections including TB in our part of the world compared to the west make it even more worthwhile to study the place of routine ileoscopy in the tropical setting. This may have a significant impact on patient management in these settings.

2. Aims

The aim of our fiststudy was to test the hypothesis that the prone position made ileal intubation easier and quicker than the standard position that is currently used – the left lateral position.

The aim of the second study was to determine if routine ileoscopy was useful.

2.1. Methods [1]

We first performed a pilot study on ten patients undergoing routine colonoscopy using fluoroscopy to determine the best patient position for the most direct (end-on) approach to the ileo-caecal valve. Confirming our clinical impressions, the prone 12 o'clock position (patient prone and the tip of the colonoscope at the 12 o'clock position in relation to the ileocaecal valve) appeared to be the best position as this brought the tip of the colonoscope in line with the ileocaecal valve (figure1). This was unlike in the 6 o'clock position (patient in left lateral position with tip of the colonoscope at the 6 o'clock position in relation to the ileocaecal valve) where the tip of the colonoscope was curved and not in the same axis (figure 2).

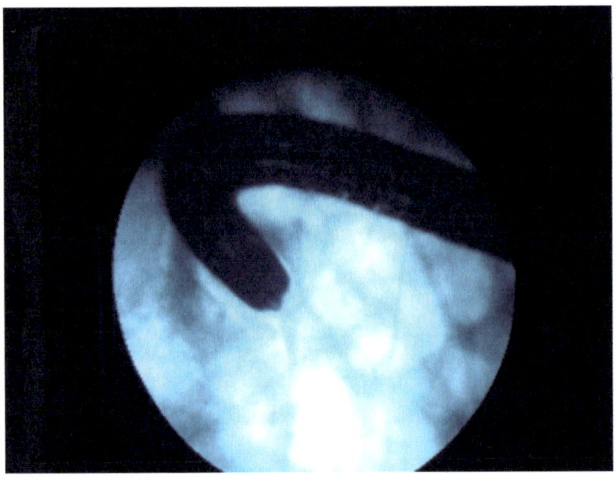

Figure 1. 6 o'clock position

We then randomized consecutive patients referred for colonoscopy to our unit between February2009 and Jan 2010 using computer generated random numbers. Patients aged between 18-80 years and who were not pregnant were recruited after obtaining their written informed consent. They were then randomized to undergo ileoscopy either in the standard position or the prone 12 o'clock position.

All patients were given four packets of polyethylene glycol (PEG) for bowel cleansing prior to colonoscopy. All patients received pre-medication with medazolam 2.5 mg i.v. and pethidine 25 mg i.v. All patients had pulse oxymetry monitoring during the procedure. None of the patients were given hyoscine-n-butyl bromide. The colonoscopes used were Olympus CF Q145L models.

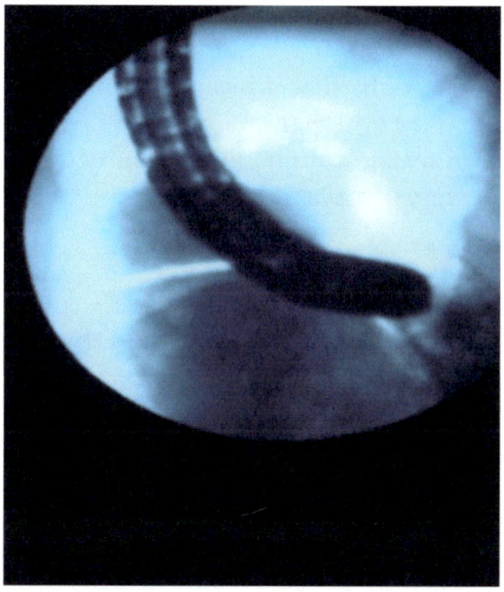

Figure 2. 12 o'clock position

All colonoscopies were performed by experienced endoscopists (MAN and KVUK). After the ileo-caecal valve was identified during colonoscopy, ileal intubation time was standardized, and defined as the time taken for the tip of the colonoscope to be maneuvered from the mid-point of the caecum to entering the terminal ileum. This was timed by an independent observer (RSK).

2.1.1. Ethical clearance

Ethical clearance for the study was obtained from the Ethics Committee of the Faculty of Medicine, University of Kelaniya, Sri Lanka. Informed written consent was obtained from all patients.

2.1.2. Statistics

Sample size calculation was done on an assumption of 75% v 95% success at ileal intubation with the PP comp, and at 90% power this required a sample of 150 patients. The data was compared using Chi squared test and the statistical difference between the two groups will compared using the program SPSS 16.

2.2. Methods [2]

A retrospective study was conducted in the University Endoscopy Unit of the Colombo North Teaching Hospital, Ragama, Sri Lanka. As a policy in the University Medical Unit all patients undergoing colonoscopy had a routine ileoscopy and biopsy. All consenting patients who underwent colonoscopy from 01 January 2008 to 31 December 2012 were included in the study. Data was obtained from the endoscopy database and patient records using a preformed data extraction form. Details of the histopathological diagnoses were obtained from the data base of the Department of Pathology, Faculty of Medicine, University of Kelaniya, Ragama.

We hypothesized patients with right iliac fossa (RIF) pain, diarrhoea, anaemia, IBD and raised inflammatory markers have a higher incidence of ileal abnormality than the patients undergoing colonoscopy for other indications. Accordingly the macroscopic and microscopic abnormalities of the ileum were compared between these two groups.

2.2.1. Ethical clearance

Ethical clearance for this study was obtained from the Ethics Committee of the Faculty of Medicine, University of Kelaniya, Ragama, Sri Lanka.

2.2.2. Statistics

All statistical analysis was done using SPSS 16.

2.3. Results [1]

Colonoscopy was performed on 150 patients [82 females, mean (SD) age 53 (16) years]. 75 patients were randomized for ileal intubation in the PP and 75 patients in the LLP. The two groups were comparable for age, sex, indication for colonoscopy and abnormalities in the ileum (Table 1). Overall, the ileum was successfully intubated in 145 (96%) patients [74 (98.7%) in the PP and71 (94.7%) in the LLP]. The median (Interquartile Range) ileal intubation time was12 (10) seconds in the PP and 87(82) seconds in the LLP ($p<0.0001$; Mann-Whitney U test). The ileum was abnormal in 11 (7.5%) patients: 6 in the PP group and 5 in the LLP group.

Indication for colonoscopy	Prone 12 (n=75)	Left lateral (n=75)
Diarrhoea	8	5
Constipation	8	12
Altered bowel habits	19	18
Abdominal pain	16	12
Iron deficiency Anaemia	9	10
Per rectal bleeding	3	6
IBD	6	8
Carcinoma of unknown primary	3	1
Loss of weight or& Loss of appetite	3	3
Number of patients with ileitis	6	5

Table 1. Indication for colonoscopy

2.4. Results [2]

A total of 2621 colonoscopies were done within the study period. Routine ileoscopy was practiced in 1096 patients who were evaluated by the University Medical Unit. Successful caecal intubation was achieved in 992 (90.51%) patients and the ileum was intubated in 832 (75.9%). 13 patients who underwent a repeat colonoscopy during the study period and 9 patients whose data records were incomplete were excluded from the final analysis Figure 3.

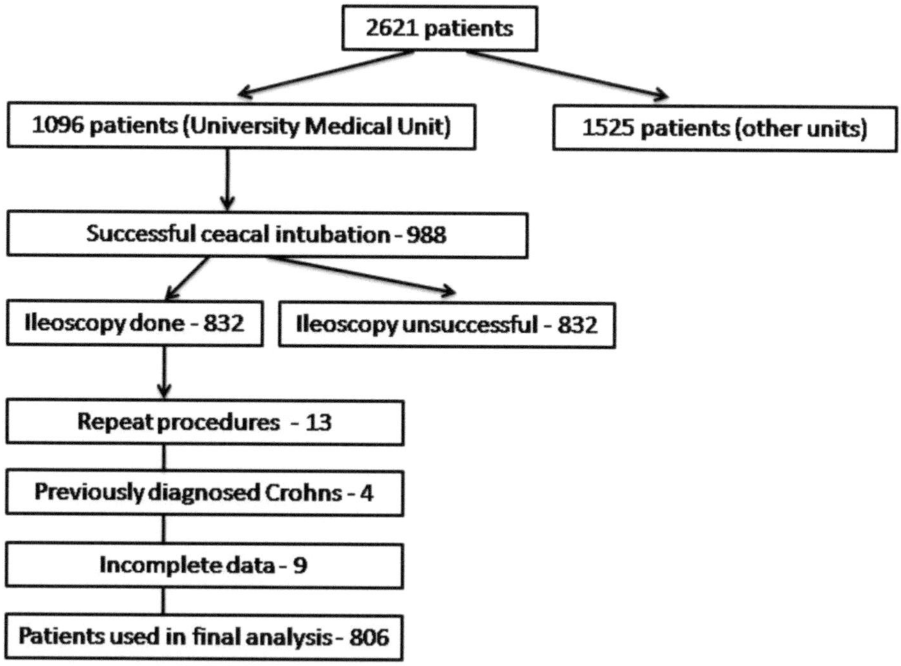

Figure 3. Trial profile

Indications for colonoscopy in patients who underwent ileal intubation were as follows (Table 2).

Four patients with Crohn disease were not analysed as they were any way expected to have ileal abnormalities. A total of 806 patients were taken in to final analysis.

These 806 patients were categorized as follows: presence of right iliac fossa (RIF) pain, diarrhoea, anaemia, ulcerative colitis (UC) and raised inflammatory markers considered as having a definite indication for ileoscopy (Group A); patients who underwent colonoscopy for any other reason as not having a definite indication for ileoscopy (Group B). Accordingly there were 593/806 (73.57%) patients with an indication for ileoscopy (Group A) and 213/806 (26.42%) patients did not have a definite indication for ileoscopy (Group B). Both groups were socio-demographically comparable to each other(Table 3).

Indication for Colonoscopy	Number of patients	Percentage (%)
RIF pain	126	15.55
Diarrhoea	238	29.38
Anaemia	80	9.88
Ulcerative colitis	89	10.98
Crohns disease	4	0.49
Polyps	7	0.86
IBS	29	3.58
Loss of weight	17	2.09
LIF pain	22	2.71
Constipation	61	7.53
Bleeding PR	47	5.80
RIF pain and Diarrhoea	18	2.22
Anaemia and Diarrhoea	6	0.74
Raised inflammatory markers	6	0.74
Bleeding PR and RIF pain	10	1.23
Bleeding PR and Diarrhoea	21	2.59
Other	29	3.58
Total	810	100.00

Table 2. Indications for colonoscopy

	Group A	Group B	P
Number	593	213	
Mean Age (SD) years	48.8 (16.5)	49.9 (15.4)	0.072
Male: Female ratio	1:1.08	1:1.05	0.818

Table 3. Demografic data of patients

137/806 patients (16.99%) studied had either macroscopic [48 (5.95%)] or microscopic [89 (11.04%)] abnormalities of the ileum. Ileum was considered macroscopically abnormal when it was described to have ulcers, strictures or evidence of inflammation by the endoscopist. Microscopic abnormalities described were Crohns disease, backwash ileitis of ulcerative colitis, tuberculosis (TB), ileitis due to resolving infection, drug induced ileitis and non specific-ileitis(Table 4,5)

Patients with macroscopic abnormalities of the ileum had significantly higher incidence of all histological abnormalities ($p<0.0001$, $\chi^2 186$) as well as histopathological diagnoses which altered the management (Crohns disease, TB, Drug induced ileitis, Ileitis due to infection) ($p<0.0001$, χ^2 119) when compared with the patients whose ileum was macroscopically normal(Table 6).

	Group A	Group B	Total (%)
Macroscopically Abnormal	41	7	48 (5.95%)
Macroscopically Normal	552	206	758 (94.05%)
Total	593	213	806 (100%)

Table 4. Macroscopic abnormalities of the ileum

Histopathological Diagnosis	Crohns	UC	TB	Drugs	Infection	Non-specific	Normal	Total
Macroscopy Abnormal	10 (20.83%)	8 (16.6%)	6 (12.5%)	01 (2.08%)	03 (6.25%)	06 (12.5%)	14 (29.16%)	48 (100%)
Macroscopy Normal	18 (2.37%)	6 (0.79%)	0	04 (0.52%)	05 (0.66%)	22 (2.9%)	703 (92.7%)	758 (100%)
Total	28 (3.47%)	14 (1.73%)	6 (0.74%)	5 (0.62%)	8 (0.99%)	28 (3.47%)	717 (88.95%)	806 (100%)

Table 5. Macroscopic and microscopic abnormalities

Histopathological Diagnosis	Group A	Group B	Total	Percentage (%)
Crohns disease	24	4	28	31.46
Tuberculosis	6	0	6	6.74
Ileitis- resolving infection	8	0	8	8.98
Drug induced ileitis	4	0	5	5.61
Back wash ileitis in UC	13	1	14	15.73
Non specific Ileitis	25	3	28	31.46
Total	80	9	89	100.00

Table 6. Histopathological abnormalities of the ileum

55 patients who had microscopic abnormalities in the ileum did not have a macroscopic abnormality of the ileum. Their histological diagnoses were Crohns disease (18), ileitis - resolving infection (5), drug induced (4), backwash ileitis in ulcerative colitis (6) and non-specific ileitis (22).

657 (81.5%) patients had no macroscopic mucosal abnormality in the colon, but 21(3.19%) of them had macroscopic ileal abnormalities. Furthermore 39(5.9%) patients with macroscopically normal colonic mucosa had histopathological abnormalities in the

ileum, namely Crohns disease (8), drug induced ileitis (2), resolving infection (2) and non specific ileitis (27).

47 (5.83%) of these microscopic abnormalities were considered to be significant ileal pathology which changed the management of the patient or provided clinically useful information, namely Crohn's disease (28), Tuberculosis(6), Ileitis due to resolving infection (8) or drug induced (5).] Such ileal abnormalities were significantly higher among patients with right iliac fossa (RIF) pain, diarrhea, anemia, ulcerative colitis (UC) and raised inflammatory markers (Group A) [43/593] when compared to the others(Group B) [4/213]: (p=0.0032, χ^2 8.23).

3. Conclusions

We have shown that during colonoscopy, the prone 12 o'clock position gives a more direct approach to the ileo-caecal valve and, although the ileum was intubated in more than 90% of cases in both positions, significantly reduces ileal intubation time when compared to the standard left lateral 6 o'clock position. The reason for this is that in the prone 12 o'clock position, the axis of the tip of the colonoscope is the same as the ileocaecal valve (as clearly demonstrated during fluoroscopy). This makes entry into the ileocaecal valve much easier. Since we use only light sedation (medazolam and pethidine) turning patients to the prone position is easy. The ileal abnormality rate was similar in both groups, and would therefore have not confounded our results.

The short coming of this study would probably be that we have not checked other positions of ileal intubation. However, we used the best position established by other studies and what is generally accepted as the best position(6 o'clock position) vs what we empirically thought was the best position (12o' clock). We also did a pilot study using fluoroscopy to establish the best possible position as well.

Although several previous studies have reported on the time taken for ileal intubation, such timings have not been standardized [5]. This has resulted in varying definitions of ileal intubation times which are not comparable, and the times reported range from seconds in some studies to more than ten minutes in some [6]. While no studies have clearly stated how to define ileal intubation time, it is assumed to be the time taken to maneuver the endoscope from the tip of the valve into the terminal ileum [4]. We felt that this does not give a true reflection of the difficulty of the procedure. We, therefore, defined it as the time taken for the tip of the colonoscope to be maneuvered from the mid-point of the caecum to entering the terminal ileum. Furthermore, we did not design our trial as a cross over study because once the ileum is intubated, the valve becomes patulous making the second intubation is easier [4].

In conclusion, during colonoscopy the prone 12 o'clock position gives a more direct approach to the ileo-caecal valve than the left lateral 6 o'clock position and significantly reduces ileal intubation time. Incorporation of this observation into one's daily practice can be considered.

In our second study we found 16.9% of our study patients had either macroscopic or microscopic abnormality in the ileum. This is a much higher figure when compared to studies conducted in western countries[5,6,9]. Such studies have shown 2%-7.2% diagnostic yield in routine ileoscopy when performed in unselected patients[6]. In one study the diagnostic yield of ileoscopy had been only 0.3%[5].Crohns ileitis had been the diagnosis made in most cases. However in most such studies, the ileum had been biopsied only when there was a macroscopic abnormality seen on endoscopy [5,6]. In our study an ileal biopsy was taken irrespective of the endoscopic findings of the ileum and we found that 55 patients with macroscopically normal ileum had microscopic abnormalities.

There were 657/806(81.5%) patients who did not have a mucosal abnormality of the colon on endoscopy. Out of this there were 21/657(3.19%) patients with macroscopic abnormalities and 39/657(5.9%) patients with histopathological abnormalities of the ileum. Among these there were 8 patients with Crohns disease who were diagnosed on ileoscopy and biopsy which would have been missed otherwise. One study conducted in India also has shown a high diagnostic yield of ileoscopy and 14 %(8/57) study participants with ileal abnormalities were found to have a normal colonoscopy and barium enema[7].

According to the literature it is clear that the yield of ileoscopy would depend on the clinical presentation of the patient. Therefore in our study we hypothesized that patients with Right iliac fossa pain (RIF pain), Diarrhea, Anemia, Inflammatory bowel disease (IBD) and Raised inflammatory markers would have a higher incidence of ileal abnormality than the patients undergoing colonoscopy for any other indication. Rationale behind this hypothesis was that it would include the patients with common conditions that would give rise to ileal abnormalities such as Crohns disease, tuberculosis and other chronic infections. Accordingly we have shown that the ileal abnormalities are significantly higher among patients with above features than those who don't have them.

Twenty eight patients were diagnosed to have Crohns disease on ileal biopsy and it is 3.4% of our total population. Even though there is no data available on population prevalence of Crohns disease in Sri Lanka, a hospital based survey carried out in two districts of Sri Lanka had found the prevalence of Crohns disease to be 1.2/100000 population[11].This study was conducted in a tertiary referral centre with a special interest in inflammatory bowel disease. Therefore it is likely that the patients undergoing colonoscopy in our unit may have a higher prevalence of Crohns disease than the general population. Same bias in the sample may have contributed to the low prevalence of ileal tuberculosis and other gastrointestinal infections.

In conclusion, ileoscopy should be an integral part of any colonoscopy and especially so in the presence of right iliac fossa pain, inflammatory bowel disease, anaemia, diarrhoea and raised inflammatory markers. It improves the diagnostic yield of the colonoscopy by giving additional information, sometimes when the macroscopic appearances of the colon and the ileum are normal.

Author details

Arjuna P. De Silva

Faculty of Medicine University of Kelaniya, Sri Lanka

References

[1] Borsh, G., & Schmidt, G. Endoscopy of the terminal ileum. Diagnostic yield in 400 consecutive examinations.Dis Colon Rectum. (1985). , 28, 499-501.

[2] Harwood GC, Mattek NC, Holub JL et al.Variation in practice of ileal intubation among diverse endoscopy settings:results from a national endoscopic database. Aliment PharmocolTher. (2005). , 22, 571-8.

[3] Seong, H. J., Kwang, J. L., & Yeong, B. K. Diagnostic value of terminal ileum intubation during colonoscopy. J Gastroenterol and Hepatol. (2008). , 23, 51-5.

[4] Ansari A, Soon SY, Saunders BP, Sanderson JD. A Prospective Study Of The Feasibility of Ileoscopy at Colonoscopy. Scand J Gastroenterol.2003; 38:1185-7.

[5] Misra SP, Dwivedi M, Misra V. Ileoscopy in 39 hematochezia patients with normal colonoscopy,World J Gastroenterol2006 May 21; 12(19): 3101-3104

[6] Cherian, S., & Singh, P. Is routine Ileoscopy useful? An observational study of procedure times, diagnostic yield, and learning curve. Am Journal of Gastroenterol (2004). , 99, 2324-2329.

[7] Bhasin, D. K., Goenka, M. K., Dhavan, S., Dass, K., & Singh, K. Diagnostic value of ileoscopy: a report from India,. J ClinGastroenterol(2000). , 31(2), 144-146.

[8] Yoong, K. K. Y., & Heymann, T. It is not worthwhile to perform ileoscopy on all patients,SurgEndosc (2006). , 20, 809-811.

[9] Kennedy, G., Larson, D., Wolff, B., Winter, D., Petersen, B., & Larson, M. Routine ileal intubation during screening colonoscopy: a useful maneuver?.SurgEndosc (2008). , 22, 2606-2608.

[10] Jeong SH, Lee KJ, Kim YB, Kwon HC, Sin SJ, Chung JY.Diagnostic value of terminal ileum intubation during colonoscopy, J. Gastroenterol. Hepatol. (2008). Jan; , 23(1), 4-5.

[11] Niriella, M. A., de Silva, A. P., Dayarathne, A. H. G. K., Ariyasinghe, M. H. A. D. P., Nawarathne, M. M. N., Pieriset, R. S. K., & al, . Prevalence of Inflammatory Bowel Disease in two districts of Sri Lanka: a hospital based survey. BMC Gastroenterology (2010).

Chapter 12

Therapeutic and Diagnostic Approaches in Colonoscopy

Naohisa Yoshida, Nobuaki Yagi, Yutaka Inada,
Munehiro Kugai, Akio Yanagisawa and Yuji Naito

Additional information is available at the end of the chapter

http://dx.doi.org/10.5772/52733

1. Introduction

Colorectal cancer is a common gastrointestinal malignancy in the USA, Europe, and Japan. Most colorectal cancers are thought to arise from preexisting adenomas based on the concept of the adenoma-carcinoma sequence [1]. Chromoendoscopy, using Kudo and Tsuruta's pit pattern classification, is an efficient tool for the differential diagnosis of colorectal polyps [2-4]. Recently, image-enhanced endoscopy (IEE) has been used for diagnosing gastrointestinal tumors [5-7]. Endoscopic therapy, including endoscopic mucosal resection (EMR) and endoscopic submucosal dissection (ESD), is used worldwide to treat adenoma and early colorectal cancer [8-10]. In this chapter, we demonstrated the effectiveness of IEE and discuss strategies of therapeutic endoscopy including EMR and ESD.

2. Image-enhanced endoscopy

Colonoscopy is accepted as an efficient examination for the detection of neoplastic colorectal lesions. However, the diagnostic capability of white-light endoscopy (WL) for the differentiation of neoplastic and non-neoplastic polyps shows low sensitivity (38–76%) and variable specificity (66–97%) [11-13]. On the other hand, chromoendoscopy has demonstrated high sensitivity (96.3–97.0%) and specificity (93.5–100%) for the differentiation of neoplastic and non-neoplastic polyps [10,11]. However, chromoendoscopy is time-consuming. Now, image-enhanced endoscopy (IEE) is used to diagnose gastrointestinal tumors. This method is a change from conventional WL endoscopy, and requires no dye. It only requires the push of a button. IEE such as narrow band imaging (NBI), flexible spectral imaging color enhancement (FICE), and autofluorescence imaging (AFI) offer many advantages for diagnosis of neoplastic tumors, evaluation of invasion depth of cancerous lesions, and detection of neoplastic lesions. We demonstrated the efficacy of IEE for diagnosis of colorectal tumors in view of endoscopic treatment options.

3. NBI, FICE, and AFI systems

With the NBI system (Olympus Medical Co., Tokyo, Japan), optical filters that allow narrow-band light to pass at wavelengths of 415 and 540 nm are mechanically inserted between a xenon lamp and a red/green/blue rotation filter [12-15]. Narrow vessels at the mucosal surface can be seen most clearly at 415 nm, which is the wavelength that corresponds to the hemoglobin absorption band, while thick vessels in the deep layer of the mucosa can be detected at 540 nm. Thus, NBI can enhance vascular patterns [Figure 1]. Moreover, NBI can detect pit like structures, which have been recognized as surface patterns by a Japanese consensus symposium [16].

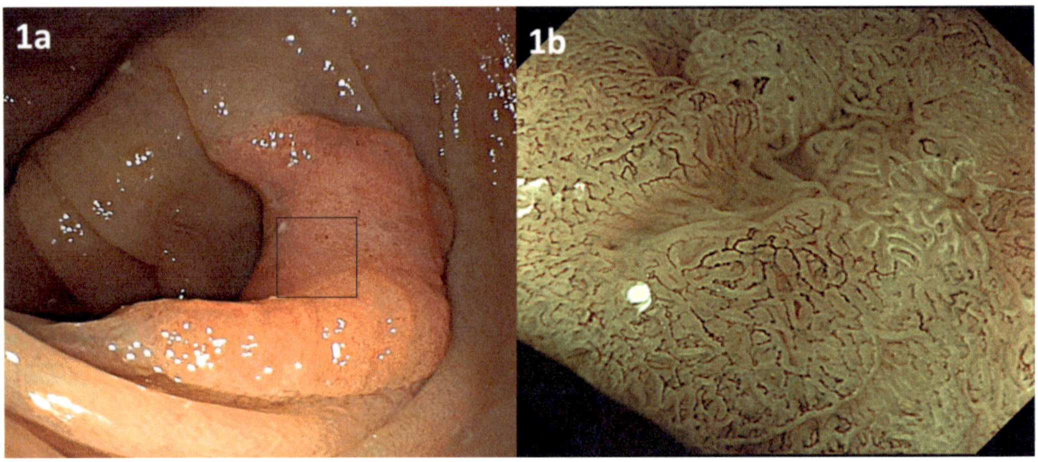

Figure 1. NBI with magnification. 1a: 0-IIa polyp, 20 mm in diameter. White-light endoscopy image. 1b: Mucosal capillary and irregular surface pattern were detected by NBI with magnification. The polyp was diagnosed as a neoplastic polyp.

The FICE system (Fujifilm Medical Co., Tokyo, Japan) is another type of IEE, but is unlike NBI. FICE was formerly known as Fuji Intelligent Color Endoscopy, but this definition has recently changed. FICE depends on optical filters and spectral-estimation technology to reconstruct images at different wavelengths based on WL images [17,18]. The suitable RGB wavelength settings and contrast levels for FICE to evaluate colorectal polyps are 540 (1) nm, 460 (4) nm, and 460 (4) nm, respectively [19,20]. FICE can display color images in real time with RGB components that have been assigned selected spectra. FICE can enhance vascular and surface patterns (Figure 2)[19-23]. AFI videoendoscopy (Olympus Medical Co., Tokyo, Japan) is comprised of a blue light to provoke emissions and a green light for hemoglobin absorption [24-26]. Neoplastic areas involve a thickening of the mucosal layer and increased hemoglobin, and so are expected to exhibit weaker autofluorescence compared to non-neoplastic areas (Figure 3).

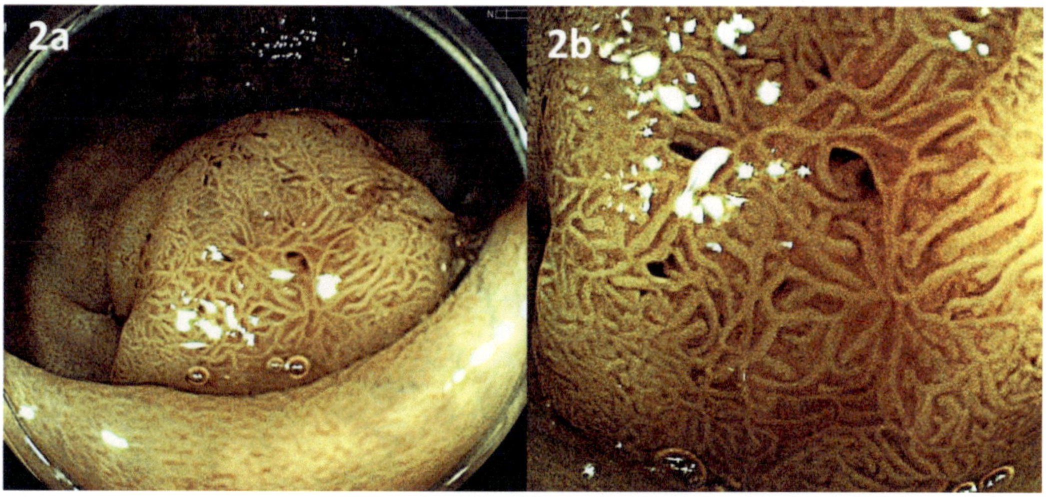

Figure 2. FICE with magnification. 2a: 0-Isp polyp 12 mm in diameter. White-light endoscopy image. 2b: Mucosal capillary and surface pattern were detected with FICE with magnification. The polyp was diagnosed as a neoplastic polyp.

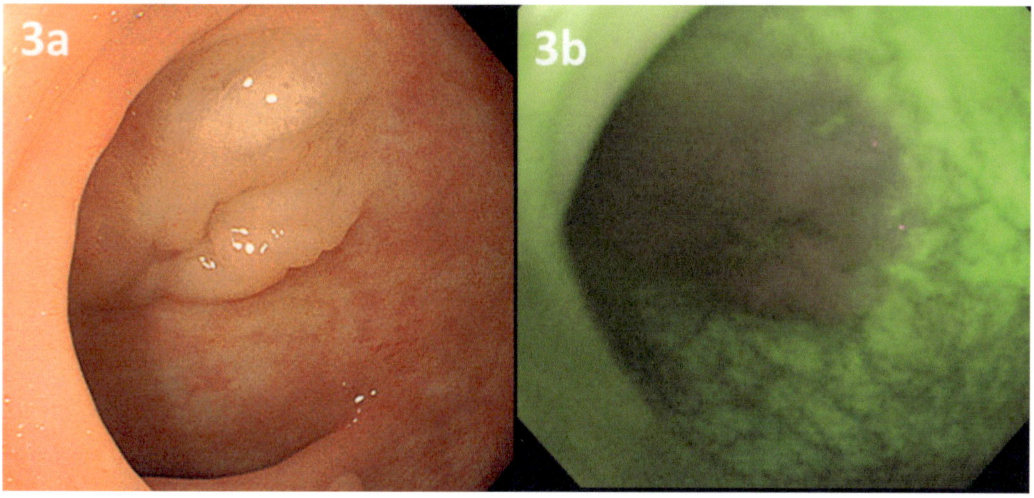

Figure 3. AFI. 3a. 0-IIa polyp 20 mm in diameter. White-light endoscoy image. 3b. In AFI, the normal mucosa is detected by green color and the neoplastic polyp was detected by magenta color.

4. Clinical advantages of NBI and FICE

Magnifying endoscopy (ME) is uncommon in the USA and Europe. Therefore, accurate diagnosis of colorectal polyps through endoscopy without magnification is required. In NBI, high-definition colonoscopy without magnification has been able to predict whether a colorectal polyp is neoplastic or non-neoplastic [26, 27]. A meshed capillary network is one of the important endoscopic features of neoplastic polyps in NBI without magnification, as described by Sano et al. [5] (Figure 4). Rex [28] adopted a surface pattern including pit and vascular pattern for neoplastic features in NBI, and Rastogi et al. used 5 different surface patterns (including mucosal, pit, and vascular patterns) to differentiate neoplastic polyps from non-neoplastic polyps [11]. In various studies, NBI without magnification had an accuracy of 89–92.7%, sensitivity of 87.9–95.7%, and specificity of 87–90.5% (Table 1) [26-30].

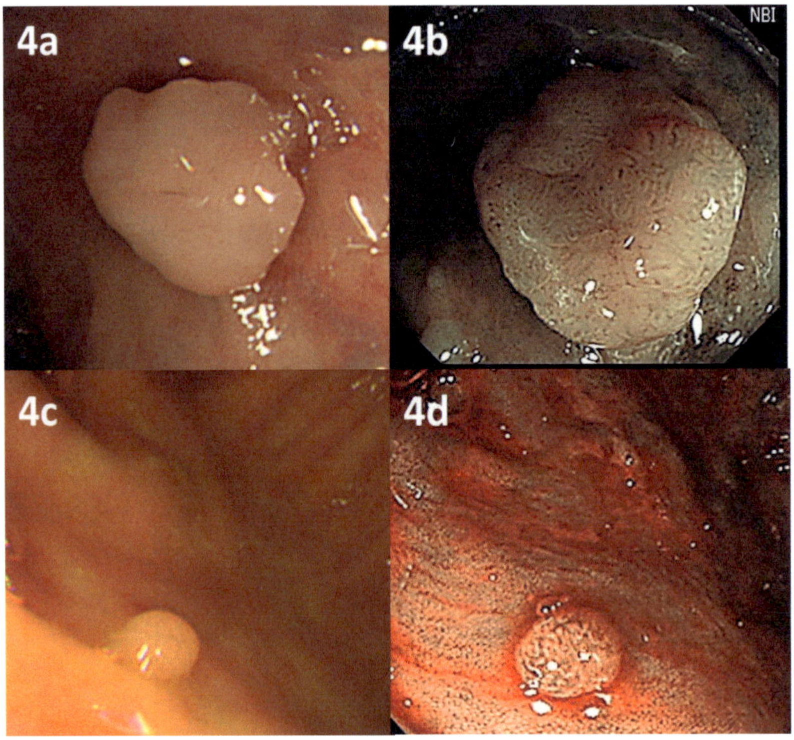

Figure 4. NBI without magnification. 4a: 0-Isp polyp 6 mm in diameter. White-light endoscopy image. 2b: Meshed capillary pattern was detected with NBI without magnification. The polyp was diagnosed as a neoplastic polyp. 4c: 0-Is polyp 3 mm in diameter. White-light endoscopy image. 4d: Meshed capillary pattern was detected with NBI without magnification. The polyp was diagnosed as a neoplastic polyp.

FICE without magnification is also reported to be useful for differentiation between neoplastic and non-neoplastic polyps. The detection of surface patterns by FICE is a reliable method to determine whether a polyp is neoplastic or non-neoplastic, and evaluation of vascular pattern has also been described (Figure 5) [19]. In various studies, FICE without magnification has demonstrated an accuracy of 84.4–89.4%, sensitivity of 89.4–93.2%, and specificity of 81.2–88%, similar to the findings for NBI (Table 1) [19,30].

Author	System	No. of cases	Accuracy (%)	Sensitivity (%)	Specificity (%)
Henry ZH et al	NBI	126	90.0	93.0	88.0
Su MY et al	NBI	110	92.7	95.7	87.5
Tischendorf JJW et al	NBI	100	89.0	87.9	90.5
Rex DK	NBI	451	89.0	92.0	87.0
Lonqcroft-Wheaton GR	FICE	232	88.0	-	-
Pohl J et al	FICE	321	84.4	93.2	61.2
Yoshida N et al	FICE	151	89.4	89.4	88.0
Sato R et al	AFI	358	91.9	92.7	92.9

NBI: narrow-band imaging, FICE: flexible spectral imaging color enhancement

Table 1. Reports of image-enhanced endoscopy without magnification for the differentiation of neoplastic and non-neoplastic polyps

When polyp size is considered, the accuracy of NBI without magnification for Polyps 10mm or greater in diameter (accuracy: 96.0%) were greater than those for polyps 5 mm or less in diameter (accuracy: 90.0%) [27]. In FICE without magnification, the accuracy, sensitivity, and specificity for polyps 6 mm or greater in diameter (97.1%, 95.2%, 90%, respectively) are greater than those for polyps 5 mm or less in diameter (82.7%, 78.0%, 87.5%) [18,32]. Diagnosis of small polyps is important for the prevention of colorectal cancer. A procedural decision to avoid resection of non-neoplastic polyps would spare patients the cost and risk of a polypectomy that serves no useful purpose.

Recently, an international cooperative group, the Colon Tumor NBI Interest Group, was formed. The group consists of members from Japan, the USA, and Europe, and it has developed the NBI international colorectal endoscopic (NICE) classification, which classifies colorectal tumors into types 1–3 and is even applicable to colorectal tumors closely observed without magnification (Table 2) [16]. NICE types 1 and 3 are mainly observed in hyperplastic polyps and massively invasive submucosal cancer, respectively. NICE Type2 is observed in various histopathological types such as adenoma, intramucosal cancer, and less invasive submucosal cancer. The NICE classification with or without magnification is considered valid in the USA, Europe, and Japan for differentiating neoplastic and non-neoplastic polyps [33].

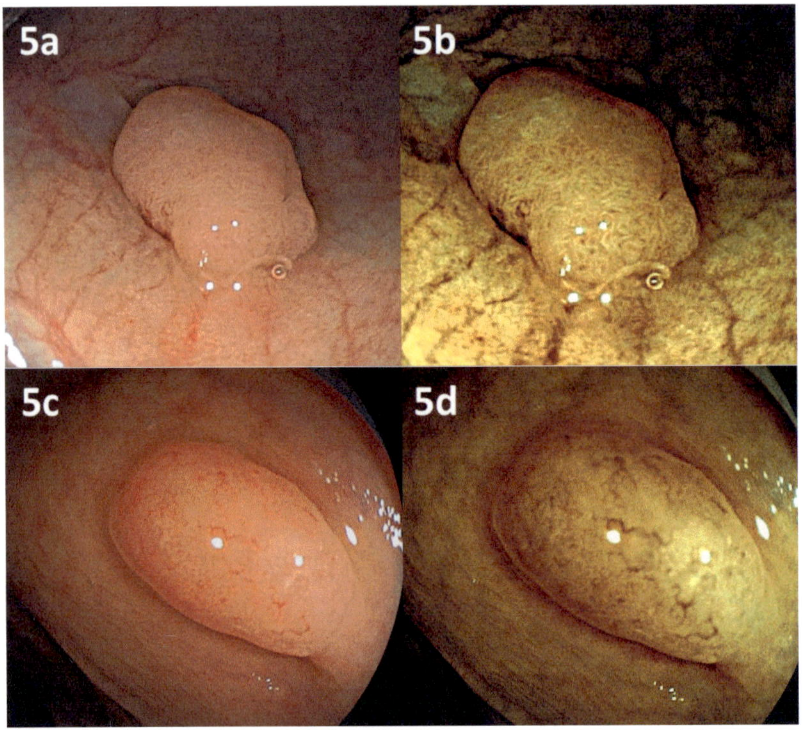

Figure 5. FICE without magnification. 5a: 0-Isp polyp 5 mm in diameter. 5b: Image of FICE without magnification. Tubular and oval pits were identified as neoplastic surface patterns. Vascular patterns were detected. 5c: 0-Is polyp 3 mm in diameter. 5d: Image of FICE without magnification. Round pits were identified as non-neoplastic surface patterns.

	Type 1	Type 2	Type 3
Color	Same or lighter than background	Browner relative to background (verify color arises from vessels)	Brown to dark brown relative to background; sometimes patchy whiter areas
Vascular pattern	None, or isolated lacy vessels may be present coursing across the lesion	Thick brown vessels surrounding white structures	Has area(s) with markedly distorted or missing vessels
Surface Pattern	Dark or white spots of uniform size, or homogenous absence of pattern	Oval, tubular or branched white structures surrounded by brown vessels	Areas of distortion or absence of pattern

Table 2. NICE classification

Regarding of IEE-ME techniques, there have been many studies on both NBI-ME and FICE-ME [12, 13, 17, 23, 34-36]. These studies have reported accuracy of 93.4–98.9%, sensitivity of 90.9–100%, specificity of 75–98.9%, PPV of 91.2–97.3%, and NPV of 90–100% for the differentiation of neoplastic and non-neoplastic lesions (Table 3). There are 4 published classifications of NBI-ME, including the Sano classification, the Hiroshima classification, the Showa Classification, and the Jikei Classification, and 1 published classification for FICE-ME [15, 16, 23, 34, 37]. In brief, the Sano classification, Showa classification, and Jikei classification are based only on vascular patterns, while the Hiroshima classification and FICE classification use surface and vascular patterns. The efficacy of surface pattern detection in NBI and FICE with magnification has been reported [16, 23].

Author	System	No. of cases	Accuracy (%)	Sensitivity (%)	Specificity (%)
Machida H et al	NBI	43	93.4	100.0	75.0
Sano Y et al	NBI	150	95.3	96.4	92.3
Wada Y et al	NBI	617	96.7	90.9	97.1
Tanaka S et al	NBI	289	98.9	100.0	98.9
Togashi K et al	FICE	107	87.0	93.0	70.0
Santos CE et al	FICE	111	92.8	97.8	79.3

NBI: narrow-band imaging, FICE: flexible spectral imaging color enhancement

Table 3. Reports of image-enhanced endoscopy with magnification for differentiation of neoplastic and non-neoplastic polyps

The accuracy, sensitivity, and specificity of each NBI and FICE classification for massively invasive submucosal cancer are described in Table 4 [15, 16, 23, 34, 37]. Accuracy of 87.7–98.3%, sensitivity of 63.8–100%, specificity of 88.7–100%, PPV of 71.8–100%, and NPV of 90–96.2% have been reported. NBI and FICE with magnification are thought to be useful for directing therapeutic strategies, including endoscopic resection by EMR, ESD, or surgery for colorectal tumors. However, the sensitivity (63.8%–100%) and specificity (88.7–100%) are not enough. Chromoendoscopy using the pit pattern classification should be performed when a lesion suspected as cancerous is detected with NBI and FICE or is diagnosed by NBI and FICE with low confidence. The following sections contain details of 2 of the published NBI classifications.

Author	System	No. of cases	Accuracy (%)	Sensitivity (%)	Specificity (%)
Wada Y et al	NBI	584	96.1	100.0	95.8
Tanaka S et al	NBI	97	94.1	63.8	100.0
Ikematsu H et al	NBI	130	87.7	84.8	88.7
Yoshida N et al	FICE	124	98.3	77.7	100.0
Saito S et al	NBI	291	88.7	95.6	77.3

NBI: narrow-band imaging, FICE: flexible spectral imaging color enhancement

Table 4. Reports of image-enhanced endoscopy with magnification for identification of massively invasive submucosal cancer

5. Sano classification (Figure 6) [5, 15]

This classification is based on the surface characteristics of the meshed capillaries. Capillary pattern (CP) type I indicates that there is no meshed capillary pattern visible, as in hyperplastic polyps. CP type II describes the regular small caliber capillaries observed in adenomatous polyps. CP type III is defined as an irregular and unarranged pattern in a mesh-like micro-vascular architecture that exhibits at least 1 of the following: irregular size, complicated branching, or disrupted irregular winding [35]. CP type III lesions are further classified into 2 groups, IIIA or IIIB, according to microvascular architecture and microvessel density with lack of uniformity and blind endings, branching and irregularly curtailed. CP type IIIA is observed mainly in adenoma, intramucosal cancer, and less invasive submucosal cancers. CP type IIIB was reported in 28% of intramucosal cancers and 72% of massively invasive submucosal cancers.

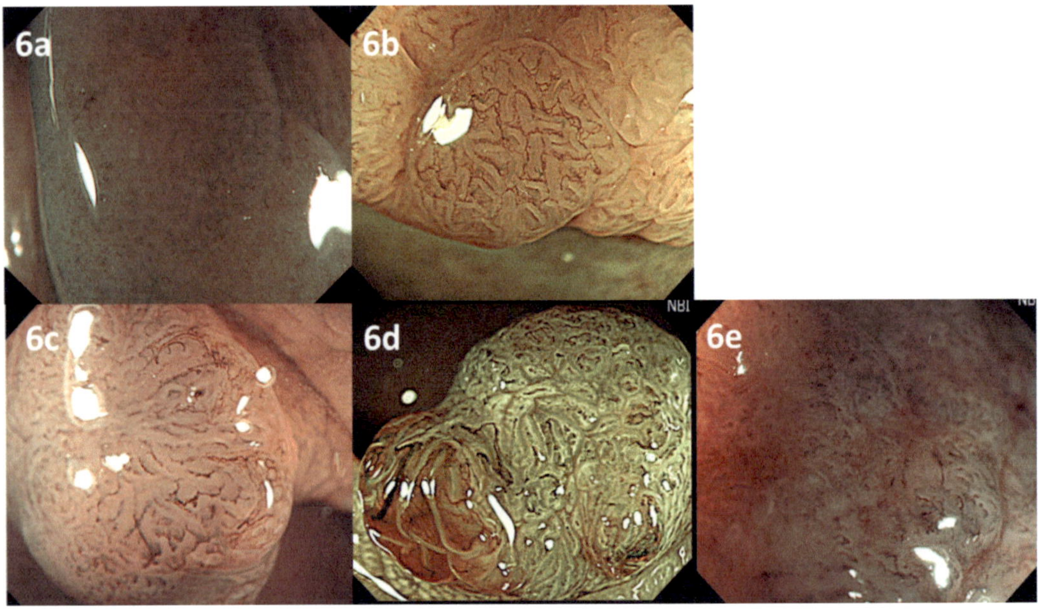

Figure 6. NBI classification. 6a. CP Type I in Sano classification. Type A in Hiroshima classification. 6b. CP Type II in Sano classification. Type B in Hiroshima classification. 6c. CP Type IIIA in Sano classification. Type C-1 in Hiroshima classification. 6d. CP Type IIIB in Sano classification. Type C-2 in Hiroshima classification. 6e. CP Type IIIB in Sano classification. Type C-3 in Hiroshima classification.

6. Hiroshima classification (Figure 6) [13]

The Hiroshima classification is based on vascular patterns and surface patterns, and includes type A, type B, or type C. Type A indicates that microvessels are not observed or are extremely opaque. In type B, fine microvessels are observed around surface patterns, and clear pits are observed via the nest of microvessels. In type C, the microvessels are irregular and the vessel diameter or distribution is heterogeneous. Type A is observed in hyperplastic polyps and type B is observed mainly in adenoma. Type C is divided into 3 subtypes (C1, C2, and C3), according to surface pattern's visibility, vessel diameter, irregularity, and distribution. In type C1, microvessels comprise an irregular network, surface patterns observed via the microvessels are slightly nondistinct, and vessel diameter or distribution is homogeneous. Type C1 has been reported in 46.7% of adenomas, 42.2% of intramucosal cancers, and 11.1% of massively invaded submucosal cancers. In type C2, microvessels comprise an irregular network, surface patterns observed via the microvessels are irregular, and vessel diameter or distribution is heterogeneous. Type C2 was observed in 45.5% of intramucosal cancers and 54.5% of massively invaded submucosal cancer. In type C3, surface patterns cannot be observed via the microvessels, irregular vessel diameter is thick, or the vessel distribution is heterogeneous, and avascular areas are seen. Type C3 is mainly found in massively invaded submucosal cancer.

7. Blue laser imaging by laser light source: A novel IEE

A newer endoscope system, "LASEREO," developed by Fujifilm, uses a semiconductor laser as a light source. It has narrow-bandwidth observation capability. The LASEREO system has 2 kinds of lasers. One laser provokes phosphor-illumination with a wavelength of 450 nm, similar to that of a xenon lamp. The combination of laser and fluorescent light provides an illumination that is almost equal to that of WL [Figure 7a]. The other laser is the "blue laser image (BLI)," which functions as a narrow-band light and has a wavelength of 410 nm [Figure 7b]. BLI is useful for acquiring mucosal surface information including surface blood vessel and structure patterns [Figure 7c]. By controlling the power of the 2 lasers, a BLI-bright mode is set by an appropriate combination of WL and BLI light. This mode is brighter than the BLI mode alone, and it is useful for tumor detection and observation of whole tumors.

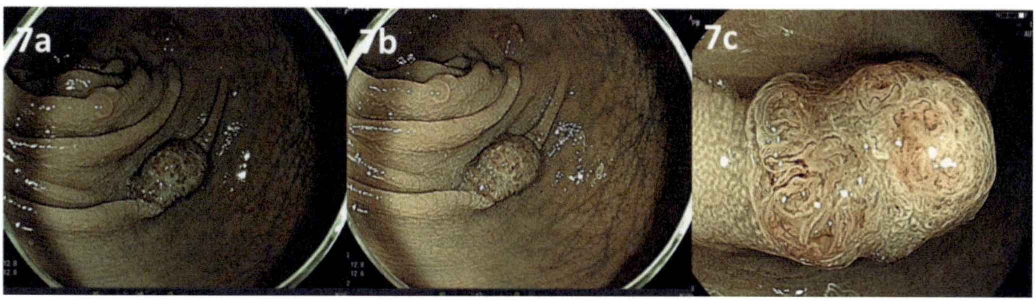

Figure 7. BLI. 7a. 0-Isp 12 mm with BLI. 7b. BLI-bright mode. 7c. Vascular pattern and surface pattern were detected clearly. CP type IIIB in Sano classification. Type C2 in the NBI classification (Hiroshima classification).

8. Adenoma detection rate

Colonoscopy is considered to be the standard examination against which the sensitivity of other colorectal cancer screening tests is compared [38,39]. A meta-analysis of 6 studies found that the missed polyp rate for polyps of any size was 22% [40]. The study also demonstrated that the missed adenoma rates were 2%, 13%, and 26% for polyp sizes of 10 mm <, 5–10 mm, and 1–5 mm respectively [41]. The reasons for missed polyps included the quality of bowel preparation, lesion characteristics (location, number, shape, and size), the endoscopist's experience, and the operator's insertion and withdrawal techniques [41-44]. Although many clinical studies, including randomized controlled trials (RCTs), have confirmed reduced missed rates in colonoscopy using NBI techniques [45-52], one recent meta-analysis revealed that there was no statistically significant difference in the rates of adenoma detection rate between NBI and WL [53], and a large-scale multicenter Japanese study did not show an improvement with NBI [54]. Moreover, another systematic review including 8 RCTs showed that NBI did not improve detection of colorectal polyps when compared to WL [55]. For FICE, 2 RCTs showed that any objective improvement of FICE was not correlated with the adenoma detection rate [56,57]. On the other hand, NBI and FICE systems have been improved recently and the recent combination of both systems and endoscopy employ high resolution and provide better contrast for vascular and surface patterns in ME than previous systems.

9. Endoscopic mucosal resection

Endoscopic mucosal resection (EMR) is now performed worldwide for early colorectal cancers. The saline injection-assisted method was first described by Rosenberg, who identified it as a safe method for the removal of rectal and sigmoid polyps, and was reintroduced by Tada et al. in 1984 [58-59]. Most adenomas and intramucosal cancers can be resected by EMR, however, tumors greater than 20 mm in diameter are considered difficult candidates for en bloc resection [60-65], and the rate of en bloc resection by EMR of tumors >20 mm in diameter is especially low (Table 5)[60-65]. While the technical feasibility of EMR for en-bloc and extended resections must still be improved, most colorectal polyps removed by EMR are <20 mm in size. EMR achieves en-bloc and complete resection of these lesions at satisfactory rates, although even some smaller lesions are difficult to resect completely, especially for less-experienced endoscopists. Many injection solutions have been used to achieve sustained mucosal elevation, definitive en-bloc resection, and complete resection while preventing perforation during EMR. Hypertonic saline, glycerol, dextrose, fibrinogen, and succinylated gelatin provide better complete resection rates and longer-lasting mucosal elevation than does normal saline (NS) [65-69]. Yamamoto et al. first reported the efficacy of hyaluronic acid (HA) for novel endoscopic resection of a large colorectal polyp, and this procedure was subsequently termed endoscopic submucosal dissection (ESD) [68]. Hyaluronic acid (HA) has been shown to create higher and more sustainable mucosal elevation than NS [68,70-72]. We have previously reported that mucosal elevation with NS dissipates within 2 min from injection, which is the median time required for most endoscopists to perform an EMR [69]. Our same study found that the viscosity of high-concentration HA can make snaring difficult. For this reason, and because HA is more expensive than NS, it is important to dilute HA prior to use. We have previously demonstrated that an HA concentration as low as 0.13% is effective for sustained mucosal elevation in resected porcine colon and in living minipig colon [69]. Moreover, we previously reported a prospective RCT concerning the efficacy of 0.13% HA in colorectal EMR that proved that using 0.13% HA instead of NS during EMR was more effective for complete resection and maintenance of mucosal elevation [73].

Author	Injection Solution	No. of cases	Rate of En bloc resection (%)	Rate of local recurrence (%)
Saito et al.	not described	228	33.0	14.0
Tanaka et al.	Glycerol	178	39.3	7.9
Tajika et al.		104	48.1	15.4
Iishi et al.	NS	56	25	not described
Kobayashi et al.		56	37.5	21.4
Uraoka et al.	NS Glycerol	44 39	20.5 23.1	18.6 15.2
Our data	HA	35	42.8	10.0

NS: normal saline, HA: hyaluronic acid

Table 5. Rates of en bloc resection and local recurrence of tumors larger than 20 mm in diameter treated by endoscopic mucosal resection (EMR)

Evaluation of en bloc resection is performed endoscopically, while complete resection is defined histopathologically based on the tumor-free lateral and vertical margins of the resected specimens. However some specimens resected by EMR have positive margins even after the tumor was grossly resected en bloc. Burning of the resected specimens may affect these results, and although most such tumors cause no local recurrence, some do recur locally. Therefore, endoscopists are obligated to perform EMR with tumor-free margins [74]. We describe a regular method of EMR to obtain complete resection of polyps. Firstly, polyp and margin are observed carefully and then injection is performed [Figure 8]. The recommended locus of injection is the proximal side of the polyp. If the injection is performed at the distal (anal) side of the polyp, the polyp may shift to a horizontal position to the endoscope. In this situation, the margin of the tumor cannot be confirmed. After injection, snaring is performed and polyp is resected with electrocautery. After resection, endoscopic clipping is sometimes performed to prevent post-operative hemorrhage and perforation.

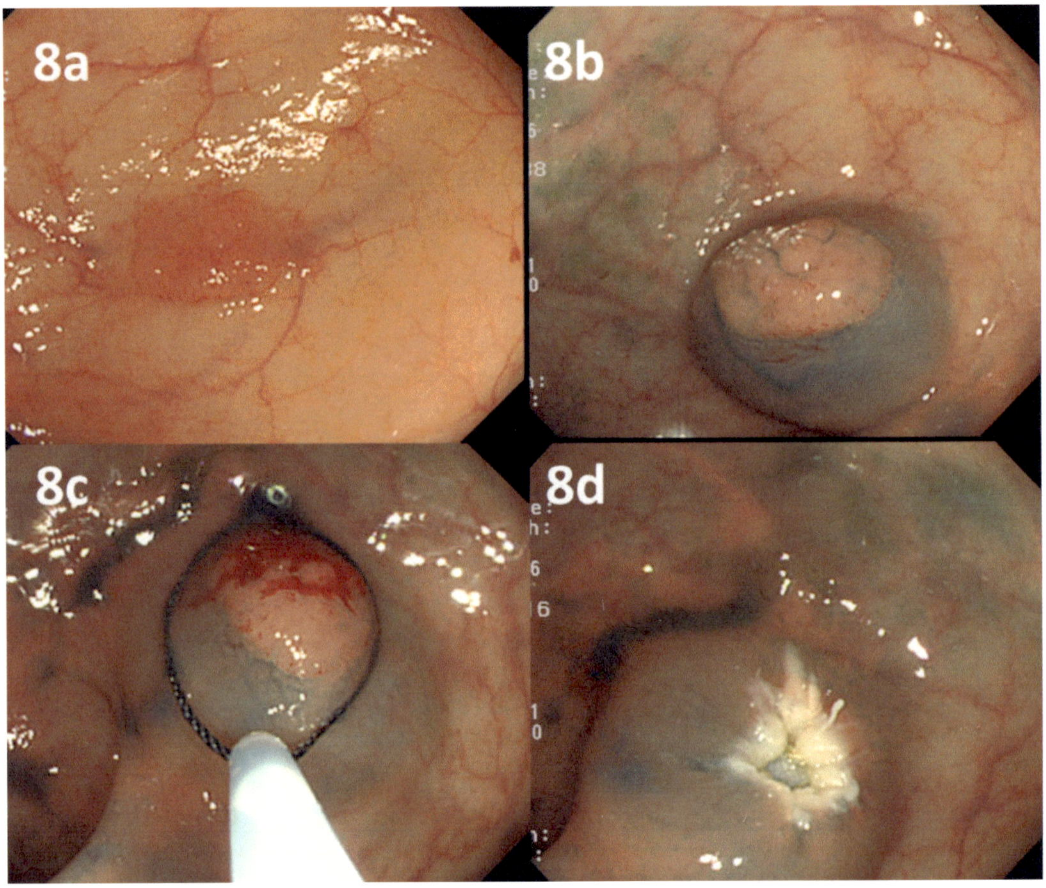

Figure 8. Strategy of EMR. 8a. Polyp and margin of it are observed carefully. 8b. Injection is performed at the oral (proximal) side of the polyp. 8c. Snaring is performed. 8d. Polyp is resected by electrocautery.

When en bloc resection of the tumor by EMR fails, piecemeal EMR is generally performed instead. Although piecemeal EMR enables the removal of large colorectal tumors, it has a high rate of local recurrence (7.9–21.4%)[60-65] (Table 5). Most recurrent adenomas, including partial intramucosal adenocarcinomas, can be cured by additional endoscopic therapy [74]. If possible, The use of piecemeal EMR should be examined carefully before endoscopic therapy by ME and IEE. In some cases, piecemeal EMR does not allow for precise histopathological evaluation. For example, partial submucosal invasion in submucosally invasive cancer can be missed in piecemeal-resected specimens. When the locus of submucosal invasion in submucosally invasive cancer is destroyed by burning, the tumor may be misdiagnosed as mucosal cancer, and when the positive vertical margin of submucosal or lymphatic-venous invasion is burned, the resection may misclassified as complete [74]. In these cases, the patient will not be advised to undergo additional surgical resection, allowing recurrence a few years later. Recurrence may occur as lung, liver, and/or lymph node metastasis, and these patients are very difficult to cure.

10. Endoscopic submucosal dissection

In Japan and some other Western and Asian countries, endoscopic submucosal dissection (ESD) is reported to be an efficient treatment with a high rate of en bloc resection for large colorectal tumors and it is considered less invasive than laparoscopic colectomy (LAC) [75-83]. However, ESD can be a time-consuming procedure and carries a higher risk of perforation than EMR [81,82]. The use of ESD was initially proposed by the Japanese special ESD group [80]. Indications in detail are, first, large lesions >20 mm in diameter for which endoscopic therapy is indicated but for which en bloc resection by snare EMR would be difficult. Second, lesions that are suspected as invasive submucosal cancer should be resected en bloc by ESD. Thirdly, lesions other than these cases can be an indication for ESD, including mucosal lesions with fibrosis caused by prolapse due to biopsy or peristalsis of the lesions, local residual early cancer after endoscopic resection, and sporadic localized tumors in chronic inflammation such as ulcerative colitis. The rate of en bloc resection for large colorectal tumors by ESD has been reported to be 80–98.9%[75-83](Table 6). However, the procedure has not been standardized because of its associated technical difficulties. The colon is winding in nature and has many folds. Moreover, the wall of the colon is thinner than the gastric wall.

Author	No. of cases	Rate of En bloc resection (%)	Perforation rate (%)	Post-operative bleeding rate (%)
Saito et al.	1111	88.0	4.9	1.5
Toyonaga et al.	468	98.9	1.5	1.5
Isomoto et al.	292	90.1	8.2	0.7
Yoshida et al.	250	86.8	6.0	2.4
Fujishiro et al.	200	91.5	10.4	1.0
Zhou et al.	74	93.2	8.1	1.3
Tanaka et al.	70	80.0	10.0	1.4
Our recent data	410	92.6	4.1	1.9

Table 6. Rates of en bloc resection and complete resection by endoscopic submucosal dissection (ESD)

We describe standard ESD devices here. ESD is performed with a regular lower gastrointestinal endoscope with a single channel. In our institution, colonoscopes with single channels such as the EC 590 MP (Fujifilm Medical, Tokyo, Japan) or the PCF Q260AI (Olympus, Tokyo, Japan) are used. With regard to the choice of endoscope, an upper gastrointestinal endoscope is preferred in some institutions because it is slim and can be used in the retroflexed position [78]. ESD requires a high-frequency generator with an automatically controlled system. A transparent short hood (Olympus Medical Systems, Co. Ltd.) is fitted at the tip of the endoscope.

This helps the easy placement of endoscope during ESD. A mixture of 0.4% hyaluronic acid solution (Mucoup; Johnson & Johnson K.K., Tokyo, Japan and Seikagaku Corporation, Tokyo, Japan) is used as the injection liquid to induce a greater elevation of the submucosa and to lengthen the duration of the continuous elevation of the submucosa [77, 82].

Various knives are used in ESD for excising colorectal tumors (Figure 9). Among the obtuse short-tipped types are included the Flush knife (Fujifilm Medical, Tokyo, Japan), Dual knife (Olympus Optical Co, Tokyo, Japan), B-knife (Zeon Medical, Tokyo, Japan), and Splash needle (Pentax Co, Tokyo, Japan) [75, 82]. The Flush knife and Splash needle are capable of submucosal injections and they allow the endoscopist to omit switching between the knife and the injection needle [75, 83]. The Dual knife, B-knife, and Flush knife all have a ball disk at the tip of the knife, enabling the operator to hook the submucosa. The insulated tipped (IT) knife (Olympus Optical Co, Tokyo, Japan), whose efficacy has been reported to be satisfactory in ESD for gastric tumors, is being used in certain institutions [84]. The IT knife allows rapid dissection. A Hook knife (Olympus Optical Co, Tokyo, Japan) is particularly useful when the dissection of the submucosa is difficult due to poor elevation of the submucosa [80]. The B-knife is the only bipolar knife, and there is thought to be less burning of the muscularis propria layer with this knife than with other monopolar knives. The clutch cutter (Fujifilm medical, Tokyo, Japan) and SB knife (Sumitomo Bakelite Co., Tokyo, Japan) are grasping-type scissor forceps [85-86]. In our institution, the Flush knife is mainly used because it can effectively administer local injections, and the clutch cutter is used when the risk of perforation is high due to the poor elevation of the submucosa [74,85].

Following are the steps of the routine ESD procedure (Figure 10) [82,87]. Before ESD, residual feces and liquid are removed from the entire colon even if the tumor is located at the rectum. Residual feces prevent smooth submucosal dissection. Moreover, it is essential to remove residual feces in order to prevent the outflow of feces into the abdomen in the case of perforation. Firstly, the border of the tumor is carefully identified using indigo carmine dye. It is generally unnecessary to mark the borders by coagulation because in the majority of cases they are clearly visible. Injection for submucosal elevation is performed with a 25G needle (8B27A, TOP, Tokyo, Japan) after visualization of the border of the tumor, and mucosal incisions are made. A partial circumferential incision is made on the distal side of the tumor [77, 80]. If the size of the tumor exceeds 50 mm, the incision is performed at the proximal side of the tumor, because in large tumors it is sometimes difficult to resect residual mucosa on the proximal side in the presence of a partially resected tumor. Mucosal incisions are made only after adequate elevation of submucosa by mucosal injection is achieved, and then, simultaneously, an incision into the deep submucosa is made. Mucosal incisions are performed with the endocut mode (output 40 W, effect 2 in ICC200; or endocut I, effect 2, duration 2, interval 1 in VIO300D).

After mucosal and submucosal incisions are made at the anal side of the tumor, the submucosa below the tumor is resected from the distal side of the tumor. Dissection of the submucosa is performed using the endocut (output 40 W, effect 2 in ICC200; endocut I, effect 2, duration 2, interval 1 in VIO300D) or coagulation mode (forced coagulation, output 40 W in ICC200 or forced coagulation, output 40 W, effect 3 in VIO300D). To achieve submucosal elevation, additional injections are performed with the injection needle or flush knife, as appropriate.

Then continuing to dissect while carefully avoiding perforation and hemorrhage, en bloc resection of the tumor is completed.

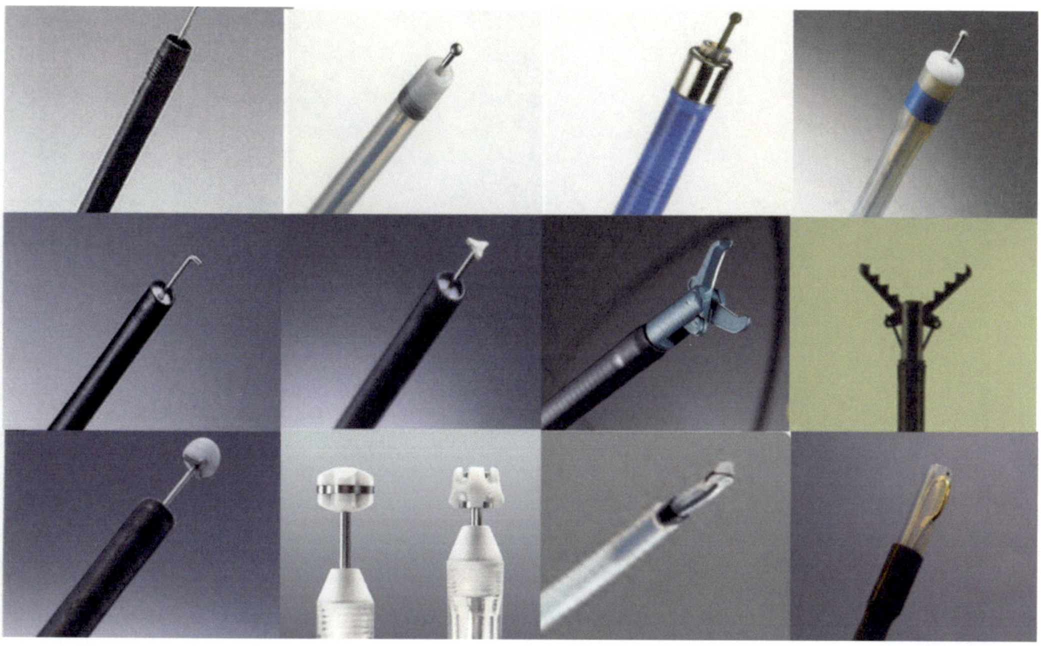

Figure 9. Various ESD knives.

The main complications of ESD are perforation and hemorrhage, similar to those of endoscopic mucosal resection (EMR). In particular, the rate of perforation is higher for ESD than for EMR (1.5–10.4%)(Table 6)[75-83]. Perforation of the colon can cause fatal peritonitis. Coagulation by knife is the most frequent cause of perforation [81]. Saito et al. showed that perforation risk was related to the number of ESD procedures, with higher risk when the endoscopist had performed fewer than 100 procedures [83]. Most cases of perforation are treated conservatively by endoscopic clipping, without need for urgent surgical intervention [40,41] (Figure 11). Carbon dioxide insufflations have been reported to be effective for the prevention of abdominal fullness [88]. They also has been reported to be effective for prevention of perforation by decreasing pressure in the colorectum. On the other hand, the rates of postoperative hemorrhage are similar for ESD and EMR. When hemorrhage occurs, endoscopic therapy, including endoscopic clipping, is performed, and most cases, can be managed conservatively and without blood transfusion. A safe strategy, suitable knife, adoption of other equipment, and training in animal models are necessary in order to minimize the complications, including perforation, of ESD [42].

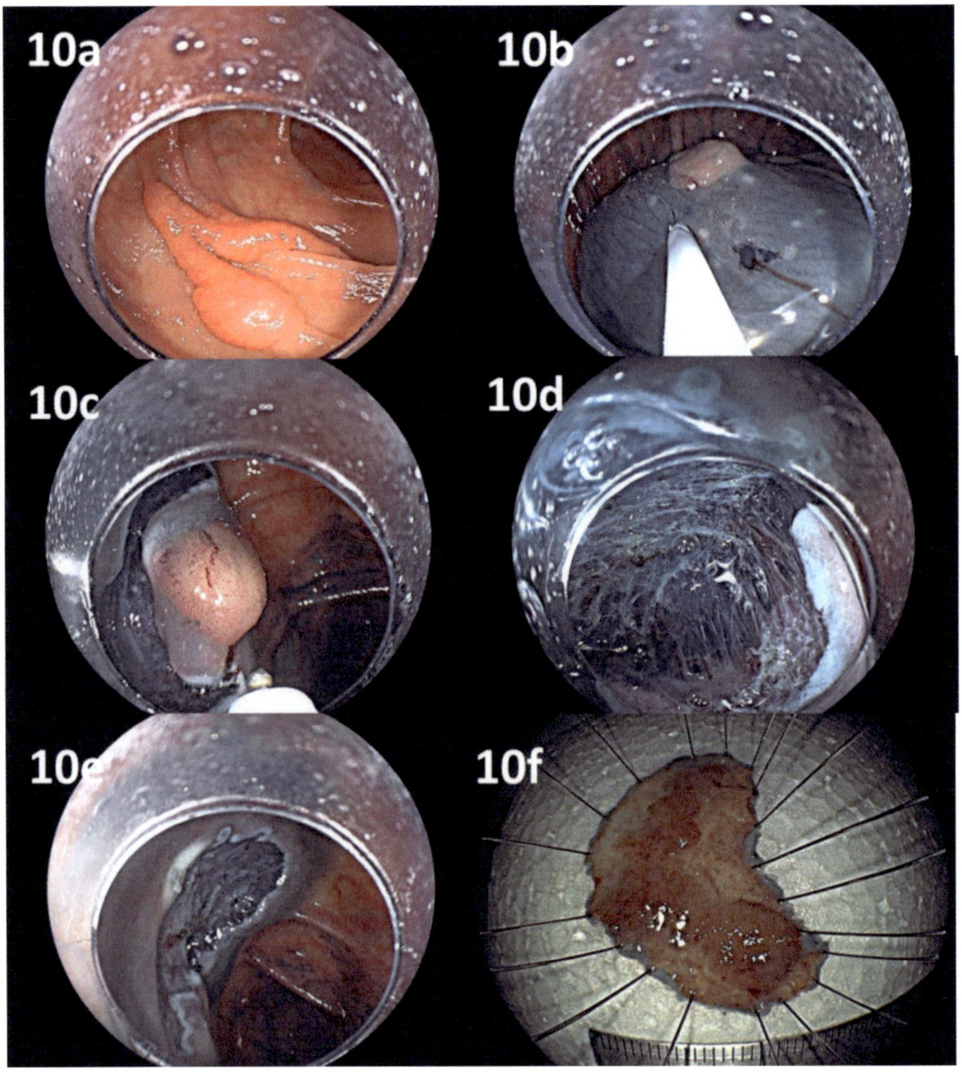

Figure 10. Strategy of ESD. 10a. 0–IIa 30 mm on the descending colon. Firstly, the tumor and margin of it are observed carefully. 10b. Injection is performed at the anal (distal) side of the tumor. 10c. A partial circumferential mucosal incision is made. 10d. Submucosal dissection is performed. 10e. The tumor is resected en-bloc. 10f. Resected specimen.

http://dx.doi.org/10.5772/52733

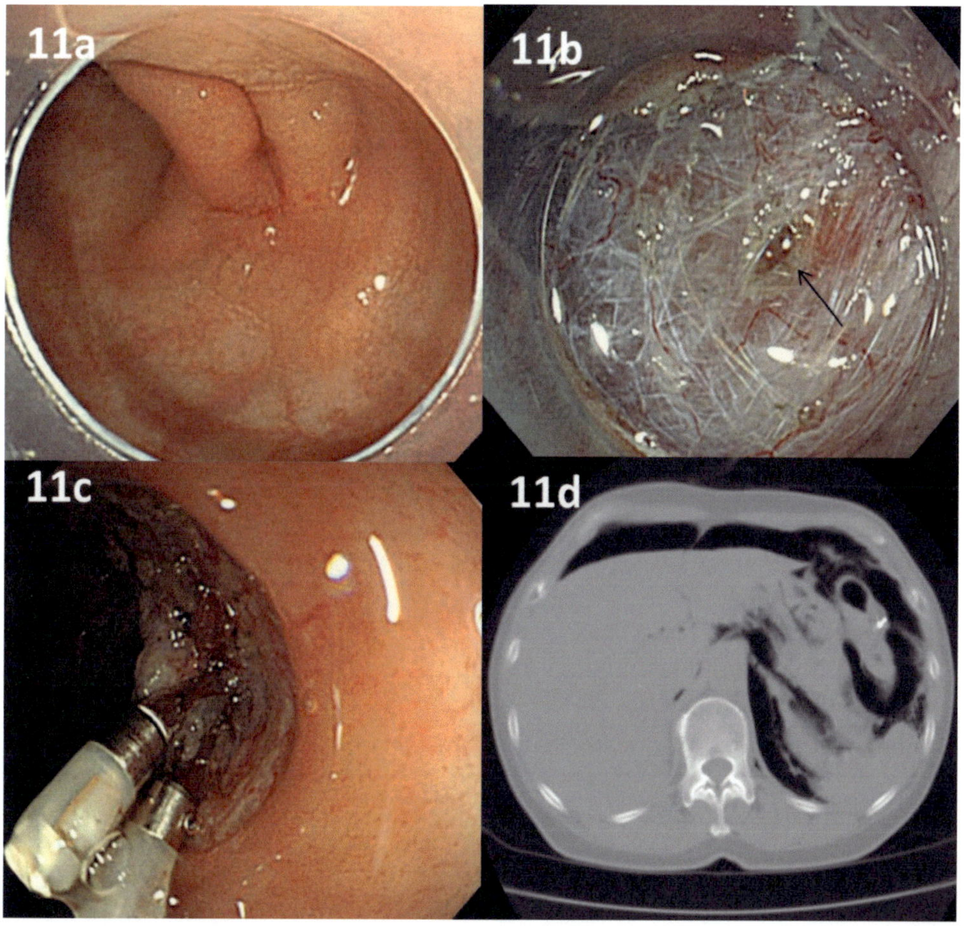

Figure 11. Perforation during ESD. 11a: 0–IIa 30 mm on the descending colon. 11b. Coagulation to submucosa during resection of submocosa below the tumor caused perforation (black arrow). 11c: The hole was closed by endoscopic clipping. 11d: CT revealed free air out side of the colorectum.

Submucosally invasive cancer can be resected by colorectal ESD. A multicenter study of 1111 colorectal ESDs showed that 213 submucosally invasive cancers (19.1%, 213/1111) were treated clinically by ESD [83]. The rate of submucosally invasive cancer in our institution is 10.2% (42/410), which is similar to the rates reported in other studies on colorectal ESD (range: 9.2%–25%)[78-80, 82]. Massively invaded submucosal cancer is not an indication for colorectal ESD and EMR, because of the possibility of lymph node metastasis. Endoscopic diagnosis of massively invasive submucosal cancer is limited even when ME for pit patterns, NBI, and FICE are available. The sensitivity of detail-magnifying observation for massively invasive submucosal cancer is only 63.8–100.0% [15, 16, 23, 34, 37] (Table 4). Therefore, some number of massively invasive submucosal cancers may be diagnosed as mucosal cancer or shallowly invaded submucosal cancer and scheduled for resection by ESD or EMR. In these cases, the probability of curative resection by ESD is influenced by various clinical features, including histopathological vertical margin, lateral margin, and venous-lymphatic invasion. The characteristics of the submucosally invasive cancers treated at our institution are shown in Table 7 [74]. The average tumor size was 26.5 mm in the submucosal cancer (SM) group and 35.1 mm in the mucosal cancer (M) group ($P < 0.01$). The proportion of tumors in the rectum was higher in the SM group than in the adenoma (A) group ($P < 0.01$). The ratio of protruding tumors to superficial tumors was significantly higher in the SM group (14:19) than in the M group (32:112) or the A group (12:145) ($P < 0.01$). The rate of severe fibrosis was higher in the SM group (18.1%) than in the M group (5.5%) ($P < 0.05$). One cause of severe fibrosis is tumor invasion. However, mucosal cancers (5.5%) and adenomas (6.0%) also showed severe fibrosis in our study. Endoscopic biopsy sometimes leads to severe fibrosis. Matsumoto et al. showed that severe fibrosis complicated ESD and was associated with perforation [89]. The median operation time for the 7 cases in the SM group with severe fibrosis was 147 min, which was longer than the M group or the A group. Severe fibrosis is difficult to dissect, and it should be cautioned that perforation may occur during dissection of severe fibrosis. In our institution, the clutch cutter, which is a scissor-shaped knife, is used to dissect severe fibrosis with minimal risk of perforation, as it can grasp, coagulate, and cut a piece of tissue without perioperative hemorrhage [74].

	SM	M	A	P-value
Number of tumors	33	144	157	
Median age (range)	65.5 (46–83)	67.9 (48–87)	67.5 (39–87)	
M/F	21/12	86/58	81/76	NS
Tumor size (mm) (range)	26.5 (10–60)	35.1 (10–130)	27.0 (10–80)	<0.01
Location (Colon/Rectum)	18: 15	87: 57	124: 33	<0.01 SM:A
Morphology (protruding/superficial)	14: 19	32: 112	12: 145	<0.01
Operation time (min) (range)	109 (20–240)	118 (30–420)	92 (10–300)	NS
Severe Fibrosis (%)	18.1(7/33)	5.5(8/144)	6.3 10/157)	<0.05 SM:M
En bloc resection (%)	90.9	90.9	89.1	NS
Complete resection (%)	72.7	84.0	81.5	NS
Perforation (%)	6.0	7.6	1.9	NS
Postoperative hemorrhage (%)	0	6.2	1.2	NS

ESD: endoscopic submucosal dissection; SM: submucosal cancer; M: mucosal cancer; A: adenoma; NS: not significant

Table 7. Characteristics of colorectal tumors resected by ESD

11. Training in EMR and ESD

Training in EMR and ESD is important for safe procedures. EMR of small polyps is considered easy and it is not rare that an inexperienced endoscopist will firstly perform EMR in these cases. Recently, animal models (Johnson & Johnson K.K., Tokyo, Japan) have become available for practicing EMR (Figure 12). Some animal model training for inexperienced endoscopists is used in our institution, and it has had positive impact on EMR in clinical cases. Colorectal ESD is difficult for less-experienced endoscopists. In general, endoscopists should acquire extensive experience with gastric ESD before performing colorectal ESD. However, different training for colorectal ESD is required when the number of patients with early gastric cancer is few, as in Western countries. In this situation, visiting ESD experts at other institutions and observing them at work are important components of training. Another expected component of ESD training is extensive practice using animal models [90-92]. Both *in vivo* animal models and *ex vivo* animal models using harvested organs have been used. Porcine and canine *in vivo* models have been reported to be useful systems for ESD training [90-92]. However, *in vivo* animal models are expensive and difficult to prepare. Hon et al. demonstrated the usefulness of a porcine colon *ex vivo* animal model for training in colorectal ESD [91]. However, training in endoscopic hemostasis is difficult in conventional *ex vivo* animal models. We have recently reported an *ex vivo* animal model with simulated blood flow (Johnson & Johnson K.K., Tokyo, Japan) [93](Figure 12). It can be made using the bovine cecum. The vessel around the cecum is detached, and red ink is injected. The mucosa shows "blood" flow after the red ink is injected (Figure 13), which can allow the endoscopist to gain whole ESD experience, including perioperative hemorrhage (Figure 14). A specific ESD training system has been implemented in some Japanese institutions, including ours. It is a step-by-step system starting with observing and assisting in ESD procedures performed by experts. Next, animal model training is performed to the extent possible. Finally, clinical practice is performed under the supervision of instructors. Generally, the clinical practice training proceeds according to the difficulty of the procedure, beginning with gastric ESD, then rectal ESD, and finally colonic ESD [93]. Regarding animal training in ESD, there are many reports on *ex vivo* animal models for gastric ESD [91, 94, 95]. There are also several reports on an *ex vivo* animal model for colorectal ESD [92, 93]. Repeated animal model training procedures have recently been proven to decrease procedure time [91-93]. For clinical colorectal ESD, Hotta et al. showed that approximately 40 procedures were sufficient to acquire skill in avoiding perforations, and the perforation rate in the first 40 cases was about 12.5% [96]. We believe that experience obtained by training on an animal model will also improve performance of clinical colorectal ESD, although the perforation rate did not decrease to zero even if the skill level improved greatly. Therefore, we believe the endoscopist must also obtain expertise in endoscopic closure. Small perforations can be closed by endoscopic clipping [81,97]. However, endoscopic clipping requires a high level of endoscopic skill and experience, and perforation is relatively rare in clinical medicine, making it difficult to gain experience in the endoscopic clipping technique in clinical practice. *Ex vivo* animal models for perforation are more useful for training in endoscopic closure than *in vivo* animal models [93] (Figure 15).

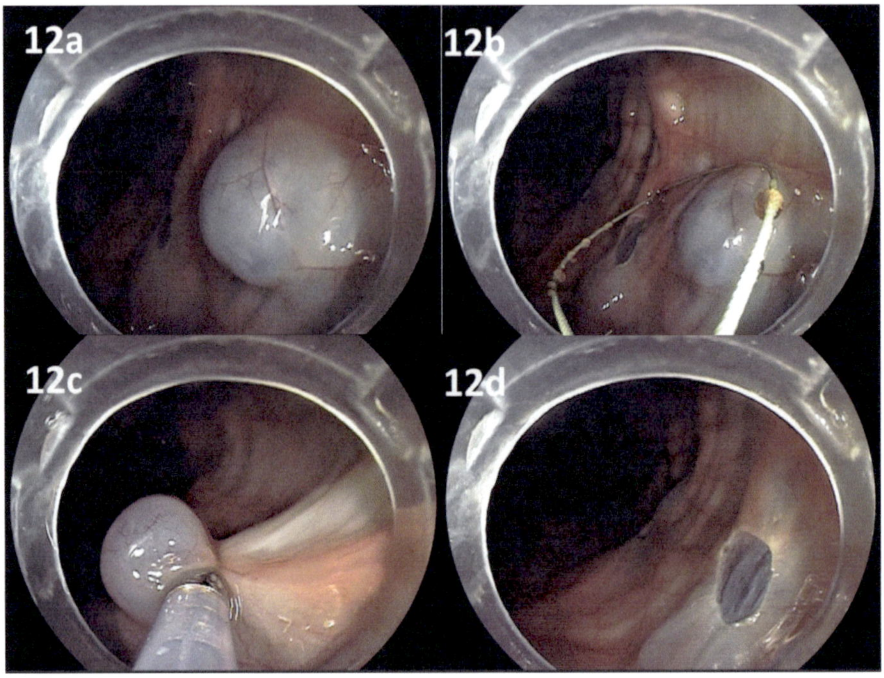

Figure 12. Animal model training for EMR. 12a. Injection is performed. 12b, 12c. Snaring is performed. 12d. Polyp is resected by electrocautery.

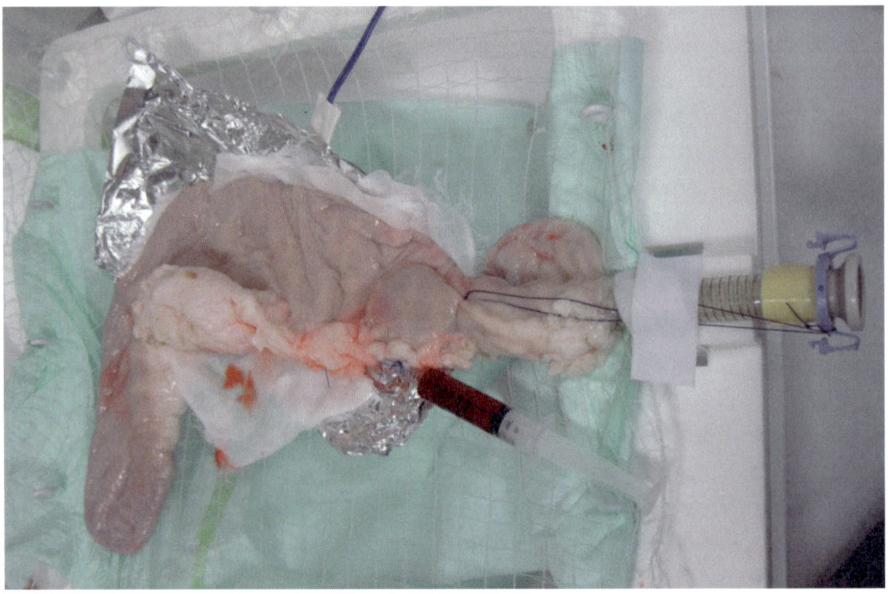

Figure 13. *Ex vivo* animal model with blood flow.

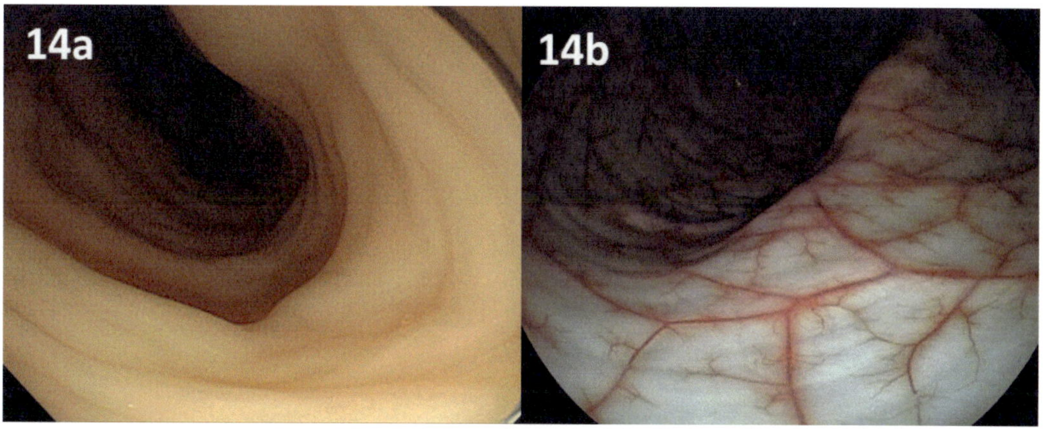

Figure 14. *Ex vivo* animal model with blood flow. 14a. The submucosal vessels were invisible before injection of red ink. 14b. The submucosal vessels were visible after injection of red ink.

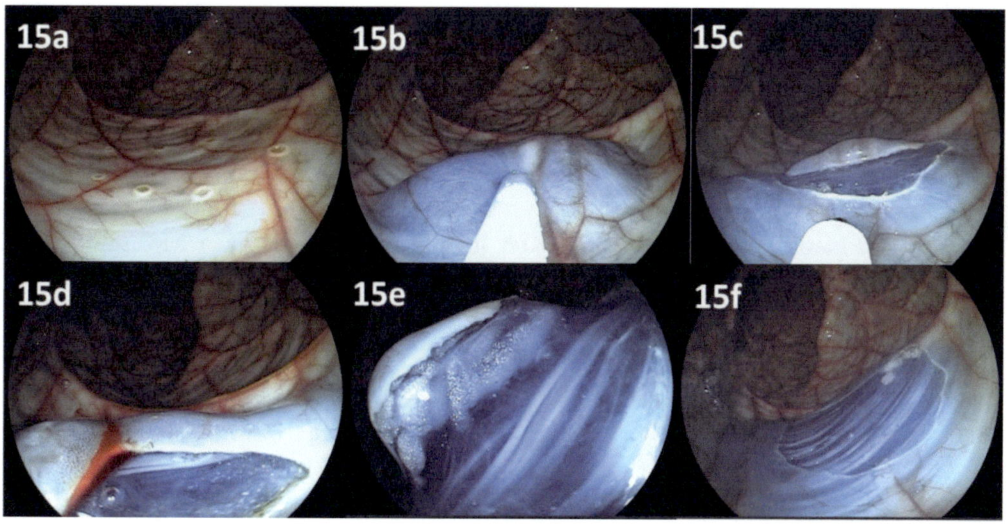

Figure 15. *Ex vivo* animal model with blood flow for whole ESD training including endoscopic hemostasis. 15a. Marking was performed to mimic the tumor. 15b. Mucosal injection was performed. 15c. Partial circumferential mucosal incision was performed. 15d. Perioperative hemorrhage was detected. 15e. Submucosal dissection was performed. 15f. En bloc resection was performed.

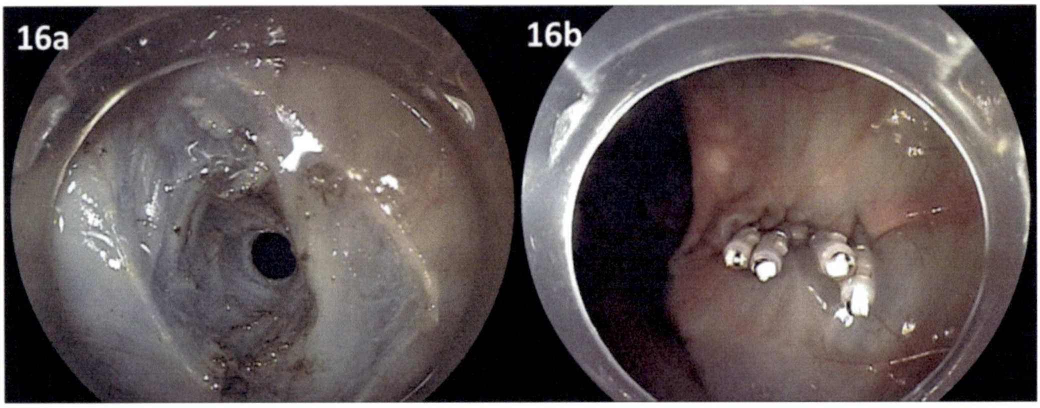

Figure 16. *Ex vivo* animal model with perforation for training of endoscopic closure 16a. After ESD, the endoscopic knife was used to make a 2–3 mm hole in the proper muscle layer of the ulceration. 16b. The endoscopic closure of the hole was performed with 4 endoscopic clips.

12. Conclusions

In this chapter, we have described the effectiveness of image-enhanced endoscopy (IEE) and the safe and definite strategies of therapeutic endoscopy, including endoscopic mucosal resection (EMR) and endoscopic mucosal dissection (ESD).

Acknowledgements

We thank Dr. Naoki Wakabayashi, Dr. Ken Inoue, and Dr. Yasutaka Morimoto and all members of the Department of Molecular Gastroenterology and Hepatology, Kyoto Prefectural University of Medicine, for helping with our study.

Author details

Naohisa Yoshida[1*], Nobuaki Yagi[1], Yutaka Inada[1], Munehiro Kugai[1], Akio Yanagisawa[2] and Yuji Naito[1]

1 Department of Molecular Gastroenterology and Hepatology, Kyoto Prefectural University of Medicine, Graduate School of Medical Science, Kyoto, Japan

2 Department of Surgical Pathology, Kyoto Prefectural University of Medicine, Graduate School of Medical Science, Kyoto, Japan

References

[1] Vogelstein B, Fearon ER, Hamilton SR et al. Genetic alterations during colorectal-tumor development. N Eng J Med 1988; 319:525-532

[2] Kudo S, Hirota S, Nakajima T et al. Colorectal tumours and pit pattern. J Clin Pathol 1994; 47:880-885

[3] Tobaru T, Mitsuyama K, Tsuruta O et al. Sub-classification of type VI pit patterns in colorectal tumors: relation to the depth of tumor invasion. Int J Oncol 2008; 33:503-508

[4] Fu KI, Sano Y, Kato S, Fujii T, Nagashima F, Yoshino T, Okuno T, Yoshida S, Fujimori T. Chromoendoscopy using indigo carmine dye spraying with magnifying observation is the most reliable method for differential diagnosis between non-neoplastic and neoplastic colorectal lesions: a prospective study. Endoscopy 2004; 36:1089-1093

[5] Sano Y, Ikematsu H, Fu KI et al. Meshed capillary vessels by use of narrow-band imaging for differential diagnosis of small colorectal polyps. Gastrointest Endosc 2009; 69:278-283

[6] Togashi K, Osawa H, Koinuma K et al. A comparison of conventional endoscopy, chromoendoscopy, and the optimal-band imaging system for the differentiation of neoplastic and non-neoplastic colonic polyps. Gastrointest Endosc 2009; 69:734-741

[7] Uedo N, Higashino K, Ishihara R, Takeuchi Y, Iishi H. Diagnosis of colonic adenomas by new autofluorescence imaging system. New autofluorescence imaging system: a pilot study. Digestive Endoscopy. 2007; 19:S134-S138

[8] Saito Y, Fukuzawa M, Matsuda T et al. Clinical outcome of endoscopic submucosal dissection versus endoscopic mucosal resection of large colorectal tumors as determined by curative resection. Surg Endosc 2010; 24:343-352

[9] Kudo S, Tamegai Y, Yamano H et al. Endoscopic mucosal resection of the colon: the Japanese technique. Gastrointest Endosc Clin N Am 2001; 11:519-535

[10] Yoshida N, Naito Y, Yagi N et al. Safe procedure in endoscopic submucosal dissection for colorectal tumors focused on preventing complications. World J Gastroenterol 2010; 16:1688-1695

[11] Rastogi A, Keighley J, Singh V et al. High accuracy of narrow band imaging without magnification for the real-time characterization of polyp histology and its comparison with high-definition white light colonoscopy: a prospective study. Am J Gastroenterol 2009; 104:2422-2430

[12] Konishi K, Kaneko K, Kurahashi T, Yamamoto T, Kushima M, Kanda A, Tajiri H, Mitamura K. A comparison of magnifying and nonmagnifying colonoscopy for diagnosis of colorectal polyps: A prospective study. Gastrointest Endosc 2003; 57:48-53

[13] Kanao H, Tanaka S, Oka S et al. Narrow-band imaging magnification predicts the histology and invasion depth of colorectal tumors. Gastrointest Endosc 2009; 69:631-636

[14] Machida H, Sano Y, Hamamoto Y et al. Narrow-band imaging in the diagnosis of colorectal mucosal lesions: a pilot study. Endoscopy 2004; 36:1094-1098

[15] Ikematsu H, Matsuda T, Emura F et al. Efficacy of capillary pattern type IIIA/IIIB by magnifying narrow band imaging for estimating depth of invasion of early colorectal neoplasms. BMC Gastroenterol 2010; 10: 33

[16] Tanaka S, Sano Y. Aim to unify the narrow band imaging (NBI) magnifying classification for colorectal tumors: current status in Japan from a summary of the consensus symposium in the 79th Annual Meeting of the Japan Gastroenterological Endoscopy Society. Dig Endosc 2011; Suppl 1:131-9. doi: 10.1111/j. 1443-1661.2011.01106.x.)

[17] Miyake Y, Sekiya T, Kubo S. et al. A new Spectrophotometer for Measuring the Spectral Reflectance of Gastric Mucous Membrane. J Photographic Science 1989; 37:134-138

[18] Pohl J, Nguyen-Tat M, Pech O et al. Computed virtual chromoendoscopy for classification of small colorectal lesions: a prospective comparative study. Am J Gastroenterol 2008; 103:562-569

[19] Yoshida N, Naito Y, Inada Y, Kugai M, Inoue K, Uchiyama K, Handa O, Takagi T, Konishi H, Wakabayashi N, Yagi N, Morimoto Y, Wakabayashi N, Yanagisawa A, Yoshikawa T. The Detection of Surface Patterns by Flexible Spectral Imaging Color Enhancement without Magnification for Diagnosis of Colorectal Polyps. Int J Colorectal Dis 2012; 27: 605-611

[20] Togashi K, Sunada K, Yoshida N, et a. Flexible spectral-imaging color enhancement: optimized settings for polyp detection? Gastrointest Endosc 2011; 74:940

[21] Santos CE, Lima JC, Lopes CV et al. Computerized virtual chromoendoscopy versus indigo carmine chromoendoscopy combined with magnification for diagnosis of small colorectal lesions: a randomized and prospective study. Eur J Gastroenterol Hepatol 2010; 22:1364-1371

[22] Parra-Blanco A, Jiménez A, Rembacken B et al. Validation of Fujinon intelligent chromoendoscopy with high definition endoscopes in colonoscopy. World J Gastroenterol 2009; 15:5266-5273

[23] Yoshida N, Naito Y, Kugai M et al. Efficacy of magnifying endoscopy with flexible spectral imaging color enhancement in the diagnosis of colorectal tumors. J Gastroenterol 2011; 46: 65-72

[24] Matsuda T, Saito Y, Fu KI, et al. Does autofluorescence imaging videoendoscopy system improve the colonoscopic polyp detection rate?—a pilot study. American Journal of Gastroenterology. 2008; 103:1926-1932

[25] McCallum AL, Jenkins JT, Gillen D, Molloy RG. Evaluation of autofluorescence colonoscopy for the detection and diagnosis of colonic polyps. Gastrointestinal Endoscopy. 2008; 68:283-290

[26] Tischendorf JJ, Schirin-Sokhan R, Streetz K et al. Value of magnifying endoscopy in classifying colorectal polyps based on vascular pattern. Endoscopy 2010; 42:22-27

[27] Henry ZH, Yeaton P, Shami VM et al. Meshed capillary vessels found on narrowband imaging without optical magnification effectively identifies colorectal neoplasia: a North American validation of the Japanese experience. Gastrointest Endosc 2010; 72:118-126

[28] Rex DK. Narrow-band imaging without optical magnification for histologic analysis of colorectal polyps. Gastroenterology 2009; 136:1174-1181

[29] Su MY, Hsu CM, Ho YP et al. Comparative study of conventional colonoscopy, chromoendoscopy, and narrow-band imaging systems in differential diagnosis of neoplastic and nonneoplastic colonic polyps. Am J Gastroenterol 2006; 101:2711-2716

[30] Yoshida N, Yagi N, Yanagisawa A, Naito Y. Imaged-enhanced endoscopy for diagnosis of colorectal tumors in view of endoscopic treatment. World J Gastrointest Endosc in press.

[31] Longcroft-Wheaton GR, Higgins B, Bhandari P. Observation of mucosal crypt pattern with magnifying colonoscopy is superior to nonmagnifying colonoscopy for distinguishing between neoplastic and non-neoplastic colorectal lesions. Eur J Gastroenterol Hepatol 2011; 23:903-911

[32] Kim YS, Kim D, Chung SJ, Park MJ, Shin CS, Cho SH, Kim JS, Song IS. Differentiating small polyp histologies using real-time screening colonoscopy with Fuji Intelligent Color Enhancement. Clin Gastroenterol Hepatol 2011; 9:744-749

[33] Hewett DG, Kaltenbach T, Sano Y, Tanaka S, Saunders B, Ponchon T, Soetikno R, Rex DK. Validation of a Simple Classification System for Endoscopic Diagnosis of Small Colorectal Polyps Using Narrow-Band Imaging. Gastroenterology. 2012 May 15. [Epub ahead of print]

[34] Wada Y, Kashida H, Kudo SE et al. Diagnostic accuracy of pit pattern and vascular pattern analyses in colorectal lesions. Dig Endosc 2010; 22:192-199

[35] Katagiri A, Fu KI, Sano Y et al. Narrow band imaging with magnifying colonoscopy as diagnostic tool for predicting histology of early colorectal neoplasia. Aliment Pharmacol Ther 2008; 27:1269-1274

[36] Singh R, Nordeen N, Mei SL, Kaffes A, Tam W, Saito Y. West meets East: preliminary results of narrow band imaging with optical magnification in the diagnosis of colorectal lesions: a multicenter Australian study using the modified Sano's classification. Dig Endosc. 2011 May; 23 Suppl 1:126-30. doi: 10.1111/j.1443-1661.2011.01107.x

[37] Saito S, Tajiri H, Ohya T, Nikami T, Aihara H, Ikegami M. Imaging by Magnifying Endoscopy with NBI Implicates the Remnant Capillary Network As an Indication for Endoscopic Resection in Early Colon Cancer. Int J Surg Oncol 2011; 2011:242608. Epub 2011 Feb 10

[38] Whitlock EP, Lin JS, Liles E, Beil TL, Fu R, O'Connor E, Thompson RN, Cardenas T. Screening for colorectal cancer: an updated systematic review. Evidence Synthesis No. 65, Part 1. AHRQ publication no. 08-05124-EF-1. Rockville, MD: Agency for Healthcare Research and Quality; 2008

[39] Whitlock E, Lin JS, Liles E, Beil TL, Fu R. Screening for colorectal cancer: a targeted systematic review for the U.S. Preventive Services Task Force. Ann Intern Med. 2008; 149

[40] van Rijn JC, Reitsma JB, Stoker J, Bossuyt PM, van Deventer SJ, Dekker E. Polyp miss rate determined by tandem colonoscopy: a systematic review. Am J Gastroenterol. 2006; 101:343-350

[41] Heresbach D, Barrioz T, Lapalus MG, Coumaros D, Bauret P, Potier P, Sautereau D, Boustière C, Grimaud JC, Barthélémy C, Sée J, Serraj I, D'Halluin PN, Branger B, Ponchon T. Miss rate for colorectal neoplastic polyps: a prospective multicenter study of back-to-back video colonoscopies. Endoscopy. 2008; 40:284-290

[42] Postic G, Lewin D, Bickerstaff C, Wallace MB. Colonoscopic miss rates determined by direct comparison of colonoscopy with colon resection specimens. Am J Gastroenterol 2002; 97:3182-3185

[43] Morini S, Hassan C, Zullo A, Lorenzetti R, de Matthaeis M, Stella F, Campo SM. Detection of colonic polyps according to insertion/withdrawal phases of colonoscopy. Int J Colorectal Dis 2009; 24:527-530

[44] Pickhardt PJ, Nugent PA, Mysliwiec PA, Choi JR, Schindler WR. Location of adenomas missed by optical colonoscopy. Ann Intern Med 2004; 7;141:352-359

[45] Adler A, Pohl H, Papanikolaou I S, et al. A prospective randomised study on narrow-band imaging versus conventional colonoscopy for adenoma detection: does narrow-band imaging induce a learning effect? Gut 2008; 57:59-64

[46] Adler A, Aschenbeck J, Yenerim T, Mayr M, Aminalai A, Drossel R. Narrow-band versus white-light high definition television endoscopic imaging for screening colonoscopy: a prospective randomized trial. Gastroenterology 2009; 136:410-416.e1

[47] Rex DK, Helbig CC. High yields of small and flat adenomas with high-definition colonoscopes using either white light or narrow band imaging. Gastroenterology 2007; 133:42-47

[48] Kaltenbach T, Friedland S, Soetikno R. A randomised tandem colonoscopy trial of narrow band imaging versus white light examination to compare neoplasia miss rates. Gut. 2008; 57:1406-1412

[49] Rastogi A, Bansal A, Wani S, Callahan P, McGregor DH, Cherian R, Sharma P. Narrow-band imaging colonoscopy--a pilot feasibility study for the detection of polyps and correlation of surface patterns with polyp histologic diagnosis. Gastrointest Endosc. 2008; 67:280-286

[50] East JE, Suzuki N, Guenther T, Palmer N, Stavrinidis M, Ignjatovic A, Saunders BP. Narrow band imaging (NBI) for adenoma detection in high risk patients: a randomised, controlled trial. Endoscopy. 2009; 41(Suppl 1):A223

[51] Uraoka T, Saito Y, Matsuda T, Sano Y, Ikehara H, Mashimo Y, Kikuchi T, Saito D, Saito H. Detectability of colorectal neoplastic lesions using a narrow-band imaging system: a pilot study. J Gastroenterol Hepatol. 2008; 23:1810-1815

[52] Inoue T, Murano M, Murano N, Kuramoto T, Kawakami K, Abe Y, Morita E, Toshina K, Hoshiro H, Egashira Y, Umegaki E, Higuchi K. Comparative study of conventional colonoscopy and pan-colonic narrow-band imaging system in the detection of neoplastic colonic polyps: a randomized controlled trial. J Gastroenterol 2008; 43:45-50

[53] Jin XF, Chai TH, Shi JW, Yang XC, Sun QY. A meta-analysis for evaluating the accuracy of endoscopy with narrow band imaging in detecting colorectal adenomas. J Gastroenterol Hepatol. 2011 Nov 18. doi: 10.1111/j.1440-1746.2011.06987.x. [Epub ahead of print]

[54] Ikematsu H, Saito Y, Tanaka S, Uraoka T, Sano Y, Horimatsu T, Matsuda T, Oka S, Higashi R, Ishikawa H, Kaneko K. The impact of narrow band imaging for colon polyp detection: a multicenter randomized controlled trial by tandem colonoscopy. J Gastroenterol. 2012 Mar 24. [Epub ahead of print]

[55] Sabbagh LC, Reveiz L, Aponte D, de Aguiar S. Narrow-band imaging does not improve detection of colorectal polyps when compared to conventional colonoscopy: a randomized controlled trial and meta-analysis of published studies. BMC Gastroenterol. 2011; 11:100

[56] Aminalai A, Rösch T, Aschenbeck J et al. Live image processing does not increase adenoma detection rate during colonoscopy: a randomized comparison between FICE

and conventional imaging (Berlin Colonoscopy Project 5, BECOP-5). Am J Gastroenterol 2010; 105:2383-2388

[57] Chung SJ, Kim D, Song JH et al. Efficacy of computed virtual chromoendoscopy on colorectal cancer screening: a prospective, randomized, back-to-back trial of Fuji Intelligent Color Enhancement versus conventional colonoscopy to compare adenoma miss rates. Gastrointest Endosc 2010; 72:136-142

[58] Tada M, Shimada, Murakami F et al. Development of the strip-off biopsy [in Japanese with English abstract]. Gastroenterol Endosc 1984; 26:833-839

[59] Karita M, Tada M, Okita K. The successive strip biopsy partial resection technique for large early gastric and colon cancers. Gastrointest Endosc 1992; 38:174-178

[60] Saito Y, Fukuzawa M, Matsuda T et al. Clinical outcome of endoscopic submucosal dissection versus endoscopic mucosal resection of large colorectal tumors as determined by curative resection. Surg Endosc 2010; 24:343-352

[61] Tanaka S, Haruma K, Oka S et al. Clinicopathological features and endoscopic treatment of superficially spreading colorectal neoplasms larger than 20 mm. Gastrointest Endosc 2001; 54:62-66

[62] Tajika M, Niwa Y, Bhatia V, et al. Comparison of endoscopic submucosal dissection and endoscopic mucosal resection for large colorectal tumors. Eur J Gastroenterol Hepatol 2011; 23:1042-1049

[63] ishi H, Tatsuta M, Iseki K, Narahara H, Uedo N, Sakai N, Ishikawa H, Otani T, Ishiguro S. Endoscopic piecemeal resection with submucosal saline injection of large sessile colorectal polyps. Gastrointest Endosc 2000; 51:697-700

[64] Kobayashi N, Yoshitake N, Hirahara Y, Konishi J, Saito Y, Matsuda T, Ishikawa T, Sekiguchi R, Fujimori T. A Matched Case-control Study Comparing Endoscopic Submucosal Dissection and Endoscopic Mucosal Resection for Colorectal Tumors. J Gastroenterol Hepatol. 2011 Oct 17. doi: 10.1111/j.1440-1746.2011.06942.x. [Epub ahead of print]

[65] Uraoka T, Fujii T, Saito Y, Sumiyoshi T, Emura F, Bhandari P, Matsuda T, Fu KI, Saito D. Effectiveness of glycerol as a submucosal injection for EMR. Gastrointest Endosc 2005; 61:736-740

[66] Lee SH, Cho WY, Kim HJ et al. A new method of EMR: submucosal injection of a fibrinogen mixture. Gastrointest Endosc 2004; 59:220-224

[67] Varadarajulu S, Tamhane A, Slaughter RL. Evaluation of dextrose 50% as a medium for injection-assisted polypectomy. Endoscopy 2006; 38:907-912

[68] Yamamoto H, Yube T, Isoda N et al. A novel method of endoscopic mucosal resection using sodium hyaluronate. Gastrointest Endosc 1999; 50:251-256

[69] Yoshida N, Naito Y, Kugai M et al. Efficacy of Hyaluronic Acid in Endoscopic Mucosal Resection for Colorectal Tumors. J Gastroenterol Hepatol 2011; 26:286-291

[70] Fujishiro M, Yahagi N, Kashimura K, Mizushima Y, Oka M, Enomoto S, et al. Comparison of various submucosal injection solutions for maintaining mucosal elevation during endoscopic mucosal resection. Endoscopy 2004; 36:579-583

[71] Hyun JJ, Chun HR, Chun HJ, Jeen YT, Baeck CW, Yu SK, et al. Comparison of the characteristics of submucosal injection solutions used in endoscopic mucosal resection. Scand J Gastroenterol 2006; 41:488-492

[72] Hirasaki S, Kozu T, Yamamoto H, Sano Y, Yahagi N, Oyama T, et al. Usefulness and safety of 0.4% sodium hyaluronate solution as a submucosal fluid "cushion" for endoscopic resection of colorectal mucosal neoplasms: a prospective multi-center open-label trial. BMC Gastroenterol 2009; 9:1

[73] Yoshida N, Naito Y, Inada Y, Kugai M, Kamada K, Katada K, et al. Efficacy of endoscopic mucosal resection with 0.13% hyaluronic acid solution for colorectal polyps: a randomized controlled trial. J Gastroenterol Hepatol. In press

[74] Naohisa Yoshida, Yuji Naito, Nobuaki Yagi, Akio Yanagisawa. Importance of Histological Evaluation in Endoscopic Submucosal Dissection and Endoscopic Mucosal Resection for Early Colorectal Cancer. World Journal of Gastrointest Pathophysiol 2012; 3:44-59

[75] Toyonaga T, Man-I M, Morita Y et al. The new resources of treatment for early stage colorectal tumors: EMR with small incision and simplified endoscopic submucosal dissection. Dig Endosc 2009; 21 Suppl 1:S31-37

[76] Isomoto H, Nishiyama H, Yamaguchi N et al. Clinicopathological factors associated with clinical outcomes of endoscopic submucosal dissection for colorectal epithelial neoplasms. Endoscopy 2009; 41:679-683

[77] Yoshida N, Naito Y, Sakai K et al. Outcome of endoscopic submucosal dissection for colorectal tumors in elderly people. Int J Colorectal Dis 2010; 25:455-461

[78] Fujishiro M, Yahagi N, Kakushima N et al. Outcomes of endoscopic submucosal dissection for colorectal epithelial neoplasms in 200 consecutive cases. Clin Gastroenterol Hepatol 2007; 5:678-683

[79] Zhou PH, Yao LQ, Qin XY. Endoscopic submucosal dissection for colorectal epithelial neoplasm. Surg Endosc. 2009; 23:1546-1551

[80] Tanaka S, Oka S, Kaneko I et al. Endoscopic submucosal dissection for colorectal neoplasia: Possibility of standardization. Gastrointest Endosc 2007; 66:100-107

[81] Yoshida N, Wakabayashi N, Kanemasa K et al. Endoscopic submucosal dissection for colorectal tumors: technical difficulties and rate of perforation. Endoscopy 2009; 41:758-761

[82] Yoshida N, Yagi N, Naito Y, Yoshikawa T. Safe Procedure in Endoscopic Submucosal Dissection for Colorectal Tumors Focused on Preventing Complications. World J Gastroenterol 2010; 16: 1688-1695

[83] Saito Y, Uraoka T, Yamaguchi Y, Hotta K, Sakamoto N, Ikematsu H, et al. A prospective, multicenter study of 1111 colorectal endoscopic submucosal dissections (with video). Gastrointest Endosc 2010; 72:1217-1225

[84] Saito Y, Fukuzawa M, Matsuda T, Fukunaga S, Sakamoto T, Uraoka T, Nakajima T, Ikehara H, Fu KI, Itoi T, Fujii T. Clinical outcome of endoscopic submucosal dissection versus endoscopic mucosal resection of large colorectal tumors as determined by curative resection. Surg Endosc 2009 Jun 11. [Epub ahead of print] PMID: 19517168

[85] Akahoshi K, Motomura Y, Kubokawa M, Matsui N, Oda M, Okamoto R, Endo S, Higuchi N, Kashiwabara Y, Oya M, Akahane H, Akiba H. Endoscopic submucosal dissection of a rectal carcinoid tumor using grasping type scissors forceps. *World J Gastroenterol* 2009;15: 2162-2165

[86] Homma K, Otaki Y, Sugawara M, Kobayashi M. Efficacy of novel SB knife Jr examined in a multicenter study on colorectal endoscopic submucosal dissection. Dig Endosc. 2012 May;24 Suppl 1:117-20. doi: 10.1111/j.1443-1661.2012.01266.x.

[87] Yoshida N, Naito Y, Kugai M, Inoue K, Wakabayashi N, Yagi N, Yanagisawa A, Yoshikawa T. Efficient hemostatic method for endoscopic submucosal dissection of colorectal tumors. World J Gastroenterol 2010; 16:4180-4186

[88] Saito Y, Uraoka T, Matsuda T, Emura F, Ikehara H, Mashimo Y, Kikuchi T, Kozu T, Saito D. A pilot study to assess the safety and efficacy of carbon dioxide insufflations during colorectal endoscopic submucosal dissection with the patient under conscious sedation. Gastrointest Endosc 2007; 65: 537-542

[89] Matsumoto A, Tanaka S, Oba S, Kanao H, Oka S, Yoshihara M, et al. Outcome of endoscopic submucosal dissection for colorectal tumors accompanied by fibrosis. Scand J Gastroenterol 2010; 45:1329-1337

[90] Tanimoto MA, Torres-Villalobos G, Fujita R, Santillan-Doherty P, Albores-Saavedra J, Gutierrez G, et al. Endoscopic submucosal dissection in dogs in a World Gastroenterology Organisation training center. World J Gastroenterol 2010; 16:1759-1764

[91] Parra-Blanco A, Arnau MR, Nicolás-Pérez D, Gimeno-García AZ, González N, Díaz-Acosta JA, et al. Endoscopic submucosal dissection training with pig models in a Western country. World J Gastroenterol 2010;16:2895-2900

[92] Hon SS, Ng SS, Lee JF, Li JC, Lo AW. In vitro porcine training model for colonic endoscopic submucosal dissection: an inexpensive and safe way to acquire a complex endoscopic technique. Surg Endosc 2010; 24:2439-2443

[93] Yoshida N, Yagi N, Inada Y, Kugai M, Kamada K, Katada K, Uchiyama K, et al. Possibility of Ex vivo Animal Training Model for Colorectal Endoscopic Submucosal Dissection. Int J Colorectal Dis 2012 in press

[94] Vazquez-Sequeiros E, de Miquel DB, Olcina JR, Martin JA, Garcia M, Lucas DJ, et al. Training model for teaching endoscopic submucosal dissection of gastric tumors. Rev Esp Enferm Dig 2009; 101:546-552

[95] Yamamoto H. Technology insight: endoscopic submucosal dissection of gastrointestinal neoplasms. Nat Clin Pract Gastroenterol Hepatol 2007; 4:511-520

[96] Hotta K, Oyama T, Shinohara T, Miyata Y, Takahashi A, Kitamura Y, et al. Learning curve for endoscopic submucosal dissection of large colorectal tumors. Digestive Endoscopy 2010; 22:302-306

[97] Fujishiro M, Yahagi N, Kakushima N, Kodashima S, Muraki Y, Ono S, et al. Successful nonsurgical management of perforation complicating endoscopic submucosal dissection of gastrointestinal epithelial neoplasms. Endoscopy 2006; 38:1001-1006

Section 4

Special Population

Chapter 13

Peculiarities of Paediatric Digestive Endoscopy

Marco Gasparetto and Graziella Guariso

Additional information is available at the end of the chapter

http://dx.doi.org/10.5772/52523

1. Introduction

1.1. What is the role of paediatric endoscopy nowadays? Which are the main indications and contra-indications?

An increased knowledge of normal and pathologic endoscopic patterns in paediatric patients has been increasing in the last decades.

Besides, the availability of flexible instruments with narrow diameter and elevate qualitative resolution allows Paediatric Gastroenterologists to investigate small infants too.

An adequate setting including endoscopic equipment, endoscopic room, support area and dedicated caregivers is fundamental to perform appropriate procedures.

Diagnostic endoscopy comprehends fiber-endoscopy, capsule endoscopy, confocal microendoscopy and echo-endoscopy.

Roles of Digestive Endoscopy

- Visualisation of the mucosa;
- Evaluation of architecture and vascularisation;
- Evaluation of mucosal secretions;
- Availability to take biopsy samples for histological examination with optic microscopy, ultra-structural examination with electronic microscopy, cultures, CRP methods, dissecting microscopy, chromo-endoscopy, vital staining, enzymatic studies, brushing;
- Endoscopic treatments.

Functions of Digestive Endoscopy

- Morphologic diagnosis of structural congenital and acquired alterations (optic microscopy, immune-histochemistry, electronic microscopy, confocal microendoscopy, brushing);
- Identification of infective processes (CRP techniques of molecular biology) and cultural examination;
- Morphological, chemical and microbiological evaluation of endoluminal secretions;
- Endoscopic treatment in case of gastrointestinal bleeding, varices, polyps, stenoses, tumors.

Appropriateness. Indications and contraindications to endoscopic examinations [1-2]

An endoscopic exam is indicated when the expected benefits (longer life survival, pain contention, reduction of anxiety, increase in functional capacity) exceed the potential negative consequences (mortality, morbidity, anxiety, pain, disability).

An endoscopic exam is necessary when it is unavoidable and mandatory for the care of the patient.

Signs and Symptoms of Indication for Upper Gastrointestinal (GI) Endoscopy

- GI bleeding;
- Disphagia, odinophagia, persistent feeding refusal, persistent chest pain;
- Upper abdominal pain with signs and symptoms suggesting organic diseases (red flags);
- Suspect of peptic disease;
- Persistent vomit;
- Suspected alterations at upper GI imaging;
- Suspected caustic ingestion;
- Iron deficiency anaemia.

Pathologic Conditions for which Diagnostic Upper GI Endoscopy is indicated:

- Peptic esophagitis, hemorrhagic gastritis, peptic ulcers in stomach, bulbus and duodenum;
- Gastrointestinal opportunistic infections i.e. Cytomegalovirus, Fungi;
- Eosinophilic esophagitis;
- Caustic ingestion;
- Atrophic gastritis;
- Helicobacter pylori (HP) gastritis;
- Coeliac disease;
- Inflammatory bowel disease (IBD) with localisation at the upper GI tract;

- Patients with liver cirrhosis, disphagia, malnutrition, oesophageal varices;
- Congestive gastropathy;
- Chronic diarrhoea of unknown nature;
- Structural alteration of the mucosa (Microvillus Inclusion Disease, Tufting Enteropathy);
- Benign or malignant lesions in common bile duct or duodenum;
- Graft Versus Host Disease (GVHD) after bone marrow transplantation;
- Lymphoproliferation after organ transplantation i.e. EBV-related gastric lymphoma after liver transplantation.

Pathologic Conditions for which Therapeutic Upper GI Endoscopy is indicated:

- Polypectomy;
- Treatment of oesophageal varices;
- Placement of ostomies;
- Treatment of GI bleeding (i.e. bleeding ulcers) non responsive to medical therapy;
- Removal of foreign bodies;
- Oesophageal stricture.

Absolute Contraindication to Upper GI Endoscopy

- Suspect of Gastrointestinal Perforation.

Relative Contraindications to Upper GI Endoscopy

- Non complicated gastro-oesophageal reflux;
- Functional uncomplicated abdominal pain;
- Congenital hypertrophic stenosis of the pylorus;
- Isolated spasm of the pylorus;
- Follow-up controls for ulcers, mucosal abnormalities, Barrett oesophagus;
- Surveillance of benign healed lesions.

Upper GI endoscopy is not appropriate for all children with dyspeptic symptoms, but only for cases [3]:

- With a family history of peptic ulcer and/or HP infection;
- Over 10 years of age;
- With symptoms persisting for more than 6 months;
- With symptoms severe enough to affect activities of daily living;

Pathologic Conditions for which Diagnostic Lower GI Endoscopy is indicated:

- Inflammatory bowel disease (IBD);
- Infective colitis;
- Allergic colitis;
- Neutrophil disfunction associated colitis i.e. Glycogenosis;
- Immune mediated diseases;
- Vascular abnormalities (venous ectasia secondary to portal hypertension, angiodysplasia, haemangiomas, vasculitis);
- Polyps and polyposes (juvenile polyps, adenomatous polyps, hyperplastic polyps, hamartomatous polyps, hereditary polyposic syndromes as Peutz-Jeghers Syndrome, Cowden Syndrome);
- Pseudopolyps of the colon;
- Neoplastic lesions i.e. leiomyosarcoma, lymphoma, carcinoma;
- Screening of displasia;
- Surveillance after bowel transplantation (rejection, complications);
- Obscure iron deficient anaemia;
- Structural alteration of the mucosa (Microvillus inclusion disease, Tufting enteropathy);
- Chronic diarrhoea of unknown nature;
- Suspect of filling defects or stenoses at radiographic-ultrasonographic images;
- Rectal trauma;
- Necessity of ileal or colonic bioptic samples.

Pathologic Conditions for which Therapeutic Lower GI Endoscopy is indicated:

- Polypectomy;
- Post-polypectomy complications;
- Mucosal resections;
- Ablation of vascular malformations (i.e. Dieulafoy Lesion);
- GI bleeding (i.e. Bleeding ulcers);
- Placement of percutaneous ostomies;
- Dilatations of colonic stenoses;
- Removal of foreign bodies;

Absolute Contraindications to Lower GI Endoscopy

- Suspected intestinal perforation;
- Severe acute colitis with toxic megacolon;

Relative Contraindications to Lower GI Endoscopy

- Acute self-limiting diarrhoea;
- Gastrointestinal bleeding with demonstrated origin at the upper GI tract;
- Recent intestinal resection;
- Irritable bowel syndrome;
- Chronic abdominal pain without significant morbidity;
- Simple constipation and encopresis.

2. The endoscopic technique in the paediatric patient: How to manage the child from pre-anestesia to the awakening

2.1. Upper gastrointestinal endoscopy [4]

Upper gastrointestinal endoscopy is a diagnostic instrumental examination which allows the physician to explore oesophagus, stomach, bulb and the first portions of duodenum.

The endoscope is a long thin flexible tube containing optic fibres. Paediatric endoscopes have diameters between 5.7 and 8 mm. An axial vision is provided.

For safety reasons, it is important for the child not to introduce solid foods since the preceding midnight whereas clear liquids (i.e. water, tea) are permitted until three hours before the procedure.

A peripheral cannula has to be placed before the exam, in order to administer in vein liquids and drugs for sedation. It will be removed after the child's awakening and after he/she will have recovered oral hydration.

An anesthetic cream will be placed in the site of venous puncture, to decrease the intensity of pain feeling.

While waiting for the procedure, the child can look to videos, listen to music or play, supported by the parents as well as by the trained staff of the endoscopic room.

To begin the exam, the child is placed on a left lateral position. The head is kept slightly lifted and inflected, in order to ensure the maximum extent of the hypo-pharynx. A mouthpiece is placed between the teeth to introduce the instrument avoiding lesions in the mouth.

The introduction of the instrument represents the most delicate part of the exam and can be performed in two ways: under strict visual control (visualisation of larynx, glottis, epiglottis and vocal chords at hours 12; visualisation of cricoid cartilage and cricoid-pharyngeal muscles in the back at hours 6) or with blind finger-directed intubation.

In case of erroneous intubation of the upper respiratory ways, the immediate removal of the instrument is indicated.

The normal oesophageal mucosa is pink; Z-line represents an important referral marker of the passage between oesophageal and gastric mucosa (more red coloured).

Just under the Z line, the oesophageal-cardiac junction appears as the confluence of mucosal plicae obliterating the lumen. Insufflation permits to overcome the cardias and enter the stomach where a sudden reduction in brightness due to the dispersion of light into the gastric cavity is observed. The pylorus need to be well visualised and overcome to enter the duodenum through an axial rotation of 90^ clockwise.

Biopsies can be taken in the return phase of the procedure. Once having reached back the gastric cavity, the manoeuvre of back-vision can be performed to visualise the gastric fundus and the oesophageal-gastric junction (an axial clockwise rotation of 180^ is required).

During the whole exam, the child is connected to a monitor for his/her vital parameters (heart rate, respiratory rate, oxygen saturation and arterial pressure) to be checked. Parents are asked to leave the room once the deep sleep has begun. They will come back inside the room at the awakening of the child, soon after the procedure has been completed.

During sedation, the endoscopist introduces the instrument through mouth, oesophagus, stomach bulb and duodenum. On a monitor, the upper GI tract mucosa being explored is visible. An appropriate orientation of the instrument needs to be maintained to obtain a real disposition of the features visualised on the monitor. The endoscopic vision is described using clock hands as spatial referral. Bioptic samples can be collected through appropriate pincers and can be sent to histological-microscopical or cultural analysis by the Pathologist and/or by the Microbiologist.

Upper GI endoscopy within its complexity offers a high diagnostic accuracy. It allows to study numerous characteristics of diseases (localisation, extension, disease activity, type of mucosal damage) and offers therapeutic possibilities too.

Upper GI endoscopy lasts 10-15 minutes but the total time for the procedure is longer, taking into consideration the initial preparation and the duration of awakening.

The Upper GI endoscopy is a safe procedure. Complications as perforation and bleeding are exceptional. Their incidence is extremely low within the paediatric population and is mainly connected to severe diseases.

The parent and the child are finally accompanied to their ward waiting for the child to be completely awaken so that he/she can start drinking. Soft and fresh or tepid tempered foods are subsequently proposed. A final clinical evaluation will be effectuated before discharge.

Lower Gastrointestinal Endoscopy [4]

Ileum-colonoscopy is an instrumental examination aimed to study the whole large bowel starting from its distal segment (the rectum) up to its proximal part (the cecum) passing through sigma, descendant colon, transverse colon and ascendant colon. Once the colonoscope has arrived to the cecum, the last tract of small bowel (terminal ileum) is also explored up to its 10-30 cm (ileal intubation).

The colonoscope is a tubular instrument provided with a video-camera and its diameter is calibrated according to the dimensions of the child. The images of the intestinal mucosa examined are viewed on a monitor being placed in front of the endoscopist.

The instrument is also equipped with a channel through which water can be introduced in order to clean any bowel content. Air can also be insufflated to distend intestinal oxbows and better introduce the instrument.

An aspirator can remove secretions and faecal remnants which prevent a complete visualisation of the mucosa. Other operative tools comprehend small pincers to collect intestinal biopsies to be analyzed by the pathologist for the histological examination, as well as therapeutic instruments (i.e. tolls for polipectomy or haemostasis).

The patient is initially placed on the left lateral position or supine. The inferior limbs are kept inflected. This position is the most approved by paediatric endoscopists because it allows the manoeuvres of abdominal compression as well as the evaluation of the trans-illumination signal thus detecting the position of the endoscope.

A lubrification of the instrument tip as well as of the anal region is effectuated before introducing the endoscope into the rectum, which is examined through a direct linear progression. Once the sigma has been reached, alternated up and down movements of the tip (hooking technique) are necessary to overcome the angle and to avoid the formation of a loop named "alpha-loop". A concomitant compression on the left abdominal quadrants is required.

Once the splenic impression is visualised from the lumen, a 180^ downward rotation has to be performed to proceed into the transverse colon and to avoid any loop formation. Parallel abdominal compressions are also needed for the manoeuvre.

The transverse and ascendant colon are differently shaped, the former being triangular whereas the latter circular.

The reaching of the cecal extremity is recognizable for the visualisation of the Bauhin valve and of the appendicular lumen. A transillumination in the right iliac quadrant is also visibile.

At the level of the valve, the circular plicae are more pronounced; a 45^ leftward rotation is required with a mild insufflation to dilate the valve and reach the lumen of the terminal ileum. Abdominal compression or the mobilisation of the patient can be of help for the manoeuvre.

Peyer's plaques are visible at the level of the terminal ileum which presents a circular shape with thickened mucosa.

The return phase need to be conducted with a carefull circular examination of the mucosa, in order to visualise any possible lesion. Bioptic samples can be taken at any examined segment.

A retro-vision manoeuvre can be performed at the rectum through a downword 180^ rotation to visualise the anal channel and sphincter from above.

Ileum-colonoscopy within its complexity offers an elevate diagnostic accuracy and permits to study several characteristics of diseases (localisation, extension, disease activity, type of damage of the intestinal mucosa) and offers therapeutic possibilities too.

A complete examination can last between 20 and 45 minutes and is performed under sedation-analgesia in children.

Complications as intestinal perforation or bleeding are very rare but need to be considered with a precise preliminary assessment of the child by the paediatric gastroenterologist and by the anaesthetist; the hematologic profile and coagulation also need to be checked.

About the presence and participation of the parents until the moment of sedation and from the initial awakening of the child soon after the procedure, the same management described in the previous paragraph for upper GI tract endoscopy is also valid for colonoscopy.

A specific paragraph dedicated to bowel preparation is following.

3. The importance of sedation-analgesia [5-8]

The endoscopic examination of upper and lower GI tracts represents a key tool for diagnosis and treatment of several GI diseases within the paediatric population.

Even though a basic diagnostic digestive endoscopy with biopsies is not necessarily a painful procedure, it frequently represents a threatening and feared event to the child and his/her family.

The introduction of the paediatric endoscope into the bowel can be annoying and requires self-control. Moreover, the approach of the child to the setting of an Hospital can be itself a cause of severe discomfort.

The sedation-analgesia has been proved to be efficacious and safe to let the child undergo endoscopic procedures with an adequate control of pain, fear and producing an amnestic effect.

Taking care of the baby implies establishing a communication with a subject whose interactions with the outside world are consolidating and growing; at the same time, the referring adults to the baby (the parents) need also to be guided. The caring team of the child is therefore aimed to create a good level of interaction around the child and his/her family.

The strategies of communication and relationship with a child are different according to the age and require flexibility by the caring team.

An adequate communication to the child of the principle steps of the endoscopic procedure is extremely useful to separate subconscious fantasies from reality. This is crucial to eliminate those fears or doubts of the child that may determine an inadequate cooperation during the procedure.

For these reasons, the importance of a setting to be conceived for the young patient and let him/her feel at ease is fundamental. The presence of an adult caring for the child (parents) is also determinant until the phase of pre-anestesia.

Even though there are no controlled randomized trials focusing on safety and efficacy, current evidences sustain Propofol as the best sedation-analgesia in the paediatric age. This drug can be safely administered by intensive care physicians even without a specialisation in anestesia, if they have an adequate experience and education thereabout.

As Upper GI endoscopy is a short lasting procedure, the baby can undergo a moderate-deep sedation with non protected airways, being placed in a comfortable position requiring the possibility of an easy access to the airways during the procedure.

During sedation-analgesia, a close monitoring of the vital parameters need to be performed (heart rate and electrocardiogram, respiratory rate, oxygen saturation, peripheral blood pressure) and the caring team needs to be necessarily trained to treat any potential emergency as well as any rare minor event or adverse effect to the drugs administered.

Level of Sedation	Definitions	Respiratory and Cardiovascular Conditions
Mild Sedation	Patients normally respond to verbal orders. A reduction in the cognitive functions and in the coordination can be attested.	Preserved cardiovascular and respiratory functions
Moderate Sedation	Patients voluntary respond to verbal orders. Reflexes are kept when evoked with a normal response to a stimulation with pain.	No need of interventions to keep the airways patent. Adequate spontaneous ventilation. Cardiovascular function maintained.
Deep Sedation	Patients can not be easily awaken but respond to pain stimulation.	The capacity to maintain the respiratory function can be compromised. An assistance to keep the airways open may be needed. Spontaneous ventilation can be inadequate and airway reflexes can be completely lost. Cardiovascular functions are generally maintained.
Anestesia	Patients cannot be awaken and do not respond to pain stimulations.	Patients require an assisted ventilation, since their cardiovascular functions can be compromised.

Table 1. Definition of the Levels of sedation (American Academy of Paediatrics, modified) [8]

Operative endoscopies or endoscopies performed on patients at risk for severe surgical complications need to be performed with protected airways and in the adequate setting of the surgery room.

4. Bowel preparation [9]

The majority of the paediatric bowel preparations available,is derived from the products existing for the adults. The process of bowel preparation in the paediatric population is age dependent, considering that the older is the child the more he collaborates.

The poor palatability of most of preparations and the need to ingest large amounts of liquid volumes, are two main limitations for the compliance of the paediatric patient.

As a consequence, it is often difficult in children to reach an adequate level of bowel cleaning.

Children do not easily tolerate the bowel preparations schedules, mainly because of the appearance of vomits, nausea and abdominal distension.

The use of an 8 French nasogastric tube is therefore often required to administer the preparation and this last procedure necessarily requires hospitalisation.

An at-home preparation would be instead ideal for paediatric patients, within a more comfortable and familial environment. A careful evaluation of the familial compliance is by the way to be firstly attested.

Since endoscopic procedures in the child require sedation, a fasting period has to be set before the examination.

The whole process of preparation can be significantly improved by an adequate involvement of parents (who are affectively closed to the child), letting one of them staying next to the child until the pre-sedation phase. A "child oriented" Endoscopic Room is also of great help to improve the child feelings and compliance.

There are currently no ideal preparations. The optimal theoretical characteristics of a bowel preparation would be safety, efficacy, tolerability and absence of contraindications.

Why is bowel cleaning important?

- Higher probability of reaching the cecum and terminal ileum through the Bauhin valve;
- A clearer and more complete vision is obtained, with an easier detection of possible lesions;
- Safety and efficacy of the examination are improved;
- An inadequate bowel cleaning relates to an increased risk of complications (i.e. bowel perforations); moreover the presence of faeces increases the infective risk during the operative procedures.

Basic instructions for bowel preparation

During the seven days preceding the endoscopic examination, a diet poor in fibers and rich in liquids should be suggested.

The day before the procedure a light breakfast (i.e. tea, milk, white bread slices with marmalade, dried biscuits, yoghurt) is indicated.

According to the scheduled timing of the endoscopic exam the day after, a light brunch can be prepared with half-liquid sugared products. The time of fasting is then programmed and the administration of the bowel preparation is then initiated. Faeces have to be viewed.

Until 3 hours before the examination, clear liquids i.e. tea and water can be introduced.

Six hours before the examination, the administration of the bowel preparation has to be interrupted.

For small infants, an adequate bowel cleaning can be obtained with enemas using small volumes of physiologic solution [20 ml/Kg) and substituting milk-feeding (breast, formulas) with clear liquids about 12-24 hours before the procedure.

Pharmacological Products: Stimulating Laxatives, Osmotic Laxatives, Solutions for Bowel Washing (Irrigation)

- Stimulating Laxatives: Bisacodyl, Senna, Sodium Picosulfate [10]

Elevated doses are required to obtain an efficacious cleaning. These products are converted by intestinal flora into active metabolites influencing the colonic motility by an acceleration of intestinal transit time. The absorption of liquids is reduced and the processes of secretion are modified.

Side effects include spastic abdominal pain, nausea and vomit.

This class of preparations is not currently indicated for the paediatric age.

- Osmotic Laxatives [11]

They represent the most indicated subclass of preparations for the paediatric age and include Lactulose, Magnesium Citrate, Polyethylene Glycol, Sodium Phosphate.

Lactulose,Mannitol and Sorbitol are sugars which are poorly absorbed by the intestinal mucosa.

They attract water within the intestinal lumen by an osmotic effect.

Side effects include:

- Significant loss of liquids and electrolytes;
- Bacterial fermentation of the non absorbed sugar with increase in the risk of infections
- Magnesium Salts are poorly tolerated and the bowel cleaning is therefore often inadequate. They are uneasily used within the paediatric population;

Sodium Phosphate is not to be used in children with chronic diarrhoea or body weight loss, intestinal obstruction, paralytic ileum, diseases of heart, kidney and liver [10-12].

It can cause aspecific erosions and ulcers on the colonic mucosa and can thus falsify the yield of the endoscopic examination, mimicking the typical lesions of IBD.

Others side effects involving mainly children and elderly people include severe electrolite alterations (hyperphosphatemia, hypocalcemia, hypokalemia), dehydration and renal failure.

It is generally orally administered with hypertonic solution, resulting palatable and efficacious for adult patients. A good safety has been also demonstrated within the adult population whereas it should be used with caution in children.

Patients willingly accept it because it requires a minor quantity of liquids with respect to other preparations.

The Food and Drug Administration of the US and Health Canada, have approved the following recommendations in terms of bowel preparation:

- The use of oral Sodium Phosphate is not recommended, whatever its indication might be, in children aging < 5 years;
- The use of oral Sodium Phosphate is not recommended for bowel preparation in children aging < 18 years;
- The use of oral Sodium Phosphate can be used in patients aging 6-18 years in case of occasional constipation only;
- The patient has to introduce a large amounts of liquids before and after bowel preparation.

PEG (Polyethylen Glycol) is a polymer with molecular weight of 3500-4000 Daltons, and cannot be absorbed by the intestinal mucosa [11].

The PEG based electrolytic solutions available have to be osmotically balanced.

The use of PEG does not determine any passage of water nor electrolytes from or towards the bowel. PEG does not undergo bacterial fermentation. Several clinical trials demonstrate its efficacy. Its palatability is however limited. The ingestion of large amounts of liquids (at least 1-2 L) is required when PEG is used.

Possible gastrointestinal side effects include nausea, vomit, abdominal distension and pain.

Useful strategies to help bowel preparation with PEG include [13]:

- Administration of prokinetic drugs (i.e. Metoclopramide, Domperidone);
- Utilization of a nasogastric-tube (8 French) is suggested in children aging < 3 years or to prevent the risk of inhaling and ab-ingestis pneumonia, particularly in those patients with altered swallowing reflex or compromised mental state. A volumetric pump may also be used;

- Suggested dosage for the paediatric patient: 30-40 ml/Kg/h

PEG is not recommended in case of [13-14]:

- Founded suspect of luminal lesions obstructing the bowel;
- Severe abdominal pain;
- Vomits;
- Acute severe colitis (a bowel preparation can increase the risk of perforation and progression to Toxic Megacolon)

Peculiar situations in bowel preparation

- Patient with diarrhoea: lower amount of preparation is indicated;
- Patient with chronic constipation: larger amount of preparation is indicated; pre-procedural enemas can be considered;
- Patient with gastrointestinal bleeding: lower amount of preparation is indicated (blood has a prokinetic effect);
- Patient with partial intestinal obstruction: larger amount of preparation is indicated and enemas of isotonic saline solution to be effectuated two hours before the procedure.

5. Endoscopy and main clinical settings in paediatrics

5.1. Gastroesophageal Reflux Disease (GERD) [15-17]

Upper digestive endoscopy represents the gold standard for detection of pathologic GER complications; a high specificity is obtainable thank to the histological analysis of the bioptic specimens.

The Savary Classification defines 4 grades of esophagitis:

1. Mucosal exudation
2. Non confluent erosions
3. Confluent erosions
4. Ulcers. Fibrosis, stenosis and/or brachi-oesophagus
5. Barrett oesophagus

Another Classification for esopghaitis is the Los Angeles Classification [18] which identifies the following 4 grades:

- **Grade A:** One (or more) mucosal break no longer than 5 mm, that does not extend between the tops of two mucosal folds (a mucosal break being defined as an area of slough or erythema with discrete demarcation from the adjacent mucosa);

- **Grade B:** One (or more) mucosal break more than 5 mm long that does not extend between the tops of two mucosal folds;
- **Grade C:** One (or more) mucosal break that is continuous between the tops of two or more mucosal folds but which involves less than 75% of the circumference;
- **Grade D:** One (or more) mucosal break which involves at least 75% of the esophageal circumference.

Barrett oesophagus can itself be subclassified within three types:

1. Defined border between oesophageal and gastric epithelia (more typical of the child);
2. Portions of oesophageal squamous epithelium are within the context of the gastric cylindrical epithelium
3. Cylindrical metaplasia with no circumferential distribution, but with stretches of tissue departing from the Z line.

Oesophageal erosions are lesions covered by fibrin and with erythematosus borders; they are confined within the tonaca mucosa and do not reach the submucosa.

Oesophageal ulcers can differently involve the deeper levels causing hemorrhagic phenomena which can be endoscopically treated.

In children with peptic esophagitis, the lower part of the oesophagus is generally involved whereas the upper tracts are mainly macroscopically normal.

Typical histological patterns in peptic esophagitis include eosinophilic infiltration (> 2 eosinophils/HPF), neutrophilic infiltration (> 2 neutrophils/HPF), basal zone hyperplasia (> 20%) and papillary hyperplasia.

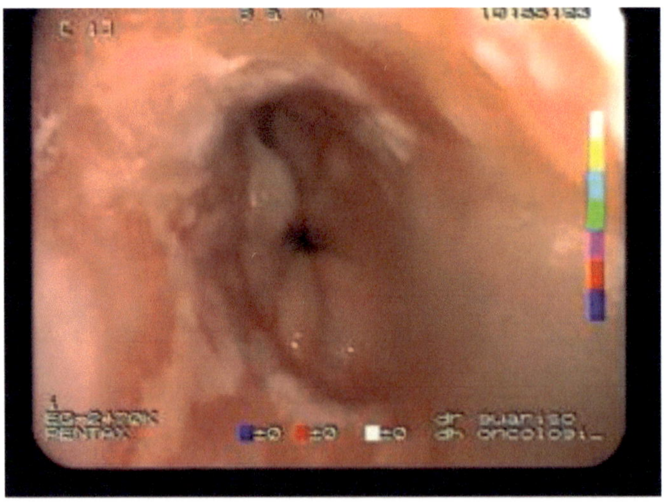

Figure 1. Peptic esophagitis (Grade 3)

http://dx.doi.org/10.5772/52523

The **Boyle Classification** associates the endoscopic and histological patterns:

- Grade 1: Extension of the papilla, increased thickening of the lamina propria; presence of eosinophils or neutrophils (1-19 cells/HPF);
- Grade 2: Same patterns as Grade 1, but with a higher number of neutrophils or eosinophils (> 20 cells/HPF);
- Grade 3: Endoscopically or histologically defined erosions (Fig. 1);
- Grade 4: Endoscopically or histologically defined ulcerations;
- Grade 5: Oesophageal stenosis or Barrett oesophagus.

5.2. Eosinophilic esophagitis [16-17-20]

Eosinophilic Esophagitis (EE) is an important disorder due to an Inflammatory condition of the esophagus that is characterized by having above normal amounts of eosinophils.

The symptoms of EE may vary with age. The clinical presentation of EE may be confused with GERD especially in younger children. Infants often present with vomiting, irritability and poor weight gain. In the older child and adolescent, difficult swallowing and food obstruction or impaction in the esophagus may be more common.

Other symptoms might include reflux not responsive to standard medical therapy, nausea, vomiting, abdominal or chest pain, poor appetite, and sleeping difficulties.

An upper endoscopy with biopsies is necessary for diagnosis of EE. The appearance of the esophagus in EE is quite characteristic (Fig. 2): a wrinkled or furrowed and ringed esophagus is covered with whitish material or exudate.

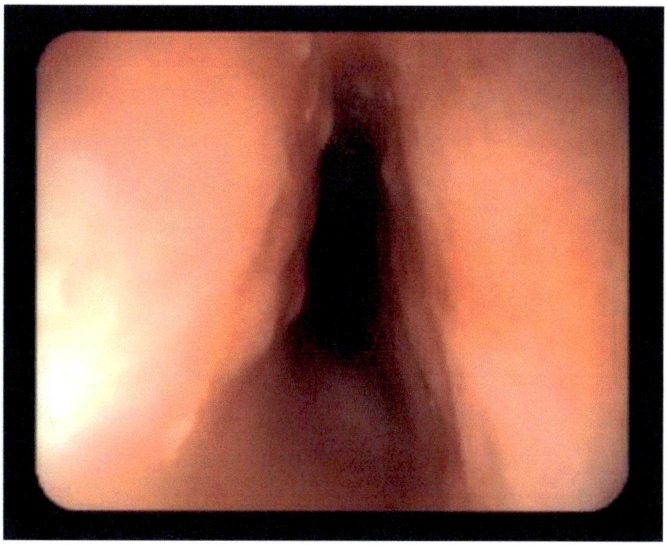

Figure 2. Eosinophilic oesophagitis

However, the esophagus may look normal.

The diagnosis of eosinophilic esophagitis is set on the histological evidence of > 15 eosinophils/HPF (normal values<3). No eosinophils are detected at gastric and duodenal biopsies.

Elevated peripheral blood levels of eosinophils as well as of total IgE are also observed.

Patients' symptoms increase to normality after a 4 week treatment with prednisone. A dietary restriction is also efficacious for these patients.

5.3. Candida associated and immunodeficiency associated esophagitis [18]

Candida associated esophagitis can be found both in immunodeficient patients (i.e. HIV affected patients, Fig. 3 and 4) as well as in basically healthy subjects. The mid oesophagus is generally the mainly involved tract. A variable endoscopic pattern can be found: the mucosa mostly appears crispy and erythematosus, and can be accompanied by plaques, erosions, ulcerations and nodularities. Lesions are mostly covered by whitish exudation.

Oesophageal candidosis can be found also in the absence of an oral localisation.

The distal oesophageal tract is often spared because of the acidic reflux protection.

Patients with immunodeficiencies (i.e. lymphoma, leukemias) can also present herpetic oesophageal lesions determining a mucosal pattern similar to the one of Candida infection, thus the histological examination is needed for the differential diagnosis. Several systemic immuno-mediated diseases can be associated with gastrointestinal involvement, also in the absence of infections [19].

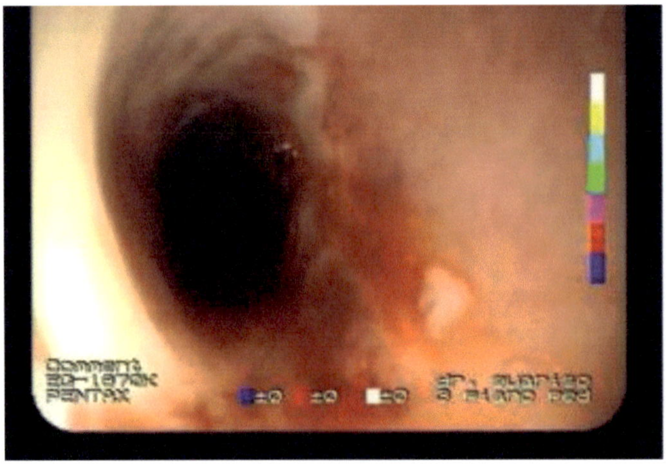

Figure 3. CMV related esophagitis in an immunodeficient patient

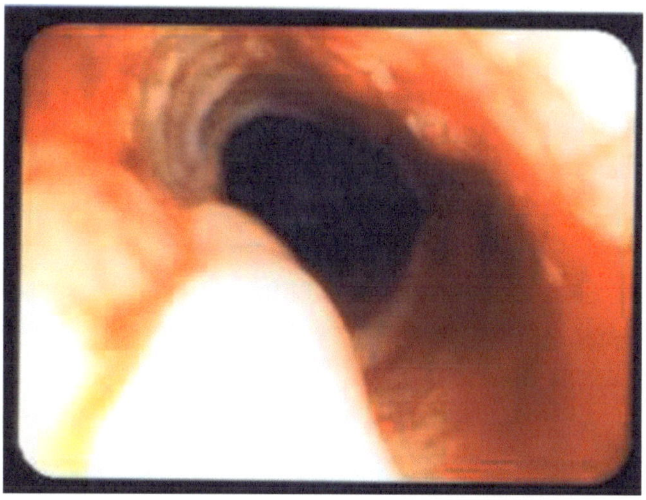

Figure 4. Oesophageal mycetomas in a child with AIDS

5.4. Oesophageal neoplasia [18]

Primitive oesophageal neoplasias are rare in the paediatric age. The most frequent type is oesophageal leiomyoma which is generally found during adolescence.

In the paediatric age all oesophageal parietal layers are infiltrated and the whole oesophageal length is involved in 30-40% of cases.

Children are often symptomatic presenting disphagia, weight loss, hematemesis, cought, dyspnea, retro-sternal pain and vomit.

A lesion protruding into the oesophageal lumen is endoscopically detected, without alterations of the oesophageal mucosa.

Differential diagnoses include mediastinal masses or achalasia.

Surgical resections represent the available treatments (tumor enucleation, oesophagectomy, oesophagus-gastrectomy).

Oesophageal adenocarcinoma and metastases are extremely rarely detected in adolescence.

5.5. Oesophageal varices [21]

Variceal bleeding as a consequence of portal hypertension is one of the complications of paediatric chronic liver diseases.

Portal hypertension is defined as portal vein pressure > 5 mmHg or a portal vein to hepatic vein gradient of > 10 mmHg.

The level of portal vein obstruction can be pre-sinusoidal (intra or extra-hepatic), sinusoidal or post-sinusoidal.

Extrahepatic portal vein obstruction is the most frequent cause of paediatric portal vein hypertension, and is mainly secondary to instrumentation of the umbilical veins in neonates, congenital malformation, omphalitis or intra-abdominal infections.

Intrahepatic presinusoidal portal hypertension is observed in congenital hepatic fibrosis and schistosomiasis.

Among the causes of post-sinusoidal portal hypertension are Budd-Chiari Syndrome, webs in the supra-hepatic vena cava, veno-occlusive disease and cardiac disease.

The management of the three levels of portal obstruction relates to the evidence that liver function is almost always normal in extra-hepatic and pre-sinusoidal obstructions whereas it is generally impaired in sinusoidal or post-sinusoidal obstructions.

Ascites is generally only present when portal hypertension is at the sinusoidal level.

Four main portal to systemic vein collateral systems become prominent in portal hypertension: the paraumbelical venous network (caput medusa), the perirectal collateral venous system, gastric varices and oesophageal varices which are best examined by endoscopy.

Once portal hypertension is suspected on clinical and US findings, elective upper endoscopy can give useful information about the size, localisation and grade of the varices.

Variceal bleeding is the most serious complication of portal hypertension, with a 30-50% mortality and high risk of rebleeding. The main factors predicting variceal bleeding are portal vein-hepatic vein gradient > 12 mmHg; large, tense varices; red wale marks, red spots on varices; severity of underlying liver disease.

In children, the risk of bleeding may change over time; in those with extra-hepatic portal vein obstruction, the development of a decompressive collateral circulation may decrease the risk with age.

Hematemesis or melena as a result of variceal bleeding is often massive, and children may present a cardiovascular shock. In these cases, resuscitation efforts and intravenous vasoconstrictor therapy are begun. Clotting factor supplementation should also be instituted immediately.

Upper-GI endoscopy is required primarily to confirm the site and cause of bleeding and to determine if treatment is indicated. A differential diagnosis of other etiologies of upper-GI bleeding includes portal hypertensive gastropathy, gastric and duodenal ulcers and Mallory-Weiss.

In most Centres, oesophageal varices are graded according to their size:

Grade 1: Small straight varices;

Grade 2: Medium enlarged tortuous varices occupying less than one third of the lumen;

Grade 3: Large coil-shaped varices occupying more than one thirs of the lumen.

A recent consensus from the American Association for the Study of Liver Diseases (AASLD) recommends to use 2 grades (small and large) with a cut-off size of 5 mm.

The North Italian endoscopic club for the study and treatment of esophageal varices indicates a classification based on variceal size (small, medium, large), severity of red wale marks (absent, mild, moderate, severe) and Child-Pugh class (A-C). A risk stratification for variceal bleeding accompanies this classification, with cumulative scores for individual features added to define a risk class.

If esophageal variceal bleeding is confirmed, therapeutic sclerotherapy or variceal ligation is indicated.

Sedation, intubation and balloon tamponade may be the only method to stabilize a patient with persistent uncontrolled bleeding: this represents by the way only a temporizing measure, since balloons can be safety left inflated for 12-24 hours.

Prevention of rebleeding and prophylaxis of first variceal bleeding include sclerotherapy, variceal ligation, vasoactive drugs and portosystemic shunts.

Sclerotherapy is the first well-established modality to control variceal bleeding in children, and has decreased the need for shunt surgery. It is now increasingly being replaced by band ligation, which appear to be safer and more effective. Both techniques usually require repetitions in order to successfully eradicate oesophageal varices in up to 90% of patients.

By the way, until the child undergoes a definitive procedure that decreases or eliminates portal hypertension (i.e. shunt operation or liver transplant), a risk of life-threatening variceal bleeding remains, often from newly formed gastric varices

Portal hypertensive gastropathy with increased bleeding risk may also be exacerbated by esophageal variceal obliteration. Gastric varices are not amenable to either sclerotherapy or ligation.

5.6. Gastritis [22-24]

Acute Gastritis

Acute gastritis can be secondary to infections (i.e. virus, Helicobacter Pylori (Fig. 5), Salmonella), drugs (i.e. NSAID, cortisone, chemotherapy), uremia (i.e. acute and chronic kidney failure), stress (i.e. surgical intervenctions, burns), shock. In adolescents mainly smoking, alcohol and drugs' assumption can relate to this kind of disease.

Three endoscopic degrees of acute gastritis are described:

- A mild form with mucosal oedema and hyperaemia;
- An intermediate form with haemorrhagic lesions (Fig. 6];
- A severe ulcerative form with extended deep erosions.

The histological pattern is characterised by leucocitary inflammation with a more frequent antral localisation

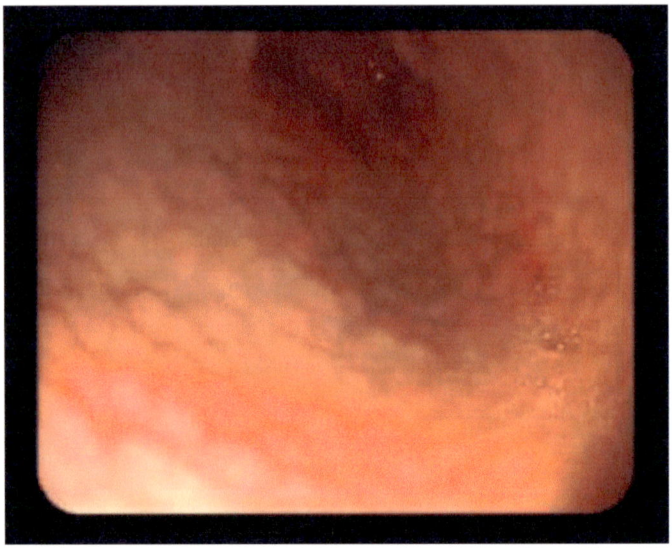

Figure 5. Helicobacter Pylori gastritis

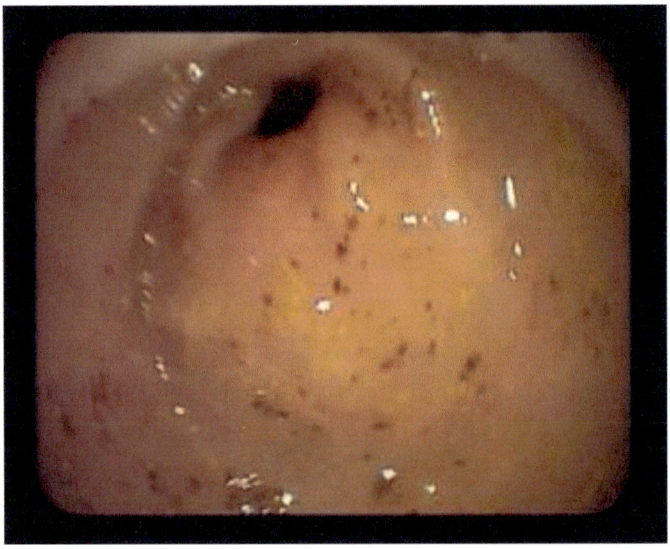

Figure 6. Haemorragic gastritis

Chronic Gastritis

Chronic gastritis represents a frequent finding in the paediatric age, and is endoscopically characterized by gastric atrophy (Fig. 7). The histological pattern shows an increased mucosal inflammatory infiltration as well as a glandular atrophy, with different degrees of severity (superficial, atrophic and gastric atrophy). Localisations at the gastric antrum, body and fundus can be detected. As regards the antral localisation, HP has a main epidemiologic role. An HP related pangastritis can also be observed. The localisation at fundus is mainly of auto-immune nature.

Atrophic gastritis can be associated to gastric metaplasia or displasia, even though this remain exceptional in the paediatric age.

Chronic gastritis can be classified as active (polimorphonucleate and eosinophilic infiltration) or quiescent (lymphocitic cell infilatration). The endoscopical pattern is characterized by hyperhaemic areas with edema and exudative secretions, alternated with opaque areas, creating a mucosal jeopardized aspect. Ulcers can also be evidenced within the inflamed areas of the mucosa.

A superficial erosive gastropathy is endoscopically characterized by minimal spotted loss of substance and whitish exudative areas with heritematosus profile.

HP related gastritis has an endoscopic pattern characterized by nodular intensively inflamed mucosal areas. Erosions and fibrine can also be found on the inflamed areas.

HP colonises the interface between gastric epithelium and mucus, and can be easily detected on gastric biopsies through specific stainings.

HP gastritis is a risk factor for development of gastric cancer in adults as well as for gastric lymphoma in children.

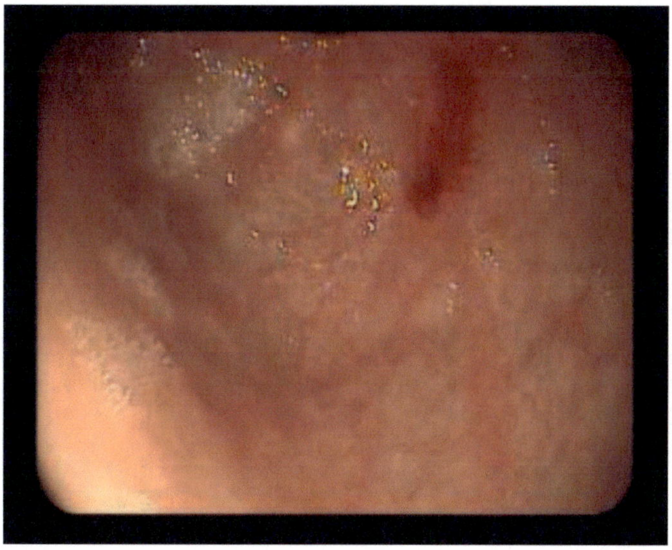

Figure 7. Atrophic gastritis

Even though peptic ulcers are rare in the paediatric age, their prevalence among children and adolescents with HP gastritis is much higher with respect to those patients without HP infection.

Haemorrhagic gastropaties are mainly secondary to stress, NSAIDs assumption or infections; the endoscopic pattern is characterised by hyperhaemic bleeding areas, sometimes with petechiae.

5.7. Gastric ulcers [22-24]

Gastric ulcers are discontinuities of the gastric mucosa with penetration to the muscolaris mucosae and exposure of the submucosa.

The Forrest Classification describes three types of peptic ulcers, basing on the characteristics of the associated upper gastrointestinal haemorrhage [25]:

Forrest Ia: Spurting arterial bleeding (Fig. 8);

Forrest Ib: Oozing arterial haemorrhage;

Forrest IIa: Large non-bleeding visible vessels (Fig. 9);

Forrest IIb: Adherent clot;

Forrest IIc: Haematin on ulcer base;

Forrest III: Lesions without signs of recent haemorrhage.

Primitive ulcers are caused by alterations of the gastric function (HCl production and pepsin function); they are mainly single lesions and are usually found at the small gastric curve and at the antrum.

Secondary ulcers are instead caused by extra-gastric pathogenic events, i.e. stress or drugs. They can be multiple and can have a spread localisation within the stomach.

HP is often involved in the pathogenesis of gastric peptic ulcers. Neoplastic ulcers are instead related to development of lymphoma.

Benign ulcers are endoscopically characterized by mild dimensions, oval or roundish shape, and by a whitish-grey base, consisting in covering fibrin and granulation tissue. Borders are thin and plane. A basal vase can be detected and represent a source of haemorrhage. Gastric plicae are usually converging to the ulcer.

Malignant ulcers generally present an irregular base, with necrotic base covered by fibrin. However, only the histological examination can differentiate the two ulcer types.

Drug-associated ulcers are mainly associated to treatments with NSAID, steroids, anti-neoplastic drugs, immunosuppressive drugs. A reduction of the protective effect of prostaglandins on gastric mucosa is considered to be the main pathogenetic mechanism.

Other stressful events (i.e. shock, sepsis, burnings, major trauma, endocranial hypertension, surgical procedures, chronic diseases) can cause acute gastric ulcers, also in the paediatric age. Lesions generally appear 3-6 days after the event and the main related symptoms are bleeding and abdominal pain. Most of times they are multiple lesions involving any part of the stomach. Intracranial illness related gastric lesions are called Cusching ulcers, whereas burning related lesions are named Curling ulcers. The endoscopic pattern is characterized by mucosal oedema, bleeding and focal erosions.

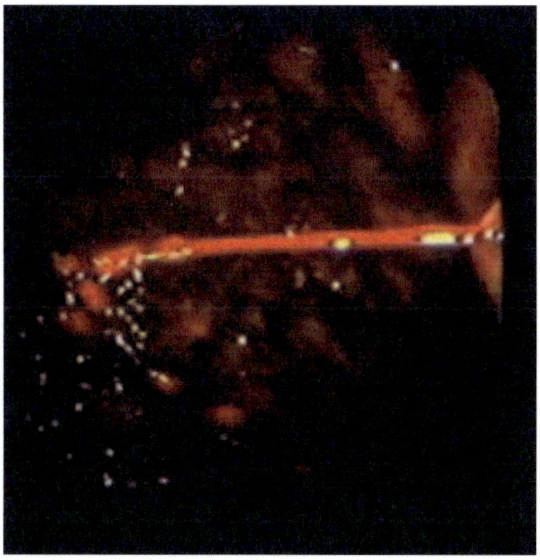

Figure 8. Peptic Ulcer (Forrest 1A)

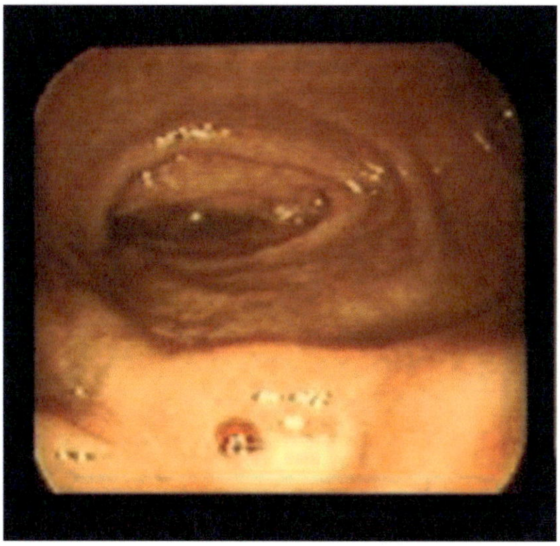

Figure 9. Peptic Ulcer (Forrest 2A)

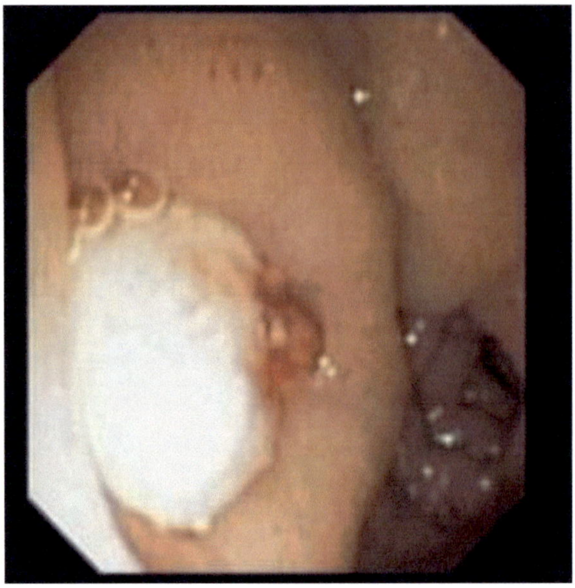

Figure 10. Bleeding bulbar ulcer

5.8. Granulomatous gastritis [22]

Several different illnesses (including Crohn's Disease) can cause granulomatous gastritis. Gastric involvement can be isolated or in association with other gastrointestinal tracts. Lesions can be found at multiple gastric localisation and can present as erythematosus-nodular gastropathy, aphthous lesions, deep linear or serpiginous ulcers. Antral pseudopolyps conferring a cobblestone pattern to the mucosa can be observed. Pyloric obstructions can be evidenced in Sarcoidosis; in those cases a nodular mucosa with thickened rigid gastric plicae can be observed, simulating the pattern of infiltrating lymphoma.

Tubercular gastritis also represents a rare but possible infection, which can be secondary to miliar diffusion of the disease as well as related to a primitive infection by mycobacterium bovis or atypical mycobacteria in immunocompromised subjects.

Mycotic infections in immunocompromised patients (including Histoplasma, Phicomyceti, Candida, Aspergillus), can also cause granulomatous gastritis, mainly when disseminated at multiple organs.

5.9. Eosinophilic gastritis [22]

This rare disease is characterised by peripheral blood hypereosinophilia, accompanied by an eosinophilic infiltration of the whole gastro-intestinal tract involving at least mucosa and submucosa. Gastric mucosa assumes a thickened nodular pattern, with bulging gastric plicae and partial obstruction of the antral-pyloric lumen. Eosinophilic granuloma appearing as polypoid lesions can be observed, as well as erosive phenomena. An involvement of duodenum can also be often attested.

Familiarity for allergies is frequently evidenced.

The disease symptoms include abdominal pain, vomit, iron-deficient anaemia, melena and protein loosing enteropathy. The involvement of the muscular tunica can cause dysmotility and sub-occlusive phenomena. The infiltration of serosa can induce formation of ascites.

5.10. Hyperplastic plical gastropathy [22]

Three variants of this disease are described: Ménétrier disease is caused by hyperplasia of superficial mucosal cells with gastric hyposecretion; Hypertrophic Hypersecretive Gastritis; Zollinger-Ellison syndrome, which is related to active gastrinoma within multiple endocrinological affections (MEN 1].

The paediatric variant of Ménétrier disease has peculiar characteristics with respect to the variant of the adult: the paediatric disease is generally CMV associated, and allergic and immune-mediated phenomena are considered to have a pathogenetic role in the disease development. The disease is generally self-limiting and with favourable prognosis in children.

Related symptoms are anorexia, body weight loss and protein loosing enteropathy.

The endoscopic pattern is characterised by giant hypertrophic plicae, conferring to the mucosa a cerebral-like pattern and without any efficacious distension with endoscopic air insufflation.

Zollinger Ellison is endoscopically characterised by multiple and persistent gastric and duodenal ulcers. A hypertrophy of the gastric plicae is observed as secondary to hypergastrinemia. Disease diagnosis requires detection of elevated blood levels of gastrine in basal condition as well as after stimulation with proteic meals or with secretine.

5.11. Gastric vascular anomalies [22]

They can be classified as non-neoplastic forms (comprehending congestive gastropathy secondary to portal hypertension, varices, teleangectasies and angiodysplasias) and neoplastic forms (angiomas, angiosarcomas and Kaposi sarcoma).

Portal hypertension can be secondary to pre-hepatic causes (i.e. portal vein cavernoma), hepatic causes (biliary cirrhosis) and post-hepatic causes (Budd-Chiari Syndrome).

The endoscopic pattern is characterised by a darker reddish colour of gastric mucosa, which appears more evident at the antrum and gastric body, with petechiae, haemorrhagic spots or with more diffuse hemorrhagic lesions (Fig. 11]. Varices of the gastric fundus can be often associated.

Gastric varices typically surround the cardial-oesophageal junction, developing in the submucosa and determining an endoscopic pattern of curved protrusions. The blue colour which is typically seen in oesophageal varices, is not generally attested in gastric varices (due to different mucosal thickening), so that they can be easily misrecognised as hypertrophic gastric plicae.

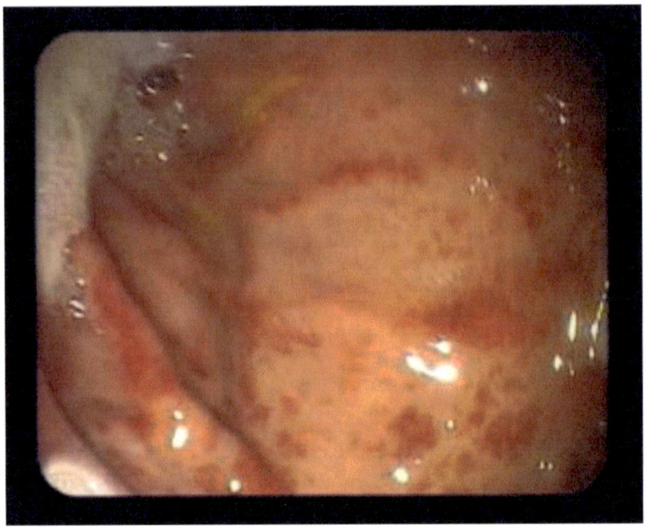

Figure 11. Congestive gastropathy

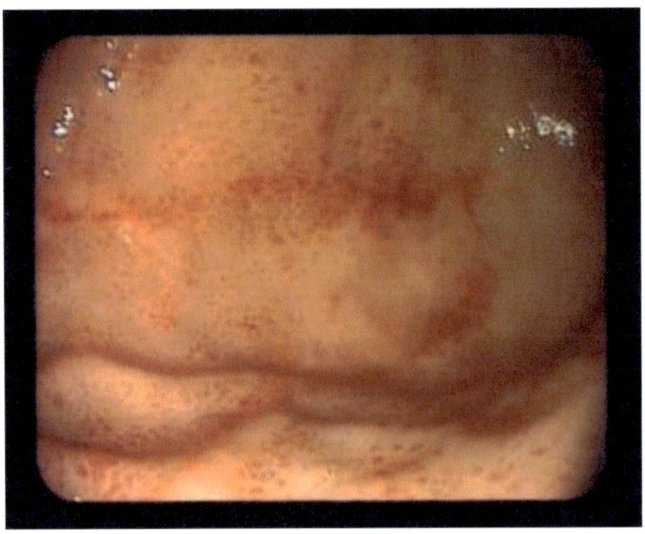

Figure 12. Gastric GVHD in a child with BMT

5.12. Graft versus Host Disease (GVHD) after Bone Marrow Transplantation (BMT)

The stomach is among the several organs which can be involved in GVHD syndrome.

The main clinical features are anorexia, nausea, vomit, watery diarrhoea, abdominal pain, gastrointestinal bleeding and body weight loss [21].

Endoscopic features include oedema, erythema, erosions, ulcerations and mucosal bleeding (Fig. 12); every portion of the stomach can be potentially involved.

The histological pattern is characterised by apoptosis of the cryptic epithelial cells, exploding crypts, lymphocytic infiltration of epithelium and lamina propria.

Rectal-sigmoid biopsies are more accurate for diagnosis of GVHD in comparison to samples from the upper GI tract *($p<0.0001$)*.

5.13. Ingestion of Caustic Substances [26-27]

In the paediatric age, caustic ingestion is still among the indications to endoscopy, which represents the most appropriate technique to evaluate mucosal lesions at the level of oesophagus and stomach.

House products are nowadays less involved in causing severe lesions thank to safer packaging and to reduced concentration of active caustic substances. On the other hand, professional and industrial caustic products still represent a concrete risk for children.

Mucosal damages determined by caustic ingestion, depend on the pH and concentration of the ingested substance.

Alcaline substances (sodium hydroxide, ammonium, sodium hypochlorite) with a concentration superior to 20% cause colliquative necrosis with deep lesions which can determine visceral perforations. When lesions involve muscular oesophageal layers in their whole circumference, stenoses and shortening of the oesophagus can be generated (Fig. 13).

Acid substances can provoke airway damages, whereas at the level of oesophagus coagulative necrosis reduces the penetration into parietal layers as well as the risk of stenoses (Fig. 14).

In the stomach, alcaline substances are neutralised by gastric acidity, but the generated exothermic reaction can cause burning lesions, mainly at the antral and pyloric regions. An accurate anamnesis is of fundamental importance to detect the nature of the ingested substance. Symptoms generally include vomit, breathing difficulty, hematemesis, excessive salivation.

The presence of lesions at the oral cavity and at hypopharynx does not relate to the severity of the oesophageal and gastric lesions.

Endoscopy represents the main diagnostic technique to evaluate the presence, severity and extension of lesions.

Before endoscopic examination, patients need to present stable general conditions and vital parameters, through correction of shock status and intubation. A chest x-ray should be performed to exclude pneumomediastinum and pneumoperitoneum which are mainly observed in adults who ingest caustics with suicidal aim.

A 12 hour time interval since ingestion, is recommended to estimate the real entity of extension and depth of caustic lesions. After 48 h since ingestion, however, the parietal colliquation can render the mucosa fragile and an excessive air inflation can cause perforations.

During the endoscopic evaluation of the oesophagus, air inflation has to be minimized. The most severe damages are generally found at the superior and intermediate oesophagus.

Caustic esophagitis is generally classified within three degrees of severity:

- 1st degree: Diffuse mucosal hyperhaemia, spotted areas of dysepithelisation without fibrin deposits;
- 2nd degree: Hyperhaemic mucosa with deep dysepithelisation and withish pseudomembranes which are typically linear and do not converge;
- 3rd degree: The whitish pseudomembranes converge and involve the entire oesophageal circumference for a variable extension from a few centimetres to the whole oesophagus;

These lesions are rare findings in the paediatric age, whereas they are more common in adults who ingest caustic substances with suicidal intents. They are severe necrotic dark lesions extended to the whole oesophageal mucosa. The surgical resection of the oesophagus can be indicated to prevent perforation and mediastinitis. In the stomach, the most active damage is localised at the body, big curve, antrum and pylorus. Duodenal lesions are generally rare.

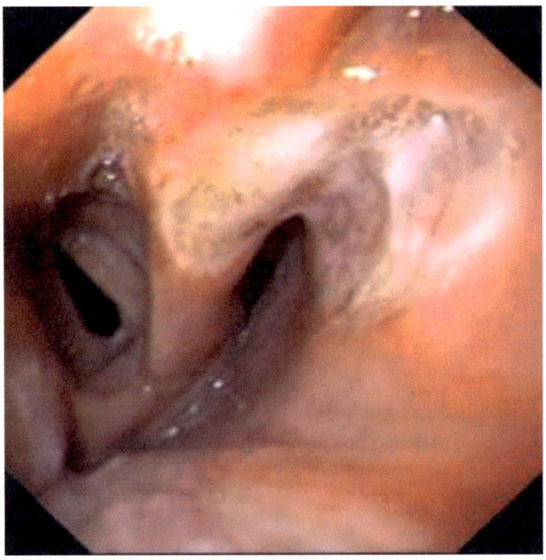

Figure 13. Caustic esophagitis

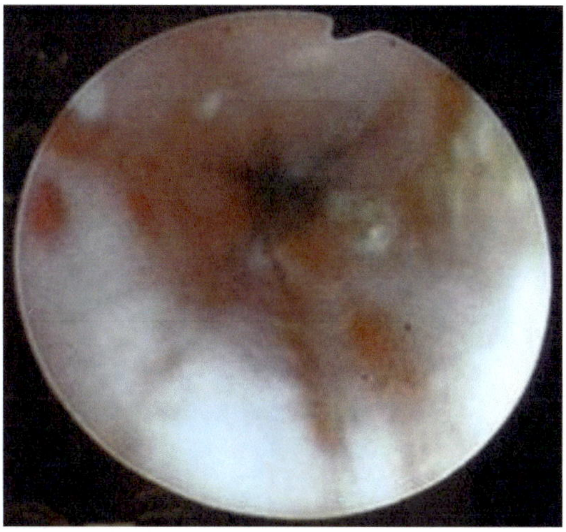

Figure 14. Esophagitis secondary to Chlore ingestion

5.14. Coeliac Disease [28]

Coeliac Disease represents one of the most common duodenal diseases in the paediatric-juvenile age.

A gluten-induced intolerance determines mucosal damage of the duodenum in genetically predisposed subjects.

Typical and atypical symptoms include malabsorption (diarrhea, body weight loss, growth deficit, dystrophia), anemia, hepatic affection, osteopoenia, neurological alteration, dental enamel dysplasia.

The diagnosis is based on the histological examination of the duodenal mucosa at the second duodenal portion. The endoscopic duodenal pattern is characterised by pale nodular mucosa, with vanishing and "scalopping" plicae.

The histological pattern evidences villous atrophy with decrease alteration of villous/cryptal ratio, and lymphocytic infiltration.

For the paediatric age, the new Guidelines of the European Society for Paediatric Gastroenterology, Hepatology, and Nutrition (ESPGHAN) state that in those cases with clear symptoms and a level of Anti Transglutaminase Antibodies IgA above 10 times the upper normal limit, a diagnosis can be set without the need of intestinal biopsy (Positivity for EMA and HLA DQ2 and/or DQ8 is also required).

5.15. Infective Colitis [29]

Infective colitis are common events at all ages, but most frequently in children aging less than 5 years.

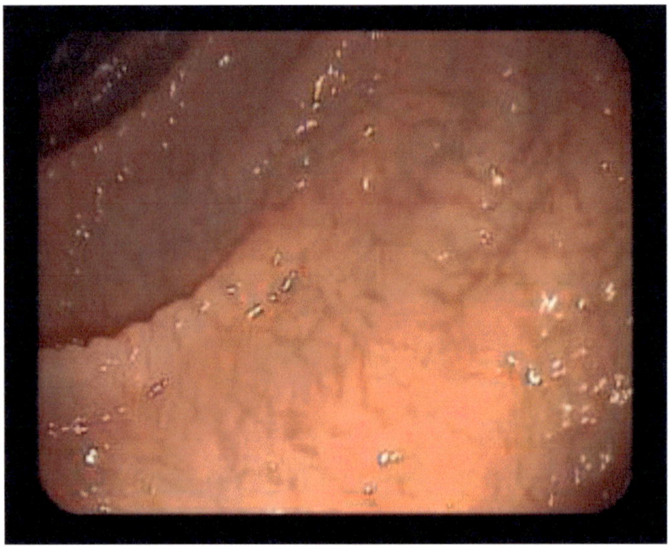

Figure 15. Scalopping of duodenal plicae in Coeliac Disease

The diagnostic ascertainments include clinical, hematochemical and cultural investigations.

Lower-GI endoscopy can have a role in the differential diagnosis, since the endoscopic pattern of infective colitis can be misrecognised as an inflammatory bowel disease, therefore the histological examination is determinant for a final diagnosis.

In the paediatric age, minor Salmonella can determine localisations at the level of the small bowel as well of the colon and rectum. The mucosa presents oedema, hyperhaemia, and in the most severe forms ulcers and bleeding or necrotic plaques.

Other bacterial infections include E. Coli, Yersinia, Campylobacter, Vibrions and Shigella.

Pseudomembranous colitis caused by Clostridium Difficile can affect paediatric patients treated with prolonged or recurrent antibiotic therapies for chronic affections.

Symptoms include bloody diarrhoea and progressive decrease in general conditions.

The endoscopic feature is characterised by aspecific inflammation (fragile mucosa with oedema, hyperhaemia, microhaemorrhagias or petechiae, superficial bleeding ulcerations) whereas the pseudomembranous lesions more classically found in adult patients are hardly detectable in children.

Among viral infections, pre-natal CMV assumes an important impact to the bowel (Fig. 16]. Other localisations can be possibly involved, including cerebral - ocular – hepatic and splenic localisations.

An involvement of the small bowel accompanying the rectal-colonic localisation can cause a severe intestinal malabsortion. A severe diarrhoea, often with bloody faeces, is clinically observed. Endoscopically, jeopardized micro-haemorrhages are seen, sometimes in association with lymphoid nodular hyperplasia.

Differential diagnoses including infections by HIV, atypical Mycobacteria, parasites (Giardia, Ameba, Schistosomes) and fungi, have to be considered in children with immune-depression.

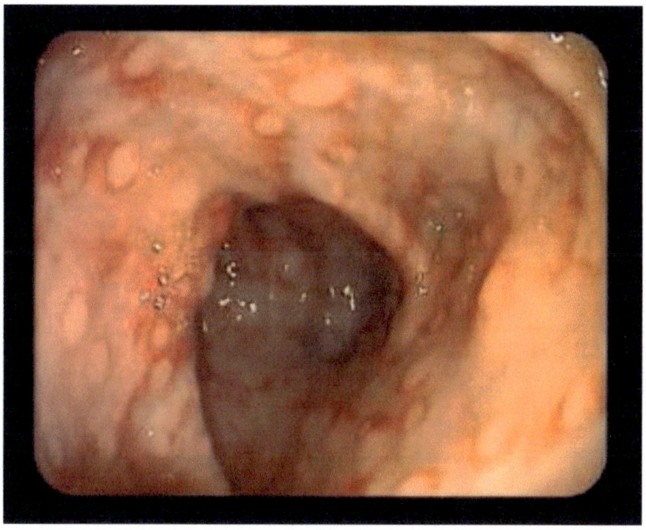

Figure 16. CMV related colitis in an immunodeficient infant

5.16. Nodular Lymphoid Hyperplasia (NLH) of the Colon-Rectum [29]

It is a very common feature in the paediatric age, in particular among newborns and toddlers. It is due to the presence of reactive hypertrophic lymphoid follicles. It is generally asymptomatic, but in some cases it can determine the appearance of bloody faeces. NLH can be related to allergic phenomena or can be expression of infective processes. In most of cases it is self-limiting and diminishes in the follow-up.

The endoscopic pattern is characterised by mucosal nodules with depressed tip (Fig. 17), sometimes associated with haemorrhage.

5.17. Allergic Colitis [29]

Colonic localisations of allergic processes in the child, are generally associated with the involvement of the upper GI segments or other organs. Allergic colitis clinically manifests with mucous bloody diarrhoea, and in those cases with important malabsorption it can determine major impairment of the general conditions. In the newborns and toddlers it is generally more frequent and related to vaccine milk proteins.

The endoscopic aspect of the colonic mucosa is characterised by inflammation of the intestinal wall of variable extension, oedema, parietal necrosis, ulcerations and bleeding, nodular lymphoid hyperplasia (Fig. 18).

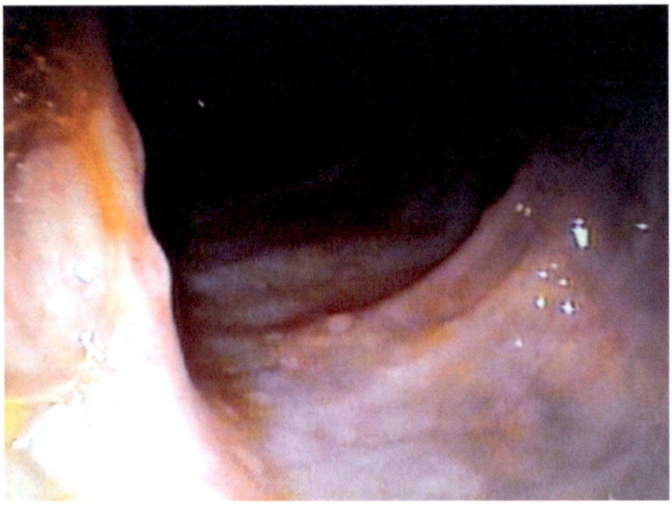

Figure 17. Lymphoid Nodular Hyperplasia of the colon

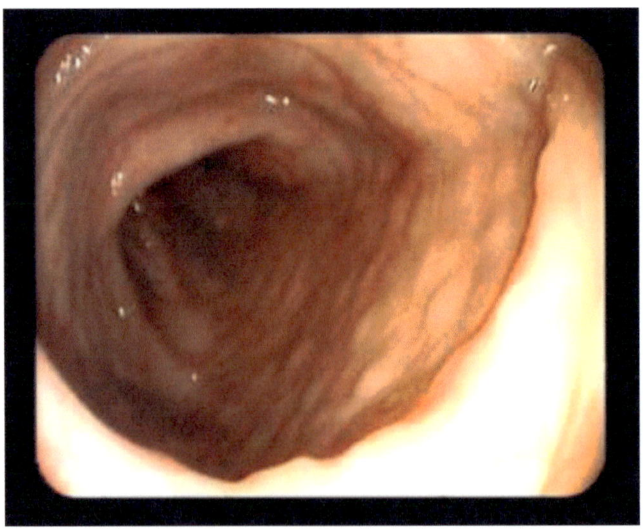

Figure 18. Allergic colitis in an infant

5.18. Inflammatory Bowel Disease [30-34]

Endoscopy is able to differentiate Crohn's Disease (CD) and Ulcerative Colitis (UC) in 89% of cases. It is, moreover, nowadays the most efficacious and diffused technique to evaluate CD localisation and activity at the level of terminal ileum and colon; its accuracy results, in fact, significantly superior with respect to bowel enema.

An immediate diagnosis with excellent accuracy is obtainable when endoscopy is associated to the histological examination of biopsy samples.

The endoscopic procedure for paediatric patients with IBD differs significantly from the modalities in use for the adults, especially as regards the use of sedation-analgesia, the number and localisation of the mucosal biopsies effectuated and the regular inclusion of terminal ileum intubation within a complete investigation.

In the paediatric age, assistance with anestesia allows to perform a complete endoscopic examination with visualisation of terminal ileum in 90% of cases.

The endoscopic evaluation of mucosal healing is important to identify the efficacy of a specific therapeutic regimen.

5.19. Crohn's Disease [30-34]

Endoscopic features in paediatric CD include aphthae (multiple, focal, surrounded by erythematosus mucosa; Fig. 19), nodules, serpiginous ulcers, cobblestone pattern of the intestinal mucosa and stenoses.

Inflammatory pseudopolips are less frequent in CD with respect to UC (Fig. 20).

According to the mucosal and phenotypical characteristics at onset, CD is classified into inflammatory, stenosing and fistulizing.

Since CD can potentially involves the whole gastrointestinal tract, the intubation of ileum and upper gastrointestinal endoscopy are always indicated for a complete staging of the disease.

At the level of the strictures, the intestinal mucosa usually appears actively inflamed, frequently ulcerated and bleeding.

In the fistulizing CD phenotype, the internal orifice of the fistula can be observed on the bowel wall, generally in correspondence of inflamed areas.

The histological pattern of CD is generally characterised by transmural inflammation, dilatation and sclerosis of the lymphatic vessels, lymphoid aggregates and non caseating granuloma.

Oesophageal localisations can be found in patients with extended and severe Crohn's disease. The finding of granuloma at the histological exam of oesophageal biopsies needs firstly tuberculosis to be excluded. Secondarily, the effectuation of a lower endoscopy is mandatory.

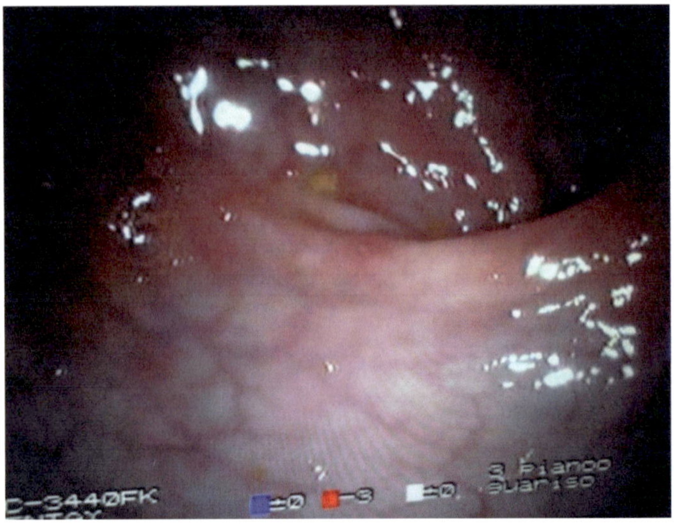

Figure 19. Crohn's Disease. Aphthae in the colonic mucosa

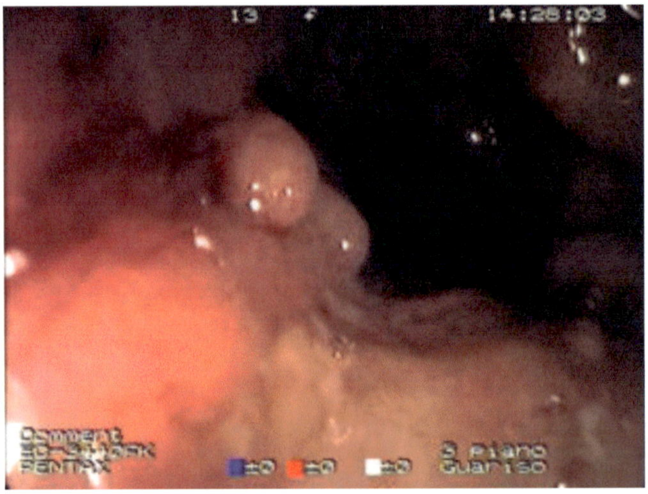

Figure 20. Colonic pseudoplyps in Ulcerative Colitis

5.20. Ulcerative Colitis [30-34]

Endoscopic features in paediatric UC include loss of normal vascular and architectural pattern, diffuse hyperhaemia, congestion, oedema, mucosal fragility and/or bleeding after contact with endoscope, mucous secretions, diffuse erosions covered by fibrin, ulcerations, aphthae, inflammatory pseudopolyps.

http://dx.doi.org/10.5772/52523

Other possible findings include loss of colonic plicae with aspect of "rigid tube", backwash ileitis (ileal extension of lesions in pancolitis), patchy colitis and relative rectal sparing

Baron and Mayo are the two principal indexes for the endoscopic grading of Ulcerative Colitis.

The histological pattern in UC is characterised by distorsion and disappearance of the mucosal glands and cryptic inflammatory infiltration.

Also villi-like profile of the mucosal surface, a high grade alteration of the mucosal architecture, Paneth cells metaplasia and decrease of the inflammation and mucosal alteration grade from the upper to the lower colonic tract are seen.

5.21. Gastrointestinal Polyps and Polyposis [35-37]

Gastrointestinal polyps are macroscopically visible protrusions of the mucosal surface which can be classified in relation to their shape as sessile, pedunculated and plane polyps. A further histological classification distinguishes adenomatous, hyperplastic, inflammatory and hamartomatous polyps (Fig. 21).

In the paediatric age, intestinal polyps are generally represented by single juvenile polyps, and more rarely by familial polyposis.

Hyperplastic polyps are generally sessile and of small dimensions (2-5 mm); they are formed by exceeding epithelial mature cells which do not separate from intestinal crypts and therefore cannot be lost in the intestinal lumen. A transformation into adenocarcinoma is attested in rare cases.

Adenomatous polyps are due to alterations in cellular proliferation and differentiation. They appear at endoscopy as sessile unique lesions, more rarely multiple, of small dimensions (2-3 cm); pedunculated and more dimensioned adenomatous polyps are more rarely found.

The covering mucosa is generally smooth and normally vascularised, with exception of bigger polyps in correspondence of which it can be hyperhaemic, spotted, lobular, ulcerated or with erosions. The histological examination of adenomatous polyps can show a tubular, villous or intermediate patterns. Adenomatous polyps are dysplastic lesions which are differentiated into mild, moderate or severe according to the relating risk of carcinomatous degeneration.

Juvenile polyps are the most frequently observed in the paediatric age (90%) and are generally isolated, exceptionally multiple and under a maximum number of 8. They are histologically characterised by an excessive development of lamina propria including crypts with cystic dilatation. The endoscopic aspect is pedunculated, roundish, with a smooth surface and a typical diameter of 1-1.5 cm (Fig. 22). A superficial ulceration and cellular inflammation are frequently found on the polyp, with regenerative epithelial hyperplasia. 70% of juvenile polyps are localised at rectum and 15% at sigma. No ileal localisations are possible. The clinical presentation is characterised by small persistent haemorrhagias, which is rarely severe to cause anemia. Associated abdominal pain is frequently observed. Alternated intestinal transit and mild diarrheal represent other possible associated clinical features.

Rectal polyps with huge dimensions can determine mucosal prolapse. Juvenile polyps are not associated with increased risk of carcinomatous transformation.

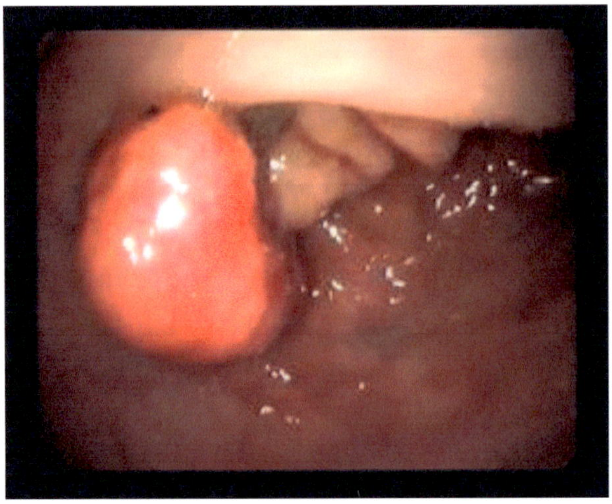

Figure 21. Hamartomatous polyp of the colon

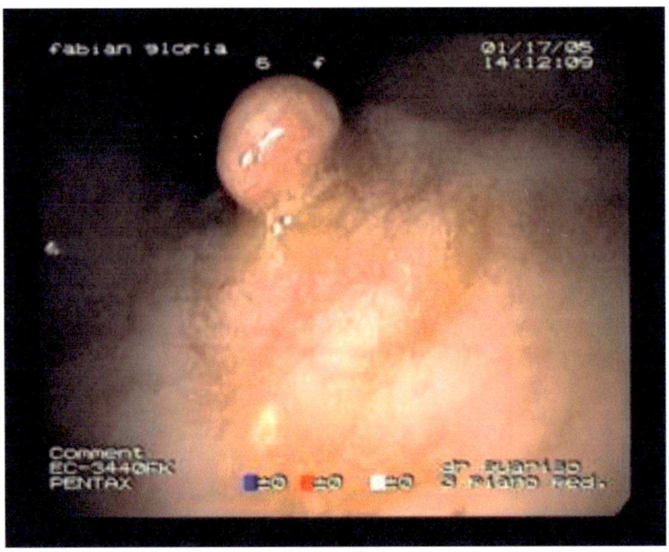

Figure 22. Juvenile rectal polyp

Principal Familial Polyposis

Familial Adenomatous Polyposis (FAP) is a disease with autosomal dominant transmimission, characterised by the formation of multiple adenomatous polyps (> 100) which can involve every GI segment, mainly the colon-rectum but also the stomach and the small bowel. Multiple extraintestinal manifestation can be associated.

The risk of neoplastic degeneration with time is of 100%. In 30% of cases there is no familiarity for the disease, so a spontaneous spot mutation is involved. The disease incidence is of 1/8.000-10.000 newborns. The responsible gene (APC) has been identified in the 5 q 21-22 region and is a "tumor suppressor gene" which encodes a protein involved in the mechanisms of intercellular connection and transmission. More than 200 mutations have been identified at present, to which disease phenotypes with different severity correspond.

A pre-symptomatic disease diagnosis as well as the development of surveillance protocols are fundamental before the disease manifests.

Polyps are not present at birth, but usually develop within the first years of life, mainly in correspondence with puberty: this suggests that other factors than genetics intervene in the manifestation of disease.

According to their degree of development, polyps can present different dimensions, shapes (plane, pedunculated or sessile), and with different histological pattern (tubular, villous, intermediate).

Gastric polyps are generally glandular and localised at the gastric fundus; antral adenoma are less frequent. At the duodenum, the risk of adenoma and adenocarcinoma at the Vater papilla is high.

The main clinical symptom is characterised by bloody faeces, both as a massive bleeding and as occult bleeding leading progressively to anemia. Intestinal intussusception or anal polyp prolapse are also possible, especially in infants. Recurrent abdominal pain is also a common symptom.

Diarrhoea, electrolytic alterations and protein-loosing enteropathy are potential consequences of an elevated number of polyps.

Screening for FAP includes faecal occult blood research, endoscopic surveillance and genetic techniques.

A number of extraintestinal manifestations can be variably attested, the most common one being an ocular disease with multiple bilateral pigmented lesions which are secondary to a hypertrophy of retinal epithelium (CHRPE). An accurate ophthalmologic exam is therefore fundamental in at-risk children.

A common FAP related manifestation is the development of desmoid tumors which is observed in 9-32% of patients: these are mesenchymal benign tumors originating from mesenter and peritoneum, and which can cause compressive phenomena on abdominal organs and on vases.

Neoplasia at the level of thyroid, pancreas, adrenal glands, urinary bladder, testicles, lipomas, myomas, fibromas and hepatoblastomas have also been found in association.

Gardner Syndrome is an autosomal dominant variant of FAP, the relative mutated gene being APC as well. This syndrome differentiates from FAP in terms of extraintestinal manifestations: in 90% of patients osteomas are observed, with localisation at teeth, jaw, other facial bones, long bones of legs and pelvis.

Over-numbered teeth and multiple tooth caries can be also associated. Desmoid tumors involve about 15-20% of affected patients.

Turcot Syndrome is a rare recessive disease, characterised by an early onset appearance of cerebral and medullar tumors in infants (glioblastomas, astrocytomas and medulloblastomas) which generally anticipate intestinal adenoma and condition the survival rate of affected patients.

Colonic adenoma evolve to cancers within the second-third decade of life.

Ruvalcaba-Myhre-Smith Syndrome is a FAP variant related to an alteration of a gene with localisation at 10q23. It is characterised by a colonic and ileal hamartomatous polyposis and associated with mental retardation, myopathy, cranial and facial dysmorphisms, macrocephaly, skeletal abnormalities and genital stains.

Peutz-Jeghers (PJS) is an autosomal dominant hereditary polyposis with a variable grade of penetration [40-50%). The mutate gene is the oncogene STK11 (19p 13.3). The distinctive elements of the syndrome are skin and mucosal pigmentation especially at the level of mouth and genitals, as well as the development of hamartomatous polyps.

Polyps can be found from stomach to anus, but their most frequent localisation is at the small bowel, especially at the jejunum and ileum. Their number is lower than in FAP, and the polyp shape also spreads from small sessile polyps to large pedunculated elements. Their histological nature is hamartomatous.

The clinical onset generally dates before adolescence, and is generally characterised by variable symptoms including recurrent abdominal pain, diarrhoea, occult bleeding, haematic faeces, intestinal obstructions or intussusceptions. Hyperpigmented (bluish-black coloured) stains are localised at the skin and mucosa of lips, cheeks, nasal orifices, eyes, genital and perianal region, hands and feet.

While skin stains can disappear, mucosal lesions are generally permanent.There are subjects who never develop skin nor mucosal stains.

An increased risk for intestinal cancers is attested in these patients, especially adenocarcinoma of jejunum and ileum. Extraintestinal manifestations include cancers at breast, uterine cervix, ovaries, testicular Sertoli's cells and thyroid. Bronchial adenomas, nasal polyps, hepatic hamartoma, pancreatic and gallbladder tumors are also possible.

Specific screening programs are therefore mandatory for PJS patients.

Cowden Syndrome is anautosomal dominant hereditary polyposis, characterised by hamartomatous lesions of ectodermal, mesodermal and endodermal origin. The responsible germinal-line mutations involve the PTEN gene (10q23) in 80% of cases, encoding a tyrosine phosphatase.

Clinical manifestations generally date at the second-third decade of life, even though earlier onsets are also possible. Abdominal pain and gastrointestinal bleeding represent the main clinical features. Polyps are generally localised at the distal colonic segments (Fig. 23). The distinctive elements of the syndrome are the skin and mucosal lesions comprehending oral papilloma, facial hamartoma and localisations at the extremities of the limbs. Narrow palate, macrocephaly and scoliosis are often found.

Benign tumors of soft tissues are common, including lipomas, angiomas and fibromas.

Malignant extraintestinal complications include breast cancer and thyroid neoplasias.

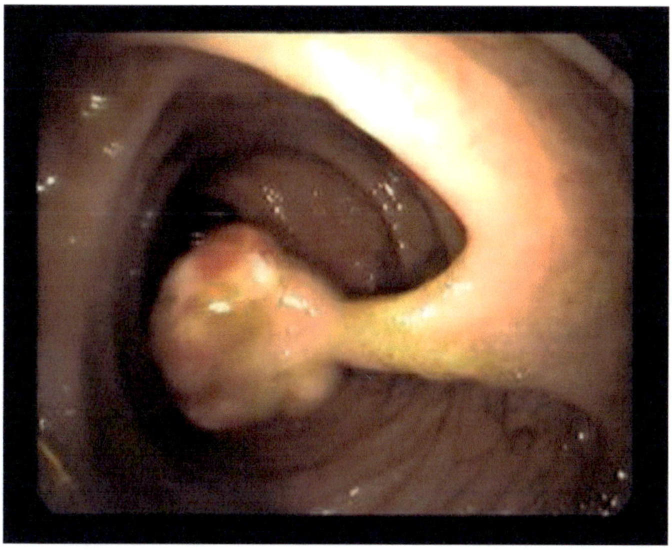

Figure 23. Polyp of the colon in Cowden Syndrome

6. Approach to children with hereditary gastrointestinal polyposis [35-36]

An accurate familial anamnesis is the first fundamental step, even though cases of spontaneous mutations [30% of FAP and PJS) are also described.

A careful clinical examination is important, especially for detection of peculiar extra-intestinal manifestations, i.e. skin and mucosal lesions in PJS, the ophthalmologic evaluation in FAP and the dental and facial bone alterations in Gardner Syndrome.

Blood tests have a role in detecting the degree of affection of general conditions, in particular the detection of anaemia. Haematic tests for liver, kidney and muscles need also to be checked as well as electrolytes and the inflammation indexes.

Genetic tests on peripheral blood lymphocytes are possible for FAP (i.e. linkage test with accuracy of 95%).

A genetic counselling needs to be considered before performing any genetic test for screening and diagnosis of polyposic syndromes. In fact, no single test is associated with a sufficient accuracy for the diagnosis of GI polyposis and more genetic alterations are usually coexisting in a single patient.

Children are generally genetically tested after 10 years of age, before the activation of an endoscopic surveillance, and once they are able to understand the implications of the diagnostic tests performed.

The fundamental priority is to characterise with the highest accuracy, the number, localisation and histological nature of the GI polyps.

Upper and lower endoscopies represent the pivotal diagnostic procedures for GI polyposes. Bioptic samples need to be taken for the histological examination of lesions and the exclusion of a malignant transformation. A collaboration between physicians and pathologists is fundamental for the diagnosis and therapeutic management of polyposes.

The performance of endoscopic polypectomies is a therapeutic option which can be considered in addition to the diagnostic role of US, CT and MRN in the detection of extraintestinal manifestations and metastases as well as in the study of those GI segment which cannot be explored with endoscopy.

Wireless capsule endoscopy permits a complete visualisation of the small bowel but does not consent the collection of bioptic samples. Barium enhanced radiologic techniques represent a less accurate and less invasive alternative for the investigation of small bowel lesions.

Polypetomy is a technique performed under sedation in children. A well conducted colonic preparation and a control of coagulation indexes are mandatory before its performance. The polyp excision is performed with a dyatermic loop.

The loop shape and kind is chosen according to the dimensional characteristics and to the localisation of the polyp.

The removed polyp will then be recuperated with a loop or with Dormia basket.

In cases of multiple polyposes, the eradications of polyps can be effectuated in repeated times.

The procedure of polypectomy results to be more feasible at the level of the stomach and duodenum with respect to colonic localisations, for technical reasons.

Potential complications of polypectomy include haemorrhage and perforation (variable incidence of 0.4-4%)

Surgical interventions of intestinal resections are indicated in subjects with FAP and comprehend total colectomy and ileal-rectal anastomosis or procto-colectomy with ileal-anal anastomosis and ileal pouch.

A multidisciplinary approach generally offers better results for patients with polyposis syndromes. Affected children should be cared by a team including a paediatric gastroenterologist, a genetist, a surgeon and a paediatric psychologist.

http://dx.doi.org/10.5772/52523

Several studies have demonstrated the importance of regional and national registers, aimed to a screening for neoplasia and to the identification of high risk relatives. These screening protocols have significantly reduced the morbidity and mortality associated to these illnesses.

Author details

Marco Gasparetto and Graziella Guariso

Department of Woman and Child Health, Unit of Gastroenterology, Digestive Endoscopy, Hepatology and Care of the Child with Liver Transplantation, University Hospital of Padova, Italy

References

[1] Squires RH Jr, Colletti RB. Indications for pediatric gastrointestinal endoscopy: a medical position statement of the North American Society for Paediatric Gastroenterology and Nutrition. J Pediatr Gastroenterol Nutr 1996;23(2): 107-10.

[2] Brook RH, Chassin MR, Fink A, Solomon DH, Kosecoff J, Park RE. A method for the detailed assessment of the appropriateness of medical technologies. Int J Technol Assess Health Care 1986;2(1):53-63.

[3] Guariso G, Meneghel A, Dalla Pozza L, et al. Indications to upper gastrointestinal endoscopy in children with dyspepsia. J Pediatr Gastroenterol Nutr 2010;50(5):493-9.

[4] De Angelis GL, Papparella A, Fornarioli F, and Torroni F. Cenni di Tecnica Endoscopica. In: L'endoscopia Digestiva in Età Pediatrica e Giovanile. De Angelis GL eds EMSI Roma 2002, pp 27-30.

[5] Van Beek EJ, Leroy PL. Safe and effective procedural sedation for gastro-intestinal endoscopy in children: a systematic review. J Pediatr Gastroenterol Nutr 2012;54(2): 171-85.

[6] Baruch K, Steven MG. Sedation and analgesia for procedures in children. N Engl J Med 2000; 342: 938-945.

[7] American Accademy of Pediatrics, Committee on Drugs. Guidelines for monitoring and management of pediatric patients during and after sedation for diagnostic and therapeutic procedures. Pediatrics 1992; 89: 1110-5.

[8] Meyer S, Grundmann U, Gottshling S, et al. Sedation and analgesia for brief diagnostic and therapeutic procedures in children. Eur J Pediatr 2007; 166: 291-302.

[9] Da Silva MM, Briars GL, Patrick MK, Cleghorn GJ, Shepherd RW. Colonoscopy preparation in children: safety, efficacy, and tolerance of high- versus low-volume cleansing methods. J Pediatr Gastroenterol Nutr 1997; 24(1):33-7.

[10] Hassal E. Risk of oral sodium phosphate for precolonoscopy bowel preparation in children. Dis Colon Rectum 2007; 50: 1099-1103.

[11] Loening-Baucke V, Krishna R, Pashankar DS. Polyethylene glycol 3350 without electrolytes for the treatment of functional constipation in infants and toddlers. J Pediatr Gastroenterol Nutr 2004; 39(5): 536-9.

[12] Dahshan A et al. A randomized, prospecitve study to evaluate the efficacy and acceptance of three bowel preparations for colonoscopy in children. Am J Gastroenterol 1999; 94: 3497-501.

[13] Gremse DA, Sacks AI, Raines S. Comparison of oral sodium phosphate to polyethylene glycol-based solution for bowel preparation for colonoscopy in children. J Pediatr Gastroenterol Nutr 1996; 23(5): 586-90.

[14] Wyllie R, Kay MH. Gastrointestinal endoscopy in infants and children. Pediatr Rev 1993; 14(9): 352-9.

[15] De Angelis GL, Bizzarri B, De Angelis N, Borrelli O: La diagnostica endoscopica. Consensus Statement SIGENP: Malattie Infiammatorie Croniche Intestinali in età pediatrica 2008; pp 23-26.

[16] Orenstein SR. Management of supraesophageal complications of gastroesophageal reflux disease in infants and children. Am J Med 2000, 108(Suppl): 139-43.

[17] Lundell LR, Dent J, Bennett JR, Blum AL, Armstrong D, Galmiche J-P et al. Endoscopic assessment of oesophagitis: clinical and functional correlates and further validation of the Los Angeles classification. Gut 1999;45:172-180.

[18] De Angelis GL, Torroni F, Bizzarri B, Manfredi M. La patologia esofagea. In: L'endoscopia Digestiva in Età Pediatrica e Giovanile. De Angelis GL eds EMSI Roma 2002, pp 37-47.

[19] Meneghel A, Zulian F, Martini G, Guariso G. Ischemic ulcerative colitis in juvenile dermatomyositis. J Pediatr Gastroenterol Nutr 2009; 49(5): 549.

[20] Walsh SV, Antonioli DA, Goldman H, et al. Allergic esophagitis in children: a clinicopathological entity. Am J Surg Pathol 1999; 23(4): 390-6.

[21] Kleinman R, Goulet OJ, Mieli-Vergani G, Sanderson I, Sherman P, Shneider B. Treatment of End-Stage Liver Disease. Walker's Pediatric Gastrointetsinal Disease, 5th Edition. Volume 2, Chapter 38: 1133-48.

[22] De Giacomo C, Bacchini PL, Lombardi M, De Angelis GL. La patologia gastrica. In: L'endoscopia Digestiva in Età Pediatrica e Giovanile. De Angelis GL eds EMSI Roma 2002, pp 49-68.

[23] Blecker U, Gold BD. Gastritis and peptic ulcer disease in childhood. Eur J Pediatr 1999; 158(7): 541-6.

[24] Imrie C, Rowland M, Bourke B, et al. Is Helicobacter Pylori infection in childhood a risk factor for gastric cancer? Paediatrics 2001; 107(2): 373-80.

[25] Heldwein W, Schreiner J, Pedrazzoli J, Lehnert P. Is the Forrestclassification a useful tool for planning endoscopic therapy of bleeding peptic ulcers? Endoscopy 1989 Nov;21(6):258-62.

[26] Gupta SK, et al. Is esophagogastroduodenoscopy necessary in all caustic ingestions? J Pediatr Gastroenterology Nutr 2001; 32: 50-53

[27] Kay M, Wyllie R. Caustic ingestions and the role of endoscopy. J Pediatr gastroenterol Nutr 2001; 32: 8-10.

[28] Husby S, Koletzko S, Korponay-Szabò IR, Mearin ML, Philips A, Shamir R, Troncone R, Giersiepen K, Branski D, Catassi C, Lelgeman M, Maki M, Ribes-Koninckx C, Ventura A, Zimmer KP. (ESPGHAN Working Group on Coeliac Disease Diagnosis).ESPGHAN Guidelines for the diagnosis of coeliac disease in children and adolescents. An evidence-based approach. In Press. 2012.

[29] De Angelis GL, Bacchini PL, Romano C, Cucchiara S. La patologia del colon. In: L'endoscopia Digestiva in Età Pediatrica e Giovanile. De Angelis GL eds EMSI Roma 2002, pp 81-91.

[30] Venkatesh K, Thomson M. Endoscopic Modalities in Pediatric Inflammatory Bowel Disease. In: Pediatric Inflammatory Bowel Diseases. Mamula P, Markowitz JE, Baldassano RN eds Springer Publ New York 2008, pp 211-35.

[31] Bourreille A et al. Role of small-bowel endoscopy in IBD: international OMED–ECCO consensus. Endoscopy 2009; 41: 618–637

[32] Venkatesh K, Thomson M. Endoscopic Modalities in Pediatric Inflammatory Bowel Disease. In: Pediatric Inflammatory Bowel Diseases. Mamula P, Markowitz JE, Baldassano RN eds Springer Publ New York 2008, pp 211-35.

[33] Venkatesh K, Thomson M. Endoscopic Modalities in Pediatric Inflammatory Bowel Disease. In: Pediatric Inflammatory Bowel Diseases. Perspectives and Consequences. Walker-Smith JA, Lebenthal E, Branski D eds Karger Publ Basel Switzerland 2009, pp 100-122.

[34] Gasparetto M, Guariso G. Endoscopy in Paediatric Inflammatory Bowel Disease (IBD). In: Gastrointestinal Endoscopy. Pascu O eds INTECH 2011, pp 237-253.

[35] Gupta SK, Fitzgerald JF. Experience with juvenile polyps in North American children: the need for pancolonoscopy. Am J Gastroenterolo 2001; 96(6): 1695-7.

[36] Olschwang S. Digestive polyposes: genetic aspects. Gastroenterol Clin Biol 2001; 25(Suppl): B26-30.

[37] Salviati L, Patricelli M, Guariso G, Sturniolo GC, Alaggio R, Bernardi F, et al. Deletion of PTEN and BMPR1A in chromosome 10q23 is not always associated with juvenile polyposis of infancy. Am J Hum Genet 2006; 79(3): 593-6.

Chapter 14

Liver Transplantation and Endoscopic Management of Bile Duct Complications

Bassam Abu-Wasel, Paul D. Renfrew and Michele Molinari

Additional information is available at the end of the chapter

http://dx.doi.org/10.5772/52630

1. Introduction

The first human liver transplant (LT) was performed in 1963 by Starzl and colleagues at the University of Colorado in Denver [1]. Since then, LT has become a life-saving procedure for patients with irreversible chronic and acute liver failure (ALF) [2-4].Only a few cases were performed during the following 15-year as the results were not satisfactory and 1-year survival rate was only 30% due to early rejection and graft failure. In the late 1970s and early 1980s, the implementation of cyclosporine-based immunosuppression led to the doubling of the 1-year survival rate and LT, from an experimental procedure, became standard of care for patients with end stage liver disease (ESLD) [5]. In the last two decades, significant advances occurred in all aspects of LT, including donor management, recipient selection, surgical techniques, immunosuppression, and postoperative care. These changes have resulted in considerable improvements in the care provided to LT recipients, and the current overall 1-year survival is now in excess of 85%, with 5- and 10-year survival ranging between 70-85% and 60-70%, respectively [6-9]. Despite all these major advances, biliary complications after LT still represent a common and challenging problem for both patients and their caregivers.

The main aim of this chapter is to inform the reader on the current indications and contraindications for LT, the risk factors associated with postoperative biliary complications and to evaluate the endoscopic techniques currently available for the diagnosis and treatment of these patients.

2. Epidemiology of liver failure

Liver disease is a common and broad definition used to describe any acute and chronic liver disorders that includes:

- Steatosis
- Fibrosis
- Cirrhosis
- Acute and chronic hepatitis (viral, metabolic, autoimmune etc.)
- Primary hepatic malignancies (hepatocellular carcinoma and cholangiocarcinoma)

ESLD encompasses all those clinical conditions characterized by the irreversible deterioration of the hepatic function and is responsible for over two million outpatient visits and over 750,000 hospitalizations per year only in the United States (US) [10]. Currently, chronic liver disease and cirrhosis are among the tenth leading causes of death, and the annual number of fatalities has remained essentially unchanged (25,000 per year) over the past two decades (Table 1).Every year in the US, over 40,000 patients develop ESLD and approximately 2,000 ALF [11]. Unfortunately, only 5,000–6,000 will undergo LT [12] and the current mismatch between the number of available grafts and the number of patients waiting for LT is responsible for 5 to 10% yearly mortality rate.

Primary Disease	% of Mortality
Heart disease	31.0
Malignant neoplasms	23.2
Cerebrovascular disease	6.8
COPD	4.8
Trauma	4.2
Pneumonia and influenza	3.9
Diabetes	2.8
Suicide	1.3
Kidney diseases	1.1
Chronic liver disease or cirrhosis	1.1

Data from Murphy S. Deaths: final data for 1998. National vital statistics reports. Hyattsville, MD: National Center for Health Statistics, 2000, Vol. 48.

Table 1. The ten leading causes of deaths in United States.

3. Indications for liver transplantation

LT is indicated for all the clinical conditions summarized in Table 2. Because LT is the only cure for ESLD, patients who develop signs of liver decompensation should be referred to transplant centers before their conditions deteriorate to a point when LT is no longer feasible (Table 3).

http://dx.doi.org/10.5772/52630

Acute Liver Failure	
Viral Hepatitis A,B,C,D	
Acetaminophen overdose and other drugs	
Autoimmune hepatitis	
Cryptogenic liver disease	
Wilson's disease	
Budd-Chiari syndrome	
Fatty infiltration—acute fatty liver of pregnancy	
Reye's syndrome	
Cirrhosis from Chronic Liver Disease	
Chronic hepatitis B and C virus infection	
Alcoholic liver disease	
Autoimmune hepatitis	
Cryptogenic liver disease	
Nonalcoholic fatty liver disease	
Metabolic Liver Disease	
Wilson's disease	
Hereditary hemochromatosis	
Alpha-1 antitrypsin deficiency	
Glycogen storage disease	
Cystic fibrosis	
Glycogen storage disease I and IV	
Crigler-Najjar syndrome	
Galactosemia	
Type 1 hyperoxaluria	
Familial homozygous hypercholesterolemia	
Hemophilia A and B	
Vascular Diseases	
Budd-Chiari syndrome	
Veno-occlusive disease	
Cholestatic Liver Diseases	
Primary biliary cirrhosis	
Primary sclerosing cholangitis	
Secondary biliary cirrhosis	
Biliary atresia	
Alagille syndrome	
Byler's disease	
Miscellaneous	
Adult polycystic liver disease	
Nodular regenerative hyperplasia	
Caroli's disease	
Severe graft-versus-host disease	
Amyloidosis	
Sarcoidosis	
Hepatic trauma	

Table 2. Main causes of irreversible liver failure.

Ascites
Coagulopathy
Encephalopathy
Jaundice
Cachexia
Hepatorenal Syndrome
Hepatopulmonary Syndrome
Pulmonary Hypertension
Persistent and intractable pruritus

Table 3. Some of the most common clinical manifestations of liver failure.

Cirrhosis is the main indication in the adult population and it accounts for more than 80% of LTs performed in the world. Other frequent indications in the US are: hepatitis C (21%), alcoholic liver disease (16%), cholestatic liver disease including primary biliary cirrhosis and sclerosing cholangitis (17%). Less frequent indications include: chronic hepatitis (hepatitis B, autoimmune hepatitis), metabolic disease (e.g. Wilson's disease, nonalcoholic steatohepatitis), fulminant hepatic failure, and non-metastatic HCC [13].

In the pediatric population the most frequent indication for LT includes biliary atresia and congenital metabolic diseases.

3.1. Acute liver failure

ALF accounts for 5% of all LT in the US. The most common causes are: toxins or drug induced liver injury (e.g., acetaminophen), viral hepatitis, or, less commonly, autoimmune hepatitis or Wilson disease [14-16]. In approximately 15-17% there are no identifiable causes [17].

3.2. Hepatocellular carcinoma

Most transplant centers would perform LT for patients with unresectable HCCs who satisfy the Milan criteria (absence of metastatic disease and one of the following two conditions: a single lesion with maximum diameter equal or smaller than 5cm in diameter or three or fewer lesions, the largest of which measures up to 3cm in diameter) [18]. The 5-year survival rate in this setting is 75-80%, which is comparable to survival rates of patients undergoing LT for benign conditions. At the University of California, San Francisco (UCSF), LT has been advocated for patients without extra-hepatic disease and affected by single tumors measuring up to 6.5 cm or by 3 or fewer lesions with the largest being equal or smaller than 4.5 cm and with a total tumor burden of 8 cm or less with similar short and long term outcomes to patients within the Milan criteria [19-22].

http://dx.doi.org/10.5772/52630

3.3. Cholangiocarcinoma

In the past, all patients with cholangiocarcinoma (CC) were thought to be poor candidates for LT due to their high rate of recurrent disease and poor survival. However, at the Mayo Clinic in Minnesota, a novel therapeutic protocol for unresectable hilar CC or CC arising in the setting of PSC combines an intensive protocol that uses neo-adjuvant chemo and radiation therapy prior to LT. Patients treated at that centre have shown excellent 1-year survival up to 82% and comparable to patients undergoing LT for other causes [16, 21]. On the other hand, patients with intrahepatic CC appear to be still poor candidates due to their poor prognosis even if treated with neo-adjuvant chemo-radiation therapy [23].

4. Contraindications to liver transplantation

Contraindications to LT can be divided in two main groups: relative contraindications and absolute contraindications. Relative contraindications are all those conditions that prevent optimal outcomes, and therefore, should be corrected whenever possible prior to transplantation (Table 4) [1 11 24]. Absolute contraindications, instead, are not reversible and lead to unsatisfactory outcomes and their presence should prevent LT if recognized in time (Table 5) [3 5].

• HIV/AIDS
• Age "/> 65 years
• Severe malnutrition
• Other irreversible organ failure
• Previous major upper abdominal surgeries
• Poor functional status
• Previous history of poor compliance

Table 4. Relative contraindications to LT.

• Severe cardiopulmonary disease
• Irreversible cerebral injury
• Sepsis or active infection
• Most of the extra-hepatic malignancies except for non-melanoma skin cancer
• Major vascular thrombosis of the arterial or venous system preventing successful arterial or venous reconstructions
• Active alcohol or drug abuse
• Sever psychological conditions

Table 5. Absolute contraindications to LT.

5. Pediatric liver transplantation

Pediatric LT is one of the most successful transplant procedures [25]. The 1-year patient survival rate is 83% to 91%, depending on the age of the child at the time of surgery [26].Five-year patient survival is also excellent, ranging from 82 to 84%. The number of pediatric LTs per year has remained steady in the last decade, averaging approximately 600 per year in the US. About 55% of these transplants are for end-stage chronic liver disease, the majority of these due to biliary atresia; about 25% are for metabolic liver diseases, 10% for ALF, and 5% for hepatic malignancies [27 28]. Underlying diagnoses of children undergoing LT are presented in Table 6. In pediatric LT, there are very few absolute contraindications. These include conditions in which LT is futile and will not improve the overall survival or quality of life, and this list of conditions has shortened dramatically over the years (Table 7).

Diagnosis	Frequency (%)
Cholestatic liver disease Biliary atresia Others: Alagille syndrome, sclerosing cholangitis, progressive familial intrahepatic cholestasis	48
Fulminant hepatic failure	11
Metabolic liver disease Primary hepatic disease: Wilson disease, a-1-antitrypsin deficiency, tyrosinemia, cystic fibrosis Primarily nonhepatic disease: ornithine transcarbamylase deficiency, primary hyperoxaluria type 1, organic academia	13
Liver tumors	4
Others	9

Data from Ng VL, Fecteau A, Shepherd R, et al. Outcomes of 5-year survivors of pediatric liver transplantation: report on 461 children from a North American multicenter registry. Pediatrics 2008;122(6):e1128–35.

Table 6. Underlying diagnoses of children undergoing liver transplantation.

Absolute contraindications:
Extrahepatic malignancy (considered incurable by standard oncologic criteria)
Sepsis
- Uncontrolled systemic infection
- Acquired immunodeficiency syndrome (AIDS)
Extrahepatic disease (incurable)
- Irreversible massive brain injury
- Uncorrectable congenital anomalies affecting major organs
Relative contraindications:
Malignancy that is considered cured or curable by standard oncologic criteria
Sepsis
- Treatable infection
- Human immunodeficiency virus
Extrahepatic disease
- Progressive extrahepatic disease
- Substance abuse

Table 7. Contraindications to pediatric liver transplantation.

6. Cadaveric graft allocation

To optimize the distribution of cadaveric grafts to patients who are in most need, the United Network for Organ Sharing (UNOS) in the US has proposed the use of the Model for End-stage Liver Disease (MELD) and Pediatric End-stage Liver Disease (PELD), which are numerical scales reflecting the degree of organ dysfunction [29]. These scores are predictive of each patient's risk of dying while waiting for a LT in 3 months period. The MELD score, used for patients aged 12 years and older, is based on serum bilirubin levels, international normalized ratio (INR), and creatinine. The PELD score, in addition to the serum levels of bilirubin, INR and albumin includes also the presence of growth failure and patients' age, which are all associated with the mortality risk in children with liver failure. Alone, these scores are not sufficient for the final allocation of liver grafts as other important factors need to be carefully evaluated such as: the compatibility between the donor's and the recipients' blood groups, the size of the graft in relation to the body size of the recipient, and finally, the fact that in some circumstances available grafts are prioritized for individuals who suffers from ALF.

7. Surgical technical aspects of liver transplantation

During LT, biliary reconstruction is the final step before the abdominal wall is closed and patients leave the operating room (Figure 1 –A,B,C,D). Biliary anastomoses are performed after all the vascular anastomoses have been successfully completed and satisfactory hemostasis is reached.

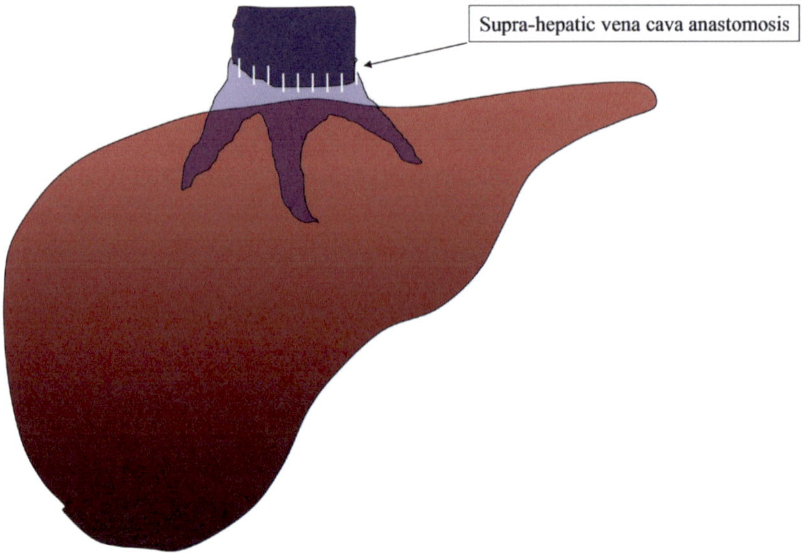

Figure 1A

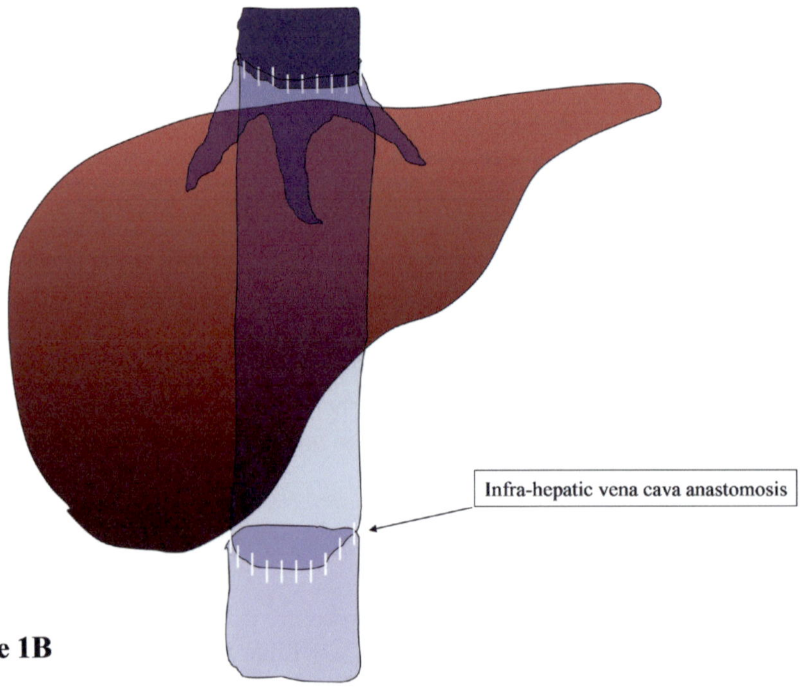

Figure 1B

http://dx.doi.org/10.5772/52630

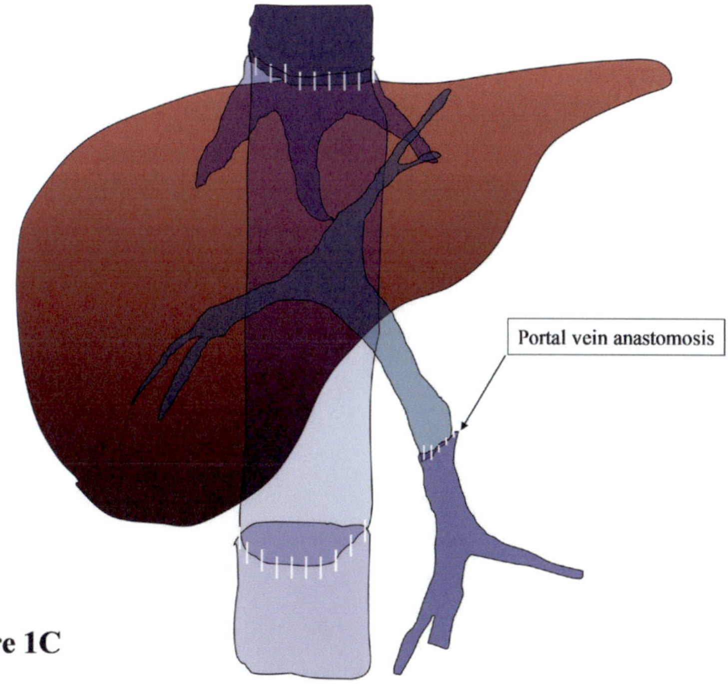

Figure 1C

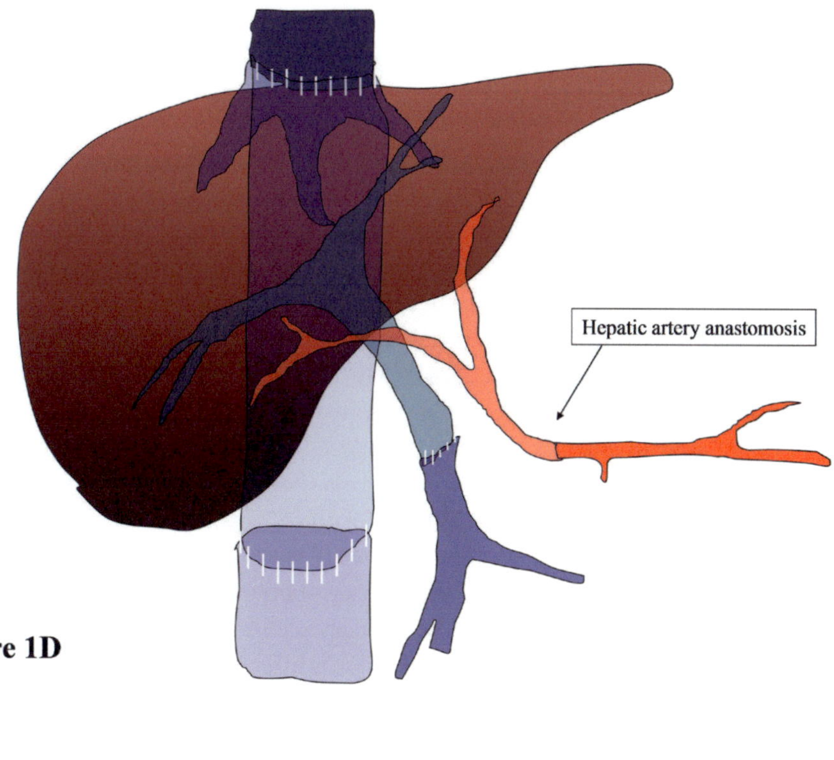

Figure 1D

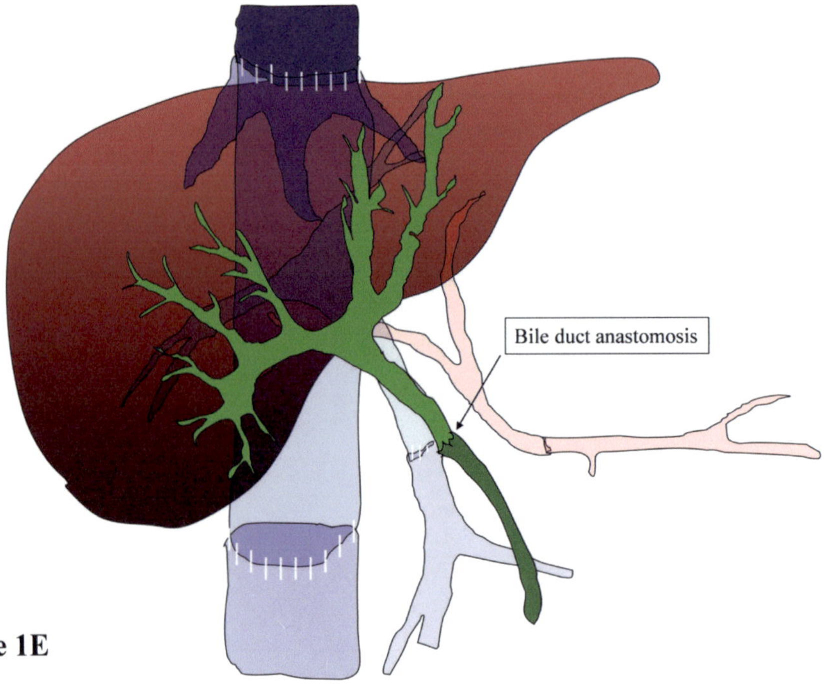

Figure 1. Temporal representation of all the necessary anastomoses performed during an orthotopic full organ LT with interposition of the donor's vena cava. After the native liver is mobilized and removed from the recipients' abdominal cavity, the liver graft is positioned in the same location (orthotopic liver transplantation) and anastomosed to the recipient's vascular and biliary structures. The first anastomosis performed is the supra-hepatic vena cava (Figure 1A), the second is the infrahepatic vena cava (Figure 1B), the third is the portal vein anastomosis (Figure 1C). After the portal vein anastomosis is completed, the liver graft is reperfused. The last vascular anastomosis is represented by the hepatic artery reconstruction (Figure 1D) followed by the biliary duct anastomosis (Figure 1E).

An end-to-end duct-to-duct anastomosis is the reconstruction of choice in patients with healthy native bile ducts of suitable caliber [30] as it reconstitutes the physiological hepato-enteric biliary cycle (Figure 1E). This technique is simpler and faster than the creation of biliary-enteric anastomoses (Figure 2A) and, when indicated, the biliary system can be investigated and treated endoscopically by retrograde cholangiography (ERCP). A side-to-side variant of the duct-to-duct anastomosis has also been used by some groups with similar good results (Figure 2B) [31, 32]. On the other hand, the surgical technique that used the gallbladder as a conduit between the donor's and the recipient's bile ducts or intestine, has been abandoned because of the associated bile stasis and stone formation causing frequent episodes of cholangitis, which lead to surgical revisions and overall inferior outcomes(Figure 2C) [33, 34, 35]. Roux-en-Y hepaticojejunostomy (Figure 2A) is utilized in cases of preexisting disease of the native biliary tract observed when patients are affected by primary sclerosing cholangitis or biliary atresia in the pediatric population. In addition, this technique is often used when there is disparity in size between the donor's and the recipient's bile ducts, when the common bile duct is very small and at risk of developing strictures at the anastomotic site and it is usually the preferred technique for the biliary reconstruction during retransplantations because of the inadequate length of the native biliary system [36, 37]. In the early years of living-donor LT and split LT, Roux-en-Y hepatico-jejunostomy was also the standard biliary reconstructive technique. With growing experience of the surgical technique and meticulous attention in preserving the blood supply around the native common bile duct [38, 39], duct-to-duct anastomosis has become the preferred reconstruction technique even during right lobe living-donor transplantation in the adult population [40, 41], as well during the right lobe split transplant [42, 43]. Initially, duct-to-duct anastomosis created during the right lobe living-donor transplants was only performed when a single donor duct was available. More recently, the use of the recipient right and left hepatic ducts, as well as the cystic duct has been reported by several authors even when facing the need of creating multiple biliary anastomoses [44, 45]. Alternatively, both duct-to-duct and bilioenteric reconstructions may also be used simultaneously in the same patient.

Left biliary-jejunostomy remains the method of choice for biliary reconstruction when using left lateral segment grafts during split livers or living related transplantations [46, 47] although, even in these circumstances, a duct-to-duct anastomosis has been recommended by some authors [48, 49].

8. Biliary complications after liver transplantation

Biliary complications after LTare relatively frequent and occur in 5-25% of patients and represent one of the major causes of morbidity and even mortality in this group of patients [50, 51, 52, 53, 54, 55].The complication rate of the biliary system varies according to the surgical techniques and nature of the graft. Biliary complications are less frequent in patients undergoing LT with the use of full size grafts (5-15%) while the incidence of biliary complications in living donor, split or reduced size grafts is much more significant and ranges between 15 to 30% [56, 57].

Biliary leaks and strictures occurring at the anastomotic site are the most common biliary complications. Other less frequent adverse events are: sphincter of Oddi dysfunction, hemobilia, biliary obstruction from cystic duct mucoceles, stones, sludge or formation of biliary duct casts that will be discussed later on in this chapter [50, 51, 58].

9. Temporal presentation of biliary complications

After LT, complications of the biliary tract can occur both in the immediate perioperative period, as well as several months or years after the procedure.

Conventionally, biliary complications are divided into three main categories:

- Early Complications (observed within 30 days after LT)
- Delayed Complications (observed during the second and third month after LT)
- Late Complications (observed after 3 months post LT)

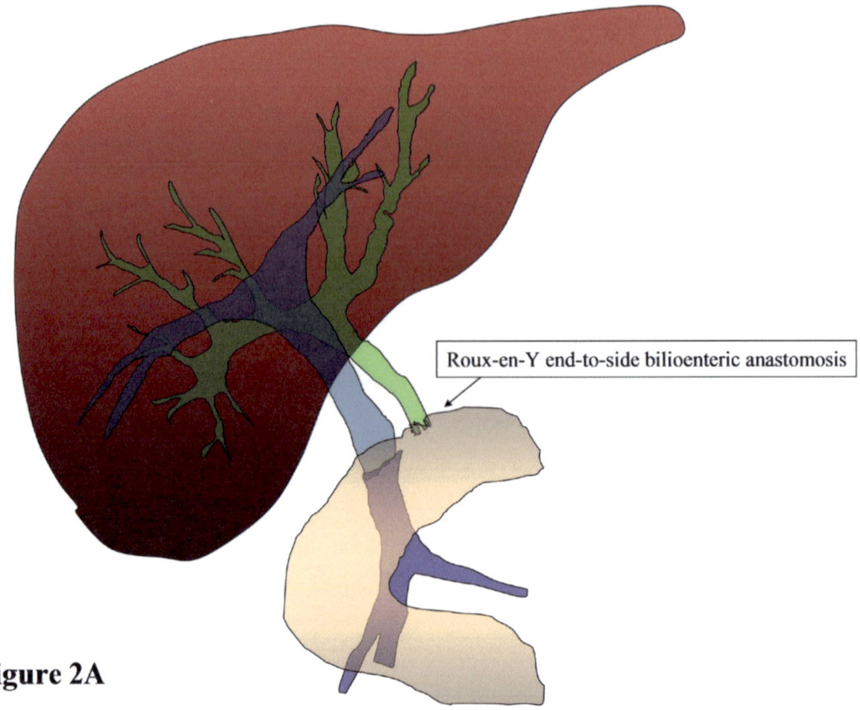

Figure 2A

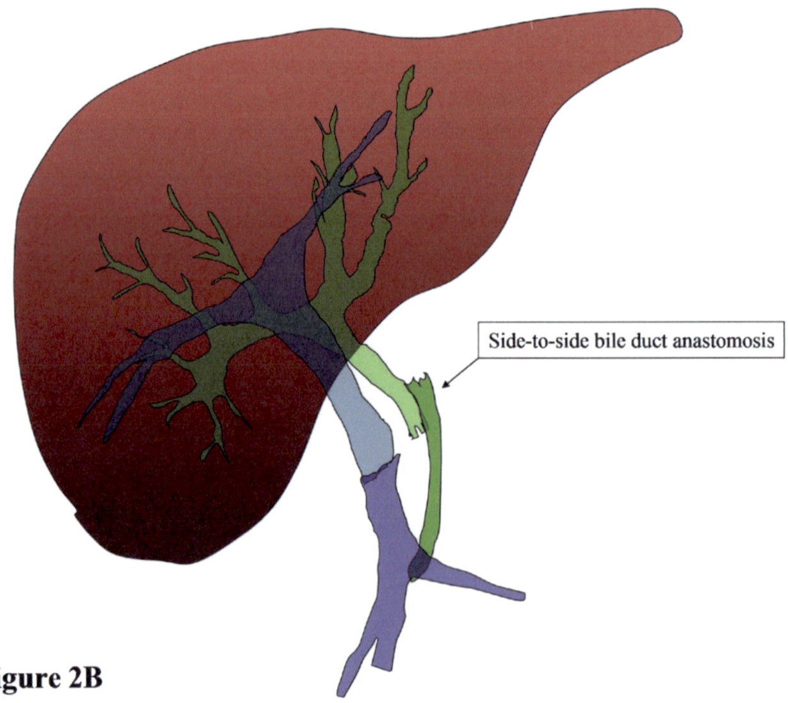

Figure 2B

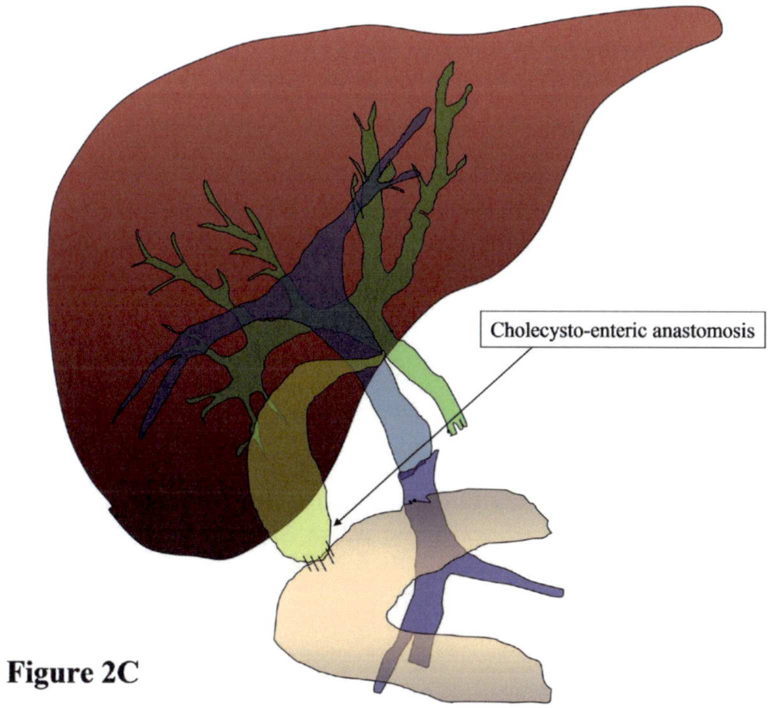

Figure 2. Graphical representation of the most common biliary reconstructions performed in liver transplantation. The most common technique is the reconstruction with an end-to-end bile duct anastomosis as represented in Figure 1E. With this technique, the two end of the donor's and the recipient's common bile ducts are anastomosed together allowing the bile to flow in a very physiologic way. Less frequently, the bile duct reconstruction is obtained by creating a Roux-en-Y bilioenteric anastomosis (Figure 2A) where the common bile duct of the donor is anastomosed to the antimesenteric wall of a loop of small intestine of the recipient, or by creating a side-to-side bile duct anastomosis (Figure 2B). In the past, a cholecysto-enteric anastomosis was often used to drain the bile but this technique has been almost completely abandoned (Figure 2C).

10. Risk factors of biliary complications

Several factors have been identified as predisposing conditions for the development of biliary complications in LT recipients. Among them the most common are: hepatic artery thrombosis, thermal and ischemic injury to the peri-biliary duct tissues, inferior quality of the liver graft, prolonged cold and warm ischemia time, blood type incompatibility between the donor and the recipient, infections and tension between the two ends of the biliary anastomosis.

10.1. Hepatic artery thrombosis or stenosis

The hepatic artery plays an important role in the blood supply of the bile duct and insufficient arterial blood flow is responsible for both acute and chronic ischemia of the biliary system. Acute ischemia can lead to anastomotic disruptions and subsequent biliary leaks in the immediate postoperative period or delayed strictures that can occur at the level of the anastomosis or in other parts of the intra and extra-hepatic ducts.

10.2. Technical factors

During surgery the most common technical factors that can result in biliary complications are: the excessive dissection of the periductal tissue during the procurement or during the mobilization of the native liver,and the excessive use of electrocautery to control bleeding from the peribiliary tissues. Another important risk factor for biliary anastomotic failures is the presence of tension between the two ends of the biliary anastomosis that can lead to an incomplete seal and subsequently to leaks and formation of peri-hepatic absesses.

10.3. Quality of the grafts and cold and warm ischemia times

Biliary complications are more frequent in recipients of grafts procured from donors after cardiac death who have an increased risk of experiencing insufficient organ perfusion or suboptimal oxigenation of the liver. This undesired warm ischemia time has been considered one of the most important risk factors for biliary complications that frequently affect recipients of livers from donors after cardiac death. In addition, biliary complications have been encountered more frequently after the use of grafts from older donors, grafts with steatosis, and in all those circumstances where the grafts experience suboptimal cold storage and prolonged cold or warm ischemia [59].

10.4. Placement of T-tubes

In the past, T-tubes were placed routinely in all patients undergoing LT to monitor the production of bile as a proxy for early graft function and, theoretically, to prevent anastomotic strictures. The role of T-tubes in LT, in the era of endoscopic therapy, is much less apparent and they have been almost unanimously abandoned. Comparative studies between post-LT patients with and without T-tubes indicate that routine T-tube placement is associated with a higher incidence of biliary complications including bile leaks and cholangitis [60, 61]. A recent meta-analysis including more than 1,000 patients indicated that those patients without a T-tube had better outcomes compared with those with a T-tube, including fewer episodes of cholangitis and fewer episodes of peritonitis [62].

10.5. Biliary reconstruction

The most common technique used for the reconstruction of the biliary system in patients undergoing cadaveric LT is the duct-to-duct choledocho-choledochostomy anastomosis (Figure 3A). When this technique is not feasible, most patients undergo a Roux-en-Y choledochojejunostomy (Figure 3B). Duct-to-duct choledochocholedochostomy has the advantage of being easier and quicker to perform, it is more physiological and prevents enteric reflux into the bile ducts, and it has also the advantage of allowing easier access to the biliay system by endoscopic means [63]. Several studies have shown that the risk of biliary complications with the Roux-en-Y reconstruction is similar, or only slightly higher compared with the duct-to-duct anastomosis [51, 64].

http://dx.doi.org/10.5772/52630

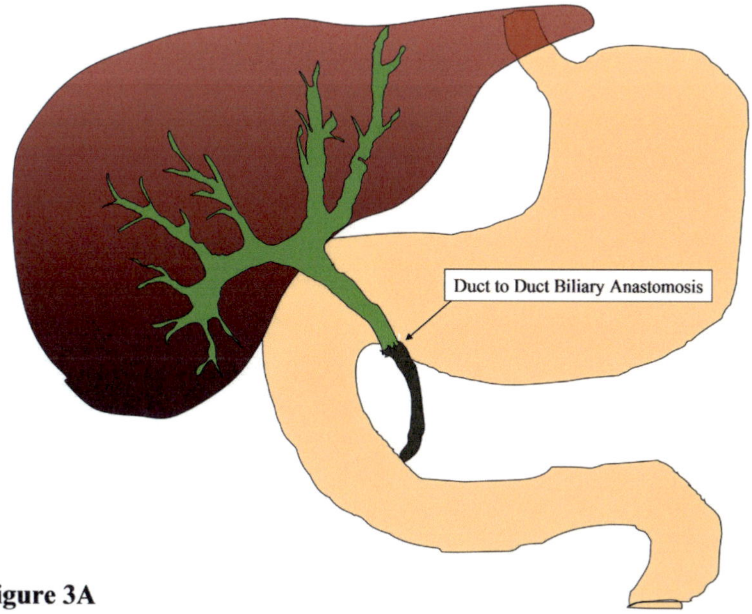

Figure 3A

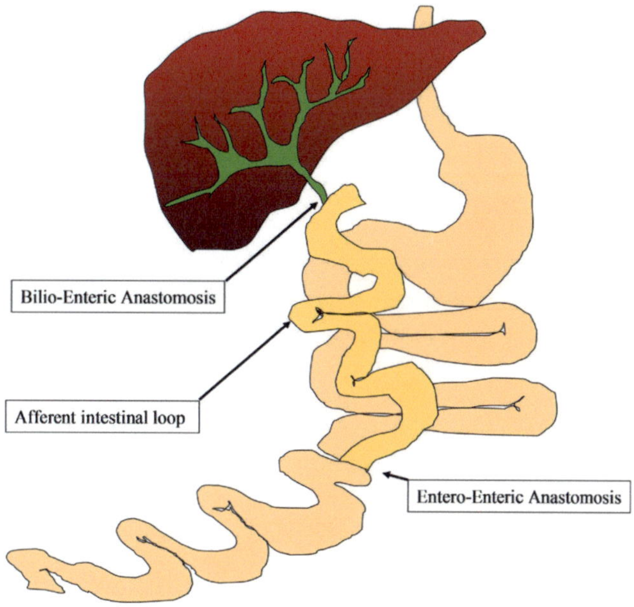

Figure 3B

Figure 3. Graphical representation of the two most common biliary reconstruction after cadaveric liver treansplantation. Figure 3A represent the classical duct-to-duct reconstruction where the donor's bile duct is anastomosed to the recipient bile duct. This anastomosis has the advantage of being less time-consuming than the biliary-enteric anastomosis (Figure 3B) and it allows a physiological flow of bile into the duodenum. Another significant advantage is that the biliary system of patients undergoing a duct-to-duct anastomosis can be reached by endoscopic means. This allows the insertion of stents or dilatation when biliary leaks or stricture develop.

10.6. Other risk factors

Several other predisposing factors for biliary complications have been identified. Among them, the most frequent are: pre-LT cytomegalovirus infection [65, 66], LT performed between donors and recipients with ABO blood group incompatibility, the diagnosis of primary sclerosing cholangitis as the primary indication for LT and intra-abdominal infections in the perioperative period.

11. Clinical presentation and diagnosis of biliary complications

The clinical presentations of biliary complications after LT can be challenging as they depend on the time of occurrence, degree of severity and patients' characteristics. Elevation of the recipient's white blood count, fever, abdominal pain, ileus and cholestasis are common findings in patients who develop early biliary complications. Often, immunosuppressed patients can be asymptomatic for a relatively long period of time before they manifest any clinical condition that can lead to the appropriate diagnosis. In asymptomatic patients, suspicion of a biliary complication should occur in the presence of any unexplained elevation of serum aminotransferases, total bilirubin, alkaline phosphatase, and gamma-glutamyltransferase levels in the absence of acute rejection. Biliary leaks are often diagnosed as fluid collections on abdominal imaging performed for unrelated reasons.

12. Non-invasive diagnostic modalities

Noninvasive radiologic investigations usually begin with a trans-abdominal ultrasound (US), which is often used in combination with Doppler examination of the flow characteristics of the hepatic artery, portal and hepatic veins. Triphasic contrast computed tomography (CT), magnetic resonance cholangiopancreatography (MRCP) and nuclear medicine HIDA scan are usually complementary investigations to the original abdominal US. Further diagnostic steps in the evaluation of these patients depend upon the initial findings. Among them, the most frequently performed are: ERCP and percutaneous transhepatic cholangiography (PTC).

13. Invasive diagnostic modalities

13.1. Endoscopic retrograde cholangiopancreatography

ERCP plays a primary role in the management of biliary complications after LT. Despite the lack of large randomized trials, ERCP has become the procedure of choice for all LT patients with their biliary tract accessible to endoscopic manipulation. Post-ERCP complications are similar to the general population and include: pancreatitis, bleeding, infec-

http://dx.doi.org/10.5772/52630

tions and perforation. Overall, the complication rate in this population ranges between 2% to 6% [67, 68, 69, 70, 71, 72] confirming that ERCP is relatively safe even in this subset of immunocompromised patients who often have persistent thrombocytopenia due to hyperspenism and transient coagulative dysfunction.

13.2. Percutaneous transhepatic cholangiography

PTC and percutaneous transhepatic biliary drainage (PTBD) are necessary when ERCP can not be performed or when it has failed. The most frequent indication for PTC in post LT patients is the presence of a Roux-en-Y biliary enteric anastomosis that prevents the access to the biliary duct by endoscopic approach. In comparison to ERCP, PTC is more hazardous in the presence of thrombocytopenia or coagulopathy and it can be technically very challenging when the intra-hepatic biliary ducts are not dilated, for example in the presence of a bile duct anastomotic leak. On the other hand, anastomotic strictures are responsible for the dilatation of the biliary ducts, making PTC easier and safer. The determination of whether to perform ERCP or PTC depends upon anatomic considerations, the diameter of the donor biliary tree, and the overall morbidity related to issues of sedation and coagulation status [73, 74].

14. Biliary stents

Endoscopic biliary stents were first introduced in 1979 [75] primarily for the palliation of malignant strictures. Until then, surgery (such as choledochojejunostomy, choledochoduodenostomy, and cholecysto-jejunostomy) had been the mainstay of treatment. Initially, interventional radiologists developed percutaneous techniques that allowed the placement of external biliary drainages. Subsequently, the introduction of new methods allowed the internalization of biliary drains that immediately became more attractive as patients did not suffer from significant fluid losses, malnutrition due to decreased intestinal absorption of lipids and fat-soluble vitamins (e.g. vitamin K, A, D, E). Plastic stents (Figure 4A and 4B) have a median duration of 3-4 months as they are subject to obstruction due to deposition of debris in their lumen and subsequent risk of ascending cholangitis. The limited long-term patency rate of plastic stents fuelled the development of metal stents that are significantly larger in diameter and have lower propensity to obstruct. Nowadays, metal stents are available in various designs. The designs differ from one another in the diameter of the expanded stent, diameter of the delivery system, length of the stent, and wall thickness [76]. Metal stents were conventionally of two types (ie, balloon-mouthed or self-expanding); however, nowadays self-expandable metallic stents (SEMS) (Figure 4C) are more commonly used, with balloon-mouthed stents having become somewhat archaic.

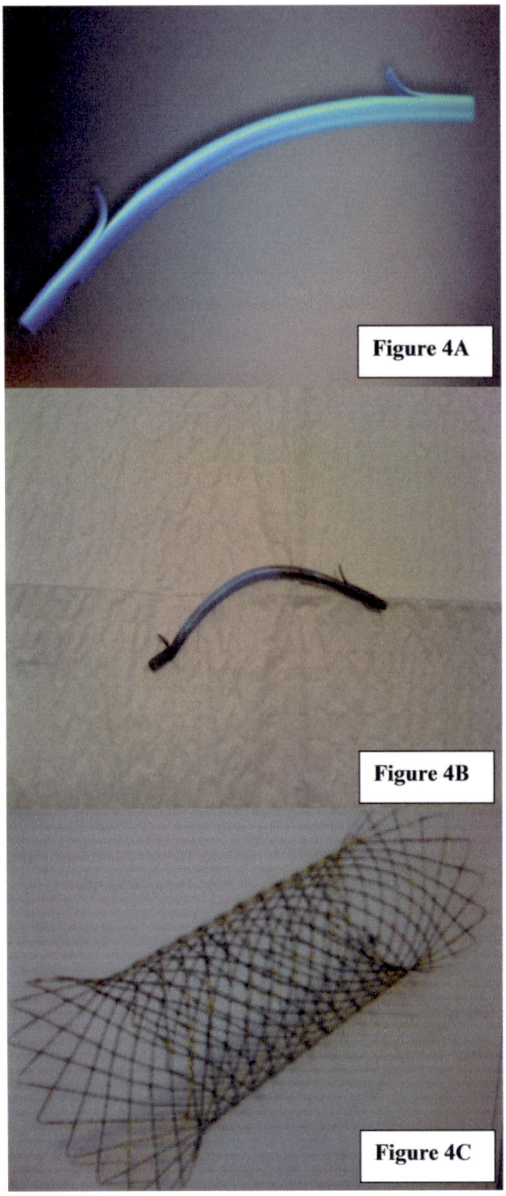

Figure 4. Plastic biliary stent inserted in a patient with anastomotic biliary leak after cadaveric liver transplantation. The patient developed leukocytosis associated with new onset of jaundice and abdominal pain. A CT scan revealed a large sub-hepatic fluid collection that was percutaneosly drained. The fluid aspirated was consistent with bile. During the following days, the 24 hours drain output was consistently above 400 ml. An ERCP confirmed the presence of a bile duct anastomotic partial dehiscence. A 10 French, 9 cm in length temporary plastic stent (Figure 4A) was inserted across the anastomosis. During the following days, the drainage output decreased and on post-ERCP day 7 the patient had no bile draining from the percutaneous drainage tha was subsequently taken out. After 3 months, the plastic stent was removed during a second ERCP (Figure 4B) and the endoscopic cholangiogram revealed a complete resolu-

tion of the leak and no anastomotic stricture. Figure 4C represents a non-covered metallic biliary stent with diameter of 10 mm and 6 cm length. These stents are usually used for malignant biliary obstructions but, when covered by a non-adsorbable layer that prevent tissue ingrowth into the stent, can be removed and are becoming popular even for the treatment of benign biliary strictures and for post liver transplant biliary leaks. The advantages of metallic stents, in comparison to plastic stents, are: larger diameters that result in longer patency rates, self-expanding material that allows constant dilatation in the areas of biliary stenosis, more flexibility and therefore better adherence to the biliary walls. This last characteristic is very important when dealing with biliary leaks as covered metallic stents are able to prevent bile extravasation and facilitate non-operative management even in severe anastomotic bile disruptions.

Metal stents can also be differentiated on the basis of stent composition, with namely stainless steel or nitinol being used. Nitinol is an example of a biocompatible, super-elastic, and shape memory alloy consisting of 55% nickel and 45% titanium. The strong inter-metallic bonds between nickel and titanium have a very low reaction rate; thus, preventing immunological responses and a decreased rate of corrosion.

Initially, SEMS featured an uncovered design but a limited patency on the account of tissue overgrowth, cancer ingrowth [77] and poor removability led to the development of covered self-expanding metal stents (CSEMS). These stents have a metallic skeleton and are covered by a biocompatible, synthetic covering, which is resistant to the effects of bile, gastric, and pancreatic secretions [78]. The increased incidence of migration associated with CSEMS, however, paved the way for the development of partially CSEMS in which the distal and proximal ends of the stent are uncovered and therefore prevent the risk of stent migration.

15. Postoperative biliary complications

15.1. Leaks

Bile leaks after LT occur in 2–25% of patients [79] and most present within one to three months after surgery. Anastomotic dehiscences are due to technical errors, tension or for ischemia of the bile duct edges due to hepatic artery thrombosis or because of devascularization of the tissue surrounding the biliary tree. In addition, bile leaks can also occur from the cystic duct remnants, the T-tube site or tract, from the gallbladder fossa or (in the case of living donor LT) from the cut surface of the liver (Table 8).

• Surgical anastomosis (duct to duct, hepaticojejunostomy)
• Cystic duct stump
• T-tube site
• Ischemic injuries of the extra-hepatic bile duct
• Gallbladder fossa
• Cut surface of the liver in LDLT

Table 8. Causes and locations of leaks following liver transplantation.

Early leaks (within 4 weeks from LT) are usually due to ischemia or technical issues [80]. Late bile leaks tend to occur following T-tube removal [80], as patients on high dose of steroids and other immunosuppressive medications have reduced ability to heal the T-tube insertion site and seal the tract around the drain. Post LT bile leaks should be suspected in patients who develop clinical deterioration, signs of peritoneal inflammation or fluid collections on cross sectional imaging tests. A bile leak should also be suspected in patients who develop persistent abdominal pain after removal of T-tube. It is very important to be aware that a relatively high proportion of patients with late bile leaks present with late biliary strictures than do those with early leaks.

Many bile leaks can be resolved non-operatively with early percutaneous or endoscopic interventions [50-52, 55].When there is a low suspicion of a biliary leak, a radionucleotide scan has reasonable accuracy for the presence of bile extravasation [81]. ERCP, though, is the gold standard diagnostic method and should be performed in all patients when there is a high suspicion for biliary leaks. Treatment for biliary leaks consists of placement of either an endoscopic stent and/or a percutaneous stent/drain. If there is an associated stricture, then both the leak and the stricture need to be bridged by the stent. Stent placement can result in up to 88% resolution of biliary leaks. Resolution of the leak occurs typically within 5 weeks but the patient's symptoms will resolve within days of stent insertion [82]. The stent should be left in place for approximately 2 to 3 months because of problems with delayed healing that may arise as a result of immunosuppression [59]. In cases where a T-tube is in place, small anastomotic leaks can be diagnosed with a T-tube cholangiogram and can be managed by leaving the tube open without further interventions. Instead of the transpapillary stent, a nasobiliary tube can be inserted. An advantage of the nasobiliary tubes is that they permit cholangiographic follow-up without the need for further endoscopies [83], however, they are often poorly tolerated and also divert bile away from the intestine, thereby decreasing the bioavailability of certain drugs.

Anastomotic leaks after Roux-en-Y choledochojejunostomies are less common. A suspected bile leak in such patients can be diagnosed with a hepatobiliaryimino-diacetic acid (HIDA) scan if patients do not have a drainage catheter in place. Standard ERC is often not feasible because of anatomic difficulties in reaching the biliary anastomosis. Management is usually performed with percutaneous internal-external drainage. Bile leaks in patients with Roux-en-Y anatomy more often require surgical management.

Bilomas occur because of bile duct rupture and extravasation of bile into the hepatic parenchyma or the abdominal cavity. Most post-LT bilomas occur in the perihepatic area. Small bilomas communicating with the biliary tree may resolve spontaneously. Large bilomas not communicating with the bile ducts should be treated with percutaneous drainage and antibiotics. Surgery is indicated only when the bile leak cannot be controlled effectively with endoscopic stenting.

15.2. Bile duct strictures

15.2.1. Introduction

Biliary strictures and bile leaks account for the majority of biliary complications after LT. The incidence of biliary strictures after cadaveric LT ranges between 5 to 15% while the incidence is much higher after living donor liver transplantation where biliary leaks occur in 28–32% of patients [84]. Although strictures can develop at any time post LT, they tend to occur in the first 5–8 months after surgery [84, 85]. Strictures that occur early after are mostly attributable to technical problems, whereas late strictures are mainly attributable to vascular insufficiency and problems with the healing of tissues and fibrosis [63, 86]. A bile leak is an independent risk factor for the development of a stricture, and for that reason, a bile leak requires emergent endoscopic therapy [66]. Strictures are classified as anastomotic (AS) or nonanastomotic (NAS), depending on the stricture site (Table 9). NAS are defined as strictures that occur more than 0.5 cm proximal to the anastomosis and tend to be multiple and longer in length (Table 9). NAS can be further classified into macroangiopathic, microangiopathic, and immunogenic be the causes determining the stenosis of the bile duct (Table 10) [84, 87].

AS tend to occur later than NAS. They are usually shorter and localized to the anastomotic site (Table 9) with an incidence of 4–9% [80, 84].Ischemic NAS usually presents within 1 year of OLT while immunological NAS usually present later than 1 year post-transplantation [88, 89]. In contrast to AS, NAS can result in graft loss [90]. AS are generally the result of scar formation (fibrosis), local ischemia, technical issues, or a bile leak in the post-operative period [89, 91].

Biliary strictures	
Anastomotic	**Non-anastomotic**
Single	Multiple
Short	Long
Anastomosis site	Intrahepatitc and proximal to anastomosis

Table 9. Classification of biliary strictures.

Macroangiopathic	**Microangiopathic**	**Immunogenic**
Hepatic artery thrombosis	Prolonged cold and warm ischemia times	Chronic rejection
	Donation after cardiac death	ABO incompatibility
	Prolonged use of vasopressors in the donor	Primary sclerosing cholangitis
		Autoimmune hepatitis

Table 10. Non-anastomotic stricture classification.

15.2.2. Anastomotic strictures

Up to 80% of biliary strictures are anastomotic, occurring either at the choledocho-choledochostomy or choledocho-jejunostomy sites [51, 55]. AS typically reflect technical problems and primarily are due to small bile leaks resulting in a peri-anastomotic fibro-inflammatory response, or ischemia at the end of the bile duct resulting in a fibro-proliferative response. By definition, they are single and short in length, making them suitable for endoscopic intervention. The characteristic cholangiographic appearance of AS is that of a thin narrowing in the area of the biliary anastomosis. In some patients, a narrowing of the anastomosis may become evident within the first 1 to 2 months after LT because of postoperative edema and inflammation [89]. This type of narrowing has an excellent response to endoscopic balloon dilation and plastic stent placement; in most patients, it resolves within 3 months and the anastomosis remains patent without further intervention. Except for the subset of patients with this early narrowing, most patients with AS require ongoing ERCP sessions (every 2 to 3 months) with balloon dilation and long-term stenting (for 12 to 24 months) (Figure 5). In most cases, an approach using balloon dilation with diameters of 6 to 8 mm and placement of 7.0- to 11.5-Fr plastic stents is more effective than balloon dilation alone [92]. Stents should be exchanged at 3-month intervals to avoid stent occlusion and the precipitation of bacterial cholangitis. Most patients require several endoscopic interventions (mean of 3 to 5) with long-term success rates in the range of 70% to 100% [52, 85, 89, 92]. The placement of a progressively increasing number of as well as diameter stents with each subsequent ERC has been shown to be a successful method of treating AS [93]. In an illustrative study, patients who developed biliary strictures after LT and who initially were treated endoscopically with balloon dilation and plastic stents had a recurrence rate of 18% with a mean time to recurrence of 110 days [94].

There is some clinical experience in temporary placement of a covered self-expanding metal stent to reduce the need for repeated stent exchanges, but data are limited [95]. The difficulty with the uncovered metallic self-expandable stent is that there is an inevitable reactive hyperplasia that can be accompanied by secondary stone formation above the stent and there may be a challenge in removing the stent once it has been in place for 6 to 9 months [96]. Fully covered stents, by contrast, almost always are able to be removed endoscopically, as they do not embed into the surrounding tissue. The data on this type of stent are limited and one article reported the stents caused strictures in the bile duct mainly secondary to the anchoring point in the distal proximal end [97]. Additionally, they may occlude secondary branch ducts, and this technical aspect might limit their use in patients with right-lobe live-donor transplants. Because of the high rates of success, endoscopic management should be considered the first choice before considering percutaneous interventions or surgical repair in patients with duct-to-duct anastomosis. In patients with Roux-en-Y choledochojejunostomy, management with balloon enteroscopy ERC or PTC and dilation followed by placement of a percutaneous transhepatic catheter is often necessary. Surgical intervention (usually a repair or conversion to a Roux-en-Y choledochojejunostomy) is required when the ERC or PTC fails to adequately treat AS.

15.2.3. Non-anastomotic strictures

NAS result mainly from hepatic artery thrombosis, increased cold ischemia time, or ABO blood-type incompatibility. Less commonly these strictures can be caused by recurrence of the underlying disease such as primary sclerosing cholangitis. They account for 10.0%to 25.0% of all stricture complications after LT, with an incidence in the range of 0.5% to 10.0% [51, 52, 53,

http://dx.doi.org/10.5772/52630

54, 55]. True ischemic strictures occur more than 0.5 cm proximal to the anastomosis and often involve the hilum and multiple separate obstructions at the level of the sectoral or segmental branch ducts. This can lead to a cholangiographic appearance that resembles primary sclerosing cholangitis. NAS tend to occur earlier than AS, with a mean time to stricture development of 3 to 6 months [55, 59].

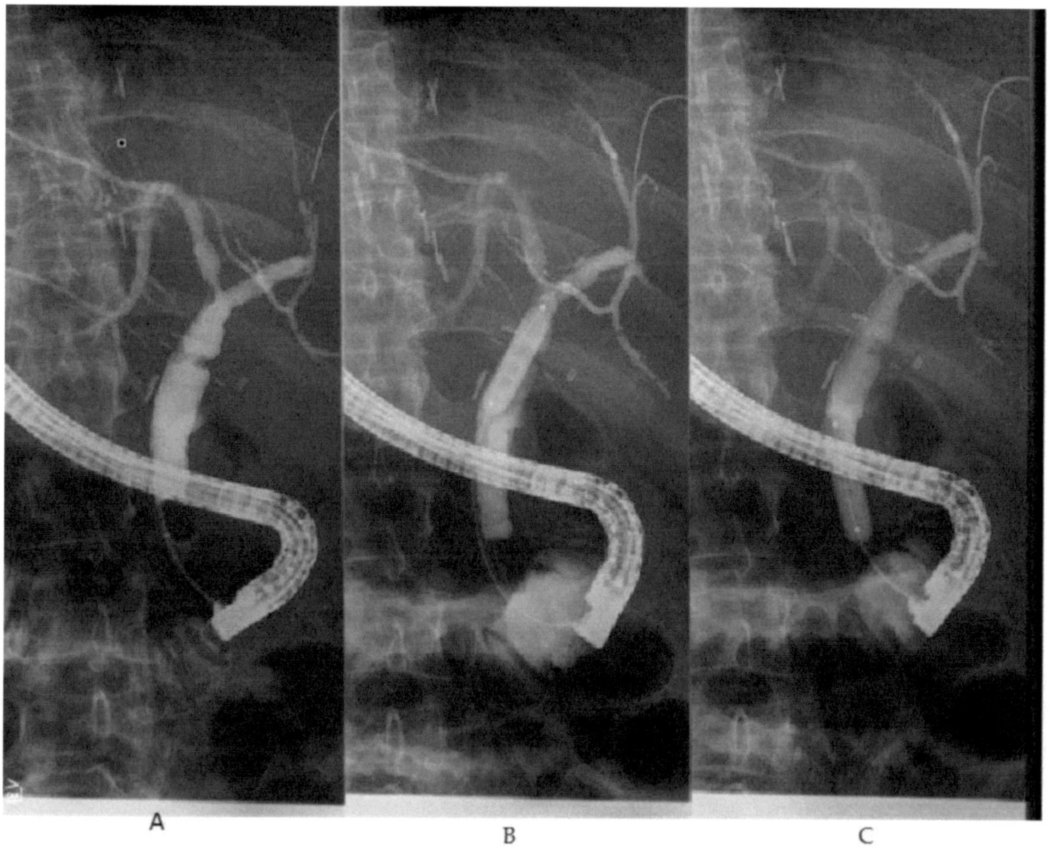

Figure 5. Example of anastomotic stricture after cadaveric liver transplantation. A 57 year old man affected by alcoholic cirrhosis underwent a liver transplant nine months before presenting with elevation of the serum total bilirubin and alkaline phosphatase. An abdominal Doppler ultrasound revealed normal portal vein, hepatic veins and hepatic artery flow with mild dilatation of the intra-hepatic bile ducts. An endoscopic retrograde cholangiography (ERCP) was ordered to assess the biliary tree and revealed the presence of a critical anastomotic stricture (Figure 5A, white arrow). An inflatable endoscopic balloon measuring 10 mm in diameter and 4 cm in length was used to dilate the anastomotic stricture for 5 minutes (Figure 5B, white triangle). After dilating the anastomotic stricture, an occlusive cholangiogram revealed an almost complete resolution of the anastomotic stenosis (Figure 5C, white arrow).

NAS are generally more difficult to treat than AS and can present with multiple episodes of cholangitis requiring hospitalizations. Endoscopic therapy of NAS typically consists of 4- to 6-mm balloon dilation (compared with 6 to 8 mm for AS) followed by sphincterotomy, and placement of a 10.0- to 11.5-Fr plastic stent with replacement every 3 months [54]. The more aggressive approach with the placement of a progressively increasing number of as well as diameter stents with each subsequent ERC has been shown to be a successful method [93]. However, time to response with NAS is more prolonged than with AS and patients with NAS, in average, require twice the number of interventions as patients with AS. The median time to resolution of the stricture is 4-6 months for NAS versus 2 months for AS [59].

Outcomes of patients with NAS are not as favorable as for patients who develop AS. The 5-year graft survival rate is 73% in patients with NAS, which is significantly lower than in matched controls without strictures [89]. Only 50% to 75% of patients have a long-term response with endoscopic therapy with dilation and stent placement [54, 59, 89, 73, 98]. Furthermore, up to 30% to 50% of patients will require re-transplantation or will die as a consequence of this complication despite endoscopic therapy [54, 55, 63]. As a general rule, ischemic events that lead to diffuse intrahepatic bile duct strictures are associated with poor graft survival and will require retransplantation for suitable candidates.

Surgical revision may ultimately be required in patients with strictures that are refractory to endoscopic or percutaneous treatment. A Roux-en-Y choledochojejunostomy is usually performed in patients with duct-to-duct anastomosis. In those who already have a Roux-en-Y anastomosis, a revision may be required by repositioning the bile duct of the graft to a more proximal vascularized area.

15.2.4. Biliary stones, sludge and casts

Biliary filling defects are identified in approximately 5% of patients undergoing radiological investigations after LT [99]. The vast majority of filling defects are caused by stones (70%) followed by sludge, debris, blood clots, casts or migration of biliary stents [54, 89]. Biliary anastomotic stenosis and intrahepatic strictures are the most frequent predisposing conditions since they cause cholestasis and bacterial overgrowth that are well known risk factors for the formation of sludge and biliary stones. Biliary duct stenoses are often caused by preservation injury or by hepatic artery insufficiency. These are the two most common causes of ischemic damage to the biliary tree that is highly dependent on the arterial blood supply for its metabolic needs. When the biliary endothelium does not receive enough arterial blood flow, it sloughs in the lumen of the biliary tree creating an optimal enviroment for the formation of crystals and early calcification of the proteinaceous debris [99].

The management of filling defects in the biliary tree of patients undergoing LT is similar to the non-transplant population and include sphincterotomy or dilatation of the sphincter of Oddi and their extraction with the use of Dormia baskets or biliary balloons with the caveat that in the presence of immunosuppressive agents, patients can have a rapid clinical decline in the presence of undrained infected biliary ducts.

Because of the denervation of the liver graft and the use of steroids and other immunosuppressive medications, LT patients affected by choledocholithiasis can be completely asymptomatic and afebrile even in the presence of bactobilia. LT patients affected by unrecognized biliary occlusion can be completely asymptomatic for a long period of time and present with

http://dx.doi.org/10.5772/52630

recurrent elevation of cholestatic serum markers that can mimick rejection, fevers of unknown etiology, pancreatitis or cholangitis leading to sepsis and multiorgan failure in a very rapid interval.

15.2.5. Stones

Stones usually form in the biliary tree of LT grafts proximally to a stricture or anastomotic stenosis. Cyclosporine is known to promote supersaturation of bile and may contribute to the formation of biliary stones in this group of patients. In one series, biliary stones were diagnosed after a median of 19 months post LT and following their successful extraction, 17% reoccurred within a median period of only 6 months [73]. In most cases (59% to 66%), a single ERCP session with biliary sphincterotomy and balloon or basket extraction was sufficient to clear the bile duct when the stones were located in the extra-hepatic system [73], while 2 or more sessions were needed in 24% of patients and 3 or more sessions may be required in 17% of patients [73]. Advanced ERC techniques, such as intraductal lithotripsy or direct choledochoscopy should be considered for all patients with large stones or for those stones located in a more proximal biliary tract [84].

15.2.6. Casts

Biliary cast are defined as the presence of hardened, often dark and calcified protenaceous material within the biliary system that takes the physical shape of the bile ducts. Biliary casts are reported in 2.5% up to 18% of LT recipients [84, 99, 100]. Acute cellular rejection, ischemia, infection, and biliary obstruction are well known risk factors for the development of casts after LT.Most commonly they develop in the setting of ischemia, for example after the development of hepatic artery thrombosis and when there is stricturing of the biliary tree at the hilum [64]. The formation of biliary casts is associated with increased morbidity, mortality, and incidence of rejection [84]. Typically it occurs within the first year after transplantation. Analysis of the casts has shown that bilirubin is the primary element along with collagen, bile acid, and cholesterol [101, 102, 103]. The true pathogenesis of biliary cast syndrome is unknown but it is believed that ischemic factors and biliary strictures play an important role in its development. Another risk factor is an increase in warm ischemia time [103]. Several endoscopic approaches have been described with variable success and often multiple procedures are required. Unfortunately it has been reported that up to 22% of patients with biliary cast syndrome will require retransplantation. Complete clearance of casts can be done in 60% of patients by ERCP or when necessary by PTC [64]. Various combinations of sphincterotomy, balloon and basket extraction, stent placement, and lithotripsy are often necessary in all those situations where casts are difficult to extract or are located in multiple branches of the biliary tree. Surgery is necessary only when endoscopic or percutaneous methods fail.

15.2.7. Sphincter of Oddi dysfunction

The sphincter of Oddi is a muscular structure that encompasses the confluence of the distal common bile and the pancreatic duct as they penetrate the wall of the duodenum. The term sphincter of Oddi dysfunction (SOD) has been used to describe a clinical syndrome of biliary or pancreatic obstruction related to mechanical or functional abnormalities of the sphincter of Oddi. The true incidence of SOD after LT is not known but appears to a relatively rare condition. It is postulated that in the posttransplant setting, denervation of the common bile duct in the ampullary region secondary to surgical intervention may lead to the development of a hypertonic sphincter causing SOD. The prevalence of SOD has been reported to be between 2% to 7% [50, 98] and should be suspected in patients with cholestasis and with a uniformly dilated bile duct without filling defects. In LT recipients affected by SOD, abdominal pain may not be present and can cause post-operative pancreatitis. SOD should be ruled out when other causes of pancreatitis have not been found. The treatment of post LT patients affected by SOD is endoscopic sphincterotomy that allows the release of the muscles of the sphincter with reduction of the intra-luminal biliary and pancreatic hypertension. As for SOD in the non-transplant setting, the risk of pancreatitis after an ERC is high and so temporary prophylactic pancreatic stents after sphincterotomy should be placed if possible to avoid this risk.

16. Biliary complications after living donation and cardiac arrest

Biliary complications after LT from living donors and grafts from donors after cardiac death are more frequent than in patients who receive full size grafts from brain dead donors. These two groups of recipients represent an increasing number of patients as the available grafts from brain dead donors have failed to match the needs of patients waiting for LT and need some considerations.

Living donor grafts are obtained by removing the right or left hepatic lobes from healthy donors. The advantages of using living donor grafts are the fact that the quality of the grafts is usually excellent, that surgery can be performed electively when the recipient is in optimal medical conditions and that the cold and warm ischemia times are minimized. On the other hand, living donor LT is technically challenging as the liver graft is only a portion of the entire liver and therefore there is an increased risk of perioperative hepatic insufficiency. The increased risk of hepatic artery thrombosis is due to the fact that the lumen of the proper hepatic artery is significantly smaller than the common hepatic artery and more prone to develop intraluminal clots. In addition, there is an increased risk for bile leaking out from the interrupted intrahepatic ducts during the dissection of the liver parenchyma and, biliary leaks at the level of the anastomoses between the right or left biliary ducts and the recipient's native common bile duct or the Roux-en-Y loop. These anastomoses are often characterized by their small caliber and the fact that, often, there are several ducts that need to be put together.

The use of donors after cardiac arrest in LT has become an acceptable strategy to increase the number of available grafts. The early experience with these grafts was considered acceptable and several programs have embraced this practice. However, recent studies have reported that the short and long term outcomes are inferior to grafts from donors who suffered brain death. Among the most common causes of perioperative complications in this group are: biliary necrosis, anastomotic and non-anastomotic strictures, anastomotic leaks and non-primary graft function. These adverse events seem to be consequences of the warm ischemic insult occurring in hemodinamically unstable patients prior and during the obervation period leading to cardiac arrest.

16.1. Recipients of living-donor liver grafts

Living-donor liver transplantation (LDLT) has been associated with a higher rate of bile leaks than in comparision to deceased-donor LT: 31.8% versus 10.2%, respectively [104]. Factors associated with increased biliary leaks are:the presence of 3 or more bile ducts, presence of hepatitis C, the experience of the transplant center at performing LDLT,long duration of surgery, donor age older than 50, and recipients with MELD greater than 35 [105, 45]. The most likely reason for these complications include a relatively smaller duct size, hence a more technically difficult anastomosis, and a higher chance of ischemic injury to the allograft [106]. Overall, biliary complications occur more frequently in recipients receiving a right graft than a left liver graft. In right liver graft recipients with single biliary reconstruction, duct-to-duct anastomosis involving a small-sized duct (<4 mm in diameter) is more of a risk for biliary complications than when a hepatico-jejunostomy is used with these duct sizes [107]. A decreased incidence of biliary complications with a Roux-en-Y reconstruction has been found in some [104], but not all, studies [108]. Endoscopic management in LDLT recipients may be quite difficult because of the complex nature of the duct-to-duct reconstruction. Patients will often require frequent endoscopic retrograde cholangiographies (ERCs) with the use of smaller caliber stents (7.0–8.5 Fr). ERC with balloon dilatation is successful in up to 65% of patients. Failure of a primary ERC with dilatation is associated with the appearance of late biliary strictures over 24 weeks from LT and more than 8 weeks between a twofold increase in serum alkaline phosphatase [109]. The relapse rate of strictures is up to 30% and occurs more in patients with shorter duration of stenting. In addition to the recipient, donors also experience biliary complications and should be made aware of this before undergoing donation. In a multicenter study that evaluated the outcome of 393 donors, bile leaks occurred in 36 patients (9%) and most of these patients required a prolonged intensive care unit stay [110]. Biliary complications in donors are seen more often with right lobe donation and the management is the same as described for the recipients.

16.2. Recipients of grafts from donation after cardiac death

The continuing shortage of organs has led to expansion of the donor pool and consideration of non-heart beating liver donation or donation after cardiac death (DCD). DCD is associated with significant risk for both early and late biliary complications. In a retrospective analysis of 20 recipients of organs from DCD in the United States, 12 out of 20 patients (60%) developed serious biliary complications [65]. Most recipients developed more than one biliary complication including bile leaks requiring liver re-transplantation, anastomotic strictures, hilar strictures, extra-hepatic donor duct stricture, stones, casts, and biliary debris. In 50% of the patients, biliary strictures were proximal to the anastomosis. Unlike conventional liver transplantation where non-anastomotic strictures (NAS)are usually attributed to ischemic preservation injury or vascular compromise due to hepatic artery failure, NAS in DCD recipients reflects ischemic injury that occurred before organ retrieval [65]. An analysis of 172

Korean recipient survivors confirmed the increased rate of biliary complications in DCD-related liver transplantation [111] and also illustrated the impact of the location of the stricture and its relation to graft survival. Patients with unilateral or at the confluence biliary strictures could be managed endoscopically with dilatation and stenting while diffuse or bilateral strictures failed endoscopic interventions [111, 112, 113]. Unilateral and bilateral or diffuse biliary strictures were associated with 86 and 0% long-term survival, respectively [111, 112, 113]. Intra-hepatic biliary strictures are also associated with increased incidence of biliary sludge, cast formation, recurrent cholangitis, and biliary fibrosis [65].

17. Future directions

Use of new intraductal endoscopy technologies such as the SpyGlass® direct visualization system (Boston Scientific®, Natick, MA, USA), which allows visualization of the inner wall of the biliary tree and can act as the guidance system for passage of the guide wire through a tight stricture, has shown some early promise in this area [84, 114, 115, 116]. New types of balloons and stents will have significant role in improvement of management of biliary stricture. Preliminary evidence shows that peripheral cutting balloons may be more effective for the treatment of benign biliary strictures not responsive to standard balloon dilatation [117]. Metal stents have been employed in an effort to reduce stricture recurrence and maintain duct patency. Traditional open-mesh metal stents are associated with occlusion, stone formation and epithelial hyperplasia that reduce their patency rate [118]. These disadvantages of metal stents have traditionally limited their use for benign biliary strictures. The drawbacks of uncovered metal stents have led to the development of covered metal stents, as they can be removed during ERCP after the resolution of the biliary complication. However, the use of covered metal stents for the management of biliary complications in LT recipients needs further evaluation, as their safety and effectiveness have not been fully established. New technologies have introduced the possibility of employing self-expanding stents made of bioabsorbable material that theoretically will offer several advantages compared to the plastic and self-expanding metal stents [119, 120]. Studies in porcine models have shown that these stents have better patency rates because of their larger diameter, lower biofilm accumulation and reduced incidence of bile duct proliferative changes that often cause occlusion of metallic stents. Furthermore, patients do not have to undergo additional procedures to remove the stents. Bioabsorbable stents can also be impregnated with pharmaceutical compounds, such as antimicrobial agents that make them an optimal choice for patients who are affected by local biliary infections. However, these stents remains investigational at the present time.

18. Summary

The overall landscape of the management of biliary complications after LT has changed rather rapidly in the past 2 decades. In the past, the conventional management of these conditions was mainly surgical. With the advancement of endoscopic equipments and accessories, therapeutic endoscopy has been playing a major role in the treatment of post-liver transplant biliary complications. Percutaneous and surgical modalities are now reserved only for patients in whom endoscopic treatment fails and for those with multiple inaccessible intrahepatic strictures or Roux-en-Y anastomoses.

Abbreviations

Liver Transplant (LT)

Acute Liver Failure (ALF)

End Stage Liver Disease (ESLD)

United States(US)

Hepatocellular Carcinoma (HCC)

University of California, San Francisco (UCSF)

Cholangiocarcinoma (CC)

United Network for Organ Sharing (UNOS)

Model for End-stage Liver Disease (MELD)

Pediatric End-stage Liver Disease (PELD)

International Normalized Ratio (INR)

Endoscopic Retrograde Cholangio-Pancreatography (ERCP)

PercutaneousTranshepatic Cholangiography (PTC)

Percutaneous Transhepatic Biliary Drainage (PTBD)

Self-Expandable Metallic Stents (SEMS)

HepatobiliaryImino-DiaceticAcid Scan (HIDA) Scan

Anastomotic Strictre(AS)

Non-anastomotic Stricture (NAS)

Sphincter of Oddi Dysfunction (SOD)

Author details

Bassam Abu-Wasel, Paul D. Renfrew and Michele Molinari*

*Address all correspondence to: michele.molinari@cdha.nshealth.ca

Department of Surgery and Transplantation, Dalhousie University, Halifax, Nova Scotia, Canada

References

[1] Starzl TE, Marchioro TL, Vonkaulla KN, Hermann G, Brittain RS, Waddell WR. Homotransplantation of the Liver in Humans. Surg Gynecol Obstet 1963;117:659-76.

[2] Yu AS, Keeffe EB, editors. "Liver transplantation," in Hepatology, 2003.

[3] Murray KCR. AASLD practice guidelines: evaluation of the patient for liver transplantation. Hepatology 2005;41(6):1407-32.

[4] Conference C. Consensus conference: indications for Liver Transplantation, Lyon-Palais Des Congr`es: text of recommendations (long version). Liver Transplantation, 2006:988-1011.

[5] Ahmed A, Keeffe EB. Current indications and contraindications for liver transplantation. Clin Liver Dis 2007;11(2):227-47.

[6] Jain A, Reyes J, Kashyap R, Dodson SF, Demetris AJ, Ruppert K, et al. Long-term survival after liver transplantation in 4,000 consecutive patients at a single center. Ann Surg 2000;232(4):490-500.

[7] Gordon RD, Fung J, Tzakis AG, Todo S, Stieber A, Bronsther O, et al. Liver transplantation at the University of Pittsburgh, 1984 to 1990. Clin Transpl 1991:105-17.

[8] Abbasoglu O, Levy MF, Brkic BB, Testa G, Jeyarajah DR, Goldstein RM, et al. Ten years of liver transplantation: an evolving understanding of late graft loss. Transplantation 1997;64(12):1801-7.

[9] Asfar S, Metrakos P, Fryer J, Verran D, Ghent C, Grant D, et al. An analysis of late deaths after liver transplantation. Transplantation 1996;61(9):1377-81.

[10] Kim WR. The burden of hepatitis C in the United States. Hepatology 2002;36(5 Suppl 1):S30-4.

[11] Brown RS, Jr., Lake JR. The survival impact of liver transplantation in the MELD era, and the future for organ allocation and distribution. Am J Transplant 2005;5(2):203-4.

[12] U.S. Department of Health and Human Services HRaSA, Healthcare Systems Bureau, Division of Transplantation, Rockville, MD., editor. Annual Report of the U.S. Organ Procurement and Transplantation Network and the Scientific Registry of Transplant Recipients: Transplant Data 1999-2008, 2009.

[13] Seaberg EC, Belle SH, Beringer KC, Schivins JL, Detre KM. Liver transplantation in the United States from 1987-1998: updated results from the Pitt-UNOS Liver Transplant Registry. Clin Transpl 1998:17-37.

[14] Ritt DJ, Whelan G, Werner DJ, Eigenbrodt EH, Schenker S, Combes B. Acute hepatic necrosis with stupor or coma. An analysis of thirty-one patients. Medicine (Baltimore) 1969;48(2):151-72.

[15] Larson AM. Diagnosis and management of acute liver failure. Curr Opin Gastroenterol 2010;26(3):214-21.

[16] Larson AM, Polson J, Fontana RJ, Davern TJ, Lalani E, Hynan LS, et al. Acetaminophen-induced acute liver failure: results of a United States multicenter, prospective study. Hepatology 2005;42(6):1364-72.

[17] Rosen CB, Heimbach JK, Gores GJ. Liver transplantation for cholangiocarcinoma. Transpl Int 2010;23(7):692-7.

[18] Mazzaferro V, Regalia E, Doci R, Andreola S, Pulvirenti A, Bozzetti F, et al. Liver transplantation for the treatment of small hepatocellular carcinomas in patients with cirrhosis. N Engl J Med 1996;334(11):693-9.

[19] Yao FY, Ferrell L, Bass NM, Watson JJ, Bacchetti P, Venook A, et al. Liver transplantation for hepatocellular carcinoma: expansion of the tumor size limits does not adversely impact survival. Hepatology 2001;33(6):1394-403.

[20] Gores GJ, Heimbach JK, Rosen CB. Liver transplantation for nonhepatocellular carcinoma malignancies. Liver Transplantation 2010;16:S22-25.

[21] Facciuto ME, Singh MK, Katta U, Samaniego S, Sharma J, Rodriguez-Davalos M, et al. Liver transplantation for hepatocellular carcinoma: defining the impact of using extended criteria liver allografts. Transplantation 2011;92(4):446-52.

[22] Rodrigue JR, Hanto DW, Curry MP. Patients' willingness to accept expanded criteria donor liver transplantation. Am J Transplant 2011;11(8):1705-11.

[23] Ali JM, Bonomo L, Brais R, Griffiths WJ, Lomas DJ, Huguet EL, et al. Outcomes and diagnostic challenges posed by incidental cholangiocarcinoma after liver transplantation. Transplantation 2011;91(12):1392-7.

[24] Mathurin P, Moreno C, Samuel D, Dumortier J, Salleron J, Durand F, et al. Early liver transplantation for severe alcoholic hepatitis. N Engl J Med 2011;365(19):1790-800.

[25] Kelly DA. Current issues in pediatric transplantation. Pediatr Transplant 2006;10(6):712-20.

[26] Berg CL, Steffick DE, Edwards EB, Heimbach JK, Magee JC, Washburn WK, et al. Liver and intestine transplantation in the United States 1998-2007. Am J Transplant 2009;9(4 Pt 2):907-31.

[27] Magee JC, Krishnan SM, Benfield MR, Hsu DT, Shneider BL. Pediatric transplantation in the United States, 1997-2006. Am J Transplant 2008;8(4 Pt 2):935-45.

[28] Martin SR, Atkison P, Anand R, Lindblad AS. Studies of Pediatric Liver Transplantation 2002: patient and graft survival and rejection in pediatric recipients of a first liver transplant in the United States and Canada. Pediatr Transplant 2004;8(3):273-83.

[29] Freeman RB, Jr., Wiesner RH, Roberts JP, McDiarmid S, Dykstra DM, Merion RM. Improving liver allocation: MELD and PELD. Am J Transplant 2004;4 Suppl 9:114-31.

[30] Verran DJ, Asfar SK, Ghent CN, Grant DR, Wall WJ. Biliary reconstruction without T tubes or stents in liver transplantation: report of 502 consecutive cases. Liver Transpl Surg 1997;3(4):365-73.

[31] Neuhaus P, Blumhardt G, Bechstein WO, Steffen R, Platz KP, Keck H. Technique and results of biliary reconstruction using side-to-side choledochocholedochostomy in 300 orthotopic liver transplants. Ann Surg 1994;219(4):426-34.

[32] Ringe B, Oldhafer K, Bunzendahl H, Bechstein WO, Kotzerke J, Pichlmayr R. Analysis of biliary complications following orthotopic liver transplantation. Transplant Proc 1989;21(1 Pt 2):2472-6.

[33] Calne RY. A new technique for biliary drainage in orthotopic liver transplantation utilizing the gall bladder as a pedicle graft conduit between the donor and recipient common bile ducts. Ann Surg 1976;184(5):605-9.

[34] Anselmi M, Sherlock D, Buist L, Zundel N, Badger I, McMaster P, et al. Gallbladder conduit vs end-to-end anastomosis of the common bile duct in orthotopic liver transplantation. Transplant Proc 1990;22(5):2295-6.

[35] Halff G, Todo S, Hall R, Starzl TE. Late complications with gallbladder conduit biliary reconstruction after liver transplantation. Transplantation 1989;48(3):537-9.

[36] Hiatt JR, Quinones-Baldrich WJ, Ramming KP, Brems J, Busuttil RW. Operations upon the biliary tract during transplantation of the liver. Surg Gynecol Obstet 1987;165(1):89-93.

[37] Vallera RA, Cotton PB, Clavien PA. Biliary reconstruction for liver transplantation and management of biliary complications: overview and survey of current practices in the United States. Liver Transpl Surg 1995;1(3):143-52.

[38] Northover JM, Terblanche J. A new look at the arterial supply of the bile duct in man and its surgical implications. Br J Surg 1979;66(6):379-84.

[39] Stapleton GN, Hickman R, Terblanche J. Blood supply of the right and left hepatic ducts. Br J Surg 1998;85(2):202-7.

[40] Azoulay D, Marin-Hargreaves G, Castaing D, ReneAdam, Bismuth H. Duct-to-duct biliary anastomosis in living related liver transplantation: the Paul Brousse technique. Arch Surg 2001;136(10):1197-200.

[41] Shokouh-Amiri MH, Grewal HP, Vera SR, Stratta RJ, Bagous W, Gaber AO. Duct-to-duct biliary reconstruction in right lobe adult living donor liver transplantation. J Am Coll Surg 2001;192(6):798-803.

[42] Rogiers X, Malago M, Gawad K, Jauch KW, Olausson M, Knoefel WT, et al. In situ splitting of cadaveric livers. The ultimate expansion of a limited donor pool. Ann Surg 1996;224(3):331-9; discussion 39-41.

[43] Azoulay D, Astarcioglu I, Bismuth H, Castaing D, Majno P, Adam R, et al. Split-liver transplantation. The Paul Brousse policy. Ann Surg 1996;224(6):737-46; discussion 46-8.

[44] Ishiko T, Egawa H, Kasahara M, Nakamura T, Oike F, Kaihara S, et al. Duct-to-duct biliary reconstruction in living donor liver transplantation utilizing right lobe graft. Ann Surg 2002;236(2):235-40.

[45] Liu CL, Lo CM, Chan SC, Fan ST. Safety of duct-to-duct biliary reconstruction in right-lobe live-donor liver transplantation without biliary drainage. Transplantation 2004;77(5):726-32.

[46] Deshpande RR, Bowles MJ, Vilca-Melendez H, Srinivasan P, Girlanda R, Dhawan A, et al. Results of split liver transplantation in children. Ann Surg 2002;236(2):248-53.

[47] Miller CM, Gondolesi GE, Florman S, Matsumoto C, Munoz L, Yoshizumi T, et al. One hundred nine living donor liver transplants in adults and children: a single-center experience. Ann Surg 2001;234(3):301-11; discussion 11-2.

[48] Soejima Y, Shimada M, Suehiro T, Kishikawa K, Minagawa R, Hiroshige S, et al. Feasibility of duct-to-duct biliary reconstruction in left-lobe adult-living-donor liver transplantation. Transplantation 2003;75(4):557-9.

[49] Kawachi S, Shimazu M, Wakabayashi G, Hoshino K, Tanabe M, Yoshida M, et al. Biliary complications in adult living donor liver transplantation with duct-to-duct hepaticocholedochostomy or Roux-en-Y hepaticojejunostomy biliary reconstruction. Surgery 2002;132(1):48-56.

[50] Stratta RJ, Wood RP, Langnas AN, Hollins RR, Bruder KJ, Donovan JP, et al. Diagnosis and treatment of biliary tract complications after orthotopic liver transplantation. Surgery 1989;106(4):675-83; discussion 83-4.

[51] Greif F, Bronsther OL, Van Thiel DH, Casavilla A, Iwatsuki S, Tzakis A, et al. The incidence, timing, and management of biliary tract complications after orthotopic liver transplantation. Ann Surg 1994;219(1):40-5.

[52] Rerknimitr R, Sherman S, Fogel EL, Kalayci C, Lumeng L, Chalasani N, et al. Biliary tract complications after orthotopic liver transplantation with choledochocholedochostomy anastomosis: endoscopic findings and results of therapy. Gastrointest Endosc 2002;55(2):224-31.

[53] Pfau PR, Kochman ML, Lewis JD, Long WB, Lucey MR, Olthoff K, et al. Endoscopic management of postoperative biliary complications in orthotopic liver transplantation. Gastrointest Endosc 2000;52(1):55-63.

[54] Thuluvath PJ, Atassi T, Lee J. An endoscopic approach to biliary complications following orthotopic liver transplantation. Liver Int 2003;23(3):156-62.

[55] Thethy S, Thomson B, Pleass H, Wigmore SJ, Madhavan K, Akyol M, et al. Management of biliary tract complications after orthotopic liver transplantation. Clin Transplant 2004;18(6):647-53.

[56] Brown RS, Jr., Russo MW, Lai M, Shiffman ML, Richardson MC, Everhart JE, et al. A survey of liver transplantation from living adult donors in the United States. N Engl J Med 2003;348(9):818-25.

[57] Reichert PR, Renz JF, Rosenthal P, Bacchetti P, Lim RC, Roberts JP, et al. Biliary complications of reduced-organ liver transplantation. Liver Transpl Surg 1998;4(5):343-9.

[58] Colonna JO, 2nd, Shaked A, Gomes AS, Colquhoun SD, Jurim O, McDiarmid SV, et al. Biliary strictures complicating liver transplantation. Incidence, pathogenesis, management, and outcome. Ann Surg 1992;216(3):344-50; discussion 50-2.

[59] Thuluvath PJ, Pfau PR, Kimmey MB, Ginsberg GG. Biliary complications after liver transplantation: the role of endoscopy. Endoscopy 2005;37(9):857-63.

[60] Scatton O, Meunier B, Cherqui D, Boillot O, Sauvanet A, Boudjema K, et al. Randomized trial of choledochocholedochostomy with or without a T tube in orthotopic liver transplantation. Ann Surg 2001;233(3):432-7.

[61] Vougas V, Rela M, Gane E, Muiesan P, Melendez HV, Williams R, et al. A prospective randomised trial of bile duct reconstruction at liver transplantation: T tube or no T tube? Transpl Int 1996;9(4):392-5.

[62] Sotiropoulos GC, Sgourakis G, Radtke A, Molmenti EP, Goumas K, Mylona S, et al. Orthotopic liver transplantation: T-tube or not T-tube? Systematic review and meta-analysis of results. Transplantation 2009;87(11):1672-80.

[63] Pascher A, Neuhaus P. Biliary complications after deceased-donor orthotopic liver transplantation. J Hepatobiliary Pancreat Surg 2006;13(6):487-96.

[64] Davidson BR, Rai R, Kurzawinski TR, Selves L, Farouk M, Dooley JS, et al. Prospective randomized trial of end-to-end versus side-to-side biliary reconstruction after orthotopic liver transplantation. Br J Surg 1999;86(4):447-52.

[65] Maheshwari A, Maley W, Li Z, Thuluvath PJ. Biliary complications and outcomes of liver transplantation from donors after cardiac death. Liver Transpl 2007;13(12):1645-53.

[66] Welling TH, Heidt DG, Englesbe MJ, Magee JC, Sung RS, Campbell DA, et al. Biliary complications following liver transplantation in the model for end-stage liver disease era: effect of donor, recipient, and technical factors. Liver Transpl 2008;14(1):73-80.

[67] Rizk RS, McVicar JP, Emond MJ, Rohrmann CA, Jr., Kowdley KV, Perkins J, et al. Endoscopic management of biliary strictures in liver transplant recipients: effect on patient and graft survival. Gastrointest Endosc 1998;47(2):128-35.

[68] Schwartz DA, Petersen BT, Poterucha JJ, Gostout CJ. Endoscopic therapy of anastomotic bile duct strictures occurring after liver transplantation. Gastrointest Endosc 2000;51(2):169-74.

[69] Mosca S, Militerno G, Guardascione MA, Amitrano L, Picciotto FP, Cuomo O. Late biliary tract complications after orthotopic liver transplantation: diagnostic and therapeutic role of endoscopic retrograde cholangiopancreatography. J Gastroenterol Hepatol 2000;15(6):654-60.

[70] Mata A, Bordas JM, Llach J, Gines A, Mondelo F, Lopez Serrano A, et al. ERCP in orthotopic liver transplanted patients. Hepatogastroenterology 2004;51(60):1801-4.

[71] Solmi L, Cariani G, Leo P, Miracolo A, Nigro G, Roda E. Results of endoscopic retrograde cholangiopancreatography in the treatment of biliary tract complications after orthotopic liver transplantation: our experience. Hepatogastroenterology 2007;54(76): 1004-8.

[72] Shastri YM, Hoepffner NM, Akoglu B, Zapletal C, Bechstein WO, Caspary WF, et al. Liver biochemistry profile, significance and endoscopic management of biliary tract complications post orthotopic liver transplantation. World J Gastroenterol 2007;13(20):2819-25.

[73] Park JS, Kim MH, Lee SK, Seo DW, Lee SS, Han J, et al. Efficacy of endoscopic and percutaneous treatments for biliary complications after cadaveric and living donor liver transplantation. Gastrointest Endosc 2003;57(1):78-85.

[74] Kim ES, Lee BJ, Won JY, Choi JY, Lee DK. Percutaneous transhepatic biliary drainage may serve as a successful rescue procedure in failed cases of endoscopic therapy for a post-living donor liver transplantation biliary stricture. Gastrointest Endosc 2009;69(1):38-46.

[75] Soehendra N, Reynders-Frederix V. [Palliative biliary duct drainage. A new method for endoscopic introduction of a new drain]. Dtsch Med Wochenschr 1979;104(6): 206-7.

[76] LaBerge JM, Doherty M, Gordon RL, Ring EJ. Hilar malignancy: treatment with an expandable metallic transhepatic biliary stent. Radiology 1990;177(3):793-7.

[77] Cantu P, Hookey LC, Morales A, Le Moine O, Deviere J. The treatment of patients with symptomatic common bile duct stenosis secondary to chronic pancreatitis using partially covered metal stents: a pilot study. Endoscopy 2005;37(8):735-9.

[78] Bezzi M, Zolovkins A, Cantisani V, Salvatori FM, Rossi M, Fanelli F, et al. New ePTFE/FEP-covered stent in the palliative treatment of malignant biliary obstruction. J Vasc Interv Radiol 2002;13(6):581-9.

[79] Londono MC, Balderramo D, Cardenas A. Management of biliary complications after orthotopic liver transplantation: the role of endoscopy. World J Gastroenterol 2008;14(4):493-7.

[80] Scanga AE, Kowdley KV. Management of biliary complications following orthotopic liver transplantation. Curr Gastroenterol Rep 2007;9(1):31-8.

[81] Roca I, Ciofetta G. Hepatobiliary scintigraphy in current pediatric practice. Q J Nucl Med 1998;42(2):113-8.

[82] Morelli J, Mulcahy HE, Willner IR, Cunningham JT, Draganov P. Long-term outcomes for patients with post-liver transplant anastomotic biliary strictures treated by endoscopic stent placement. Gastrointest Endosc 2003;58(3):374-9.

[83] Saab S, Martin P, Soliman GY, Machicado GA, Roth BE, Kunder G, et al. Endoscopic management of biliary leaks after T-tube removal in liver transplant recipients: nasobiliary drainage versus biliary stenting. Liver Transpl 2000;6(5):627-32.

[84] 84. Sharma S, Gurakar A, Jabbour N. Biliary strictures following liver transplantation: past, present and preventive strategies. Liver Transpl 2008;14(6):759-69.

[85] Pasha SF, Harrison ME, Das A, Nguyen CC, Vargas HE, Balan V, et al. Endoscopic treatment of anastomotic biliary strictures after deceased donor liver transplantation: outcomes after maximal stent therapy. Gastrointest Endosc 2007;66(1):44-51.

[86] Testa G, Malago M, Broelseh CE. Complications of biliary tract in liver transplantation. World J Surg 2001;25(10):1296-9.

[87] Moench C, Moench K, Lohse AW, Thies J, Otto G. Prevention of ischemic-type biliary lesions by arterial back-table pressure perfusion. Liver Transpl 2003;9(3):285-9.

[88] Buis CI, Verdonk RC, Van der Jagt EJ, van der Hilst CS, Slooff MJ, Haagsma EB, et al. Nonanastomotic biliary strictures after liver transplantation, part 1: Radiological features and risk factors for early vs. late presentation. Liver Transpl 2007;13(5):708-18.

[89] Verdonk RC, Buis CI, van der Jagt EJ, Gouw AS, Limburg AJ, Slooff MJ, et al. Nonanastomotic biliary strictures after liver transplantation, part 2: Management, outcome, and risk factors for disease progression. Liver Transpl 2007;13(5):725-32.

[90] Guichelaar MM, Benson JT, Malinchoc M, Krom RA, Wiesner RH, Charlton MR. Risk factors for and clinical course of non-anastomotic biliary strictures after liver transplantation. Am J Transplant 2003;3(7):885-90.

[91] Ostroff JW. Post-transplant biliary problems. Gastrointest Endosc Clin N Am 2001;11(1):163-83.

[92] Zoepf T, Maldonado-Lopez EJ, Hilgard P, Malago M, Broelsch CE, Treichel U, et al. Balloon dilatation vs. balloon dilatation plus bile duct endoprostheses for treatment of anastomotic biliary strictures after liver transplantation. Liver Transpl 2006;12(1): 88-94.

[93] Holt AP, Thorburn D, Mirza D, Gunson B, Wong T, Haydon G. A prospective study of standardized nonsurgical therapy in the management of biliary anastomotic strictures complicating liver transplantation. Transplantation 2007;84(7):857-63.

[94] Alazmi WM, Fogel EL, Watkins JL, McHenry L, Tector JA, Fridell J, et al. Recurrence rate of anastomotic biliary strictures in patients who have had previous successful endoscopic therapy for anastomotic narrowing after orthotopic liver transplantation. Endoscopy 2006;38(6):571-4.

[95] Kahaleh M, Behm B, Clarke BW, Brock A, Shami VM, De La Rue SA, et al. Temporary placement of covered self-expandable metal stents in benign biliary strictures: a new paradigm? (with video). Gastrointest Endosc 2008;67(3):446-54.

[96] Larghi A, Tringali A, Lecca PG, Giordano M, Costamagna G. Management of hilar biliary strictures. Am J Gastroenterol 2008;103(2):458-73.

[97] Wang AY, Ellen K, Berg CL, Schmitt TM, Kahaleh M. Fully covered self-expandable metallic stents in the management of complex biliary leaks: preliminary data - a case series. Endoscopy 2009;41(9):781-6.

[98] Sawyer RG, Punch JD. Incidence and management of biliary complications after 291 liver transplants following the introduction of transcystic stenting. Transplantation 1998;66(9):1201-7.

[99] Sheng R, Sammon JK, Zajko AB, Campbell WL. Bile leak after hepatic transplantation: cholangiographic features, prevalence, and clinical outcome. Radiology 1994;192(2):413-6.

[100] Barton P, Maier A, Steininger R, Muhlbacher F, Lechner G. Biliary sludge after liver transplantation: 1. Imaging findings and efficacy of various imaging procedures. AJR Am J Roentgenol 1995;164(4):859-64.

[101] Waldram R, Williams R, Calne RY. Bile composition and bile cast formation after transplantation of the liver in man. Transplantation 1975;19(5):382-7.

[102] Canete JJ, Aidlen JT, Uknis ME, Cicalese L. Images of interest. Hepatobiliary and pancreatic: biliary cast syndrome. J Gastroenterol Hepatol 2005;20(5):791.

[103] Shah JN, Haigh WG, Lee SP, Lucey MR, Brensinger CM, Kochman ML, et al. Biliary casts after orthotopic liver transplantation: clinical factors, treatment, biochemical analysis. Am J Gastroenterol 2003;98(8):1861-7.

[104] Freise CE, Gillespie BW, Koffron AJ, Lok AS, Pruett TL, Emond JC, et al. Recipient morbidity after living and deceased donor liver transplantation: findings from the A2ALL Retrospective Cohort Study. Am J Transplant 2008;8(12):2569-79.

[105] Shah SA, Grant DR, McGilvray ID, Greig PD, Selzner M, Lilly LB, et al. Biliary strictures in 130 consecutive right lobe living donor liver transplant recipients: results of a Western center. Am J Transplant 2007;7(1):161-7.

[106] Gondolesi GE, Varotti G, Florman SS, Munoz L, Fishbein TM, Emre SH, et al. Biliary complications in 96 consecutive right lobe living donor transplant recipients. Transplantation 2004;77(12):1842-8.

[107] Hwang S, Lee SG, Sung KB, Park KM, Kim KH, Ahn CS, et al. Long-term incidence, risk factors, and management of biliary complications after adult living donor liver transplantation. Liver Transpl 2006;12(5):831-8.

[108] Soejima Y, Taketomi A, Yoshizumi T, Uchiyama H, Harada N, Ijichi H, et al. Biliary strictures in living donor liver transplantation: incidence, management, and technical evolution. Liver Transpl 2006;12(6):979-86.

[109] Seo JK, Ryu JK, Lee SH, Park JK, Yang KY, Kim YT, et al. Endoscopic treatment for biliary stricture after adult living donor liver transplantation. Liver Transpl 2009;15(4):369-80.

[110] Ghobrial RM, Freise CE, Trotter JF, Tong L, Ojo AO, Fair JH, et al. Donor morbidity after living donation for liver transplantation. Gastroenterology 2008;135(2):468-76.

[111] Hwang S, Lee SG, Joh JW, Suh KS, Kim DG. Liver transplantation for adult patients with hepatocellular carcinoma in Korea: comparison between cadaveric donor and living donor liver transplantations. Liver Transpl 2005;11(10):1265-72.

[112] Huang J. Ethical and legislative perspectives on liver transplantation in the People's Republic of China. Liver Transpl 2007;13(2):193-6.

[113] 113. Fung JJ, Eghtesad B, Patel-Tom K. Using livers from donation after cardiac death donors--a proposal to protect the true Achilles heel. Liver Transpl 2007;13(12):1633-6.

[114] Chen YK, Pleskow DK. SpyGlass single-operator peroral cholangiopancreatoscopy system for the diagnosis and therapy of bile-duct disorders: a clinical feasibility study (with video). Gastrointest Endosc 2007;65(6):832-41.

[115] Judah JR, Draganov PV. Intraductal biliary and pancreatic endoscopy: an expanding scope of possibility. World J Gastroenterol 2008;14(20):3129-36.

[116] Wright H, Sharma S, Gurakar A, Sebastian A, Kohli V, Jabbour N. Management of biliary stricture guided by the Spyglass Direct Visualization System in a liver transplant recipient: an innovative approach. Gastrointest Endosc 2008;67(7):1201-3.

[117] Atar E, Bachar GN, Bartal G, Mor E, Neyman H, Graif F, et al. Use of peripheral cutting balloon in the management of resistant benign ureteral and biliary strictures. J Vasc Interv Radiol 2005;16(2 Pt 1):241-5.

[118] 118. Silvis SE, Sievert CE, Jr., Vennes JA, Abeyta BK, Brennecke LH. Comparison of covered versus uncovered wire mesh stents in the canine biliary tract. Gastrointest Endosc 1994;40(1):17-21.

[119] Ginsberg G, Cope C, Shah J, Martin T, Carty A, Habecker P, et al. In vivo evaluation of a new bioabsorbable self-expanding biliary stent. Gastrointest Endosc 2003;58(5): 777-84.

[120] Meng B, Wang J, Zhu N, Meng QY, Cui FZ, Xu YX. Study of biodegradable and self-expandable PLLA helical biliary stent in vivo and in vitro. J Mater Sci Mater Med 2006;17(7):611-7.